Insulin, Insulin-like Growth Factors, and Their Receptors in the Central Nervous System

Finally, since insulin is a member of a family of closely related peptide hormones, the book would be incomplete without reference to the insulin-like growth factors (IGF I and IGF II) and their receptors in the central nervous system. Insulin may exert some of its physiological effects via these related receptors. These and other pertinent aspects of IGFs are discussed in the third section. This includes an indepth and updated discussion of distributions of IGF and their receptors in the central nervous system and the role of IGF receptors in mammalian brain in general and neurite formation in particular.

The decision to publish these contributions follows a successful symposium on "Functional Aspects of Insulin and Insulin-Related Peptides: Implications for the Central Nervous System" held at the University of Florida College of Medicine in Gainesville, Florida in January, 1987. This symposium was primarily supported by the KROC Foundation and various departments in the College of Medicine. The editors wish to thank the authors for their time and energy in making this book a reality. Sincere thanks are also extended to Dr. Noel Maclaren, Professor and Chairman, Department of Pathology for support and encouragement, and Diane Childs, Mr. Kevin Fortin and Mrs. Carolyn Gabbard for invaluable assistance in the preparation and editing of manuscripts.

Mohan K. Raizada
M. Ian Phillips
Derek LeRoith

PREFACE

Traditionally, intercellular communication and the regulation of biological functions of the body have been considered the role of two major and distinct systems: the nervous system and the endocrine system. The classic nervous system transmitted its signal rapidly by using electrical currents, whereas the signals used by the endocrine system were hormones produced by endocrine glands which reached the target tissues via the blood stream. During the past few decades, it has become apparent that these systems of intercellular communication are not distinct and the signal messenger molecules are not unique to one or the other system. Many classic endocrine hormones are found in and act on nervous tissues and evidence exists for their *de novo* synthesis by neural-related tissues. An exciting development in this area is the possibility that insulin and insulin-like growth factors (IGF) are not only produced by neural tissues but also exert profound physiological and biochemical effects on these tissues.

The area of investigation of CNS insulin and IGF has been expanding rapidly and the availability of this book complete with up-to-date reviews on the subject by leaders in the field allows other scientists to utilize the knowledge in planning and adapting the latest ideas for future experiments. In addition, the book provides a collection of up-to-date articles for teachers to be used for the latest instructional material.

The first section of the book covers general aspects of insulin receptors and insulin action. These include recent studies demonstrating the role of insulin and insulin receptor internalization in signaling of insulin's actions on glucose transport. In addition, there are articles demonstrating that some of insulin's actions may be mediated by the phospholipid-intermediates whereas others may involve tyrosine-specific substrates. Also, an up-to-date progress on glucose transporters and their implications for the brain is covered.

Next, the discussion turns specifically to the possible production of insulin and related molecules by the brain. These studies include measurement of insulin in the brain tissues by radioimmunoassay, immunohistochemistry, *in situ* hybridization of the insulin mRNA and northern blot analysis of the insulin mRNA. In addition, neuronal cells in culture, devoid of any influence of pancreatic insulin, have been used to provide transcriptional and translational evidence of insulin's synthesis and release by the brain. Whether insulin is produced in the brain or reaches it from the plasma is of secondary importance when considering insulin actions on neural tissues. The interaction of insulin with various brain regions including the circumventricular organs in the physiology of regulation of appetite and body weight have been discussed. Insulin receptors are widespread throughout the brain and are physiologically and biochemically unique when compared with peripheral and non-neuronal insulin receptors. The role of insulin receptors in the development of the brain and in neuromodulation is also described.

Library of Congress Cataloging in Publication Data

Insulin, insulin-like growth factors, and their receptors in the central nervous system.

Proceedings of a symposium held Jan. 19–20, 1987 in Gainesville, Fla.
Includes bibliographies and index.
1. Insulin—Physiological effect—Congresses. 2. Insulin—Receptors—Congresses. 3. Somatomedin—Physiological effect—Congresses. 4. Somatomedin—Receptors—Congresses. 5. Central nervous system—Congresses. I. Raizada, Mohan K. II. Phillips, M. Ian. III. LeRoith, Derek, 1945- . [DNLM: 1. Insulin—congresses. 2. Receptors, Insulin—Congresses. 3. Receptors, Neurohumor—congresses. 4. Somatomedins—congresses. WK 820I582 1987]
QP572.I5I55 1987 615′.365 87-20337
ISBN 0-306-42666-8

Proceedings of a symposium entitled Functional Aspects of Insulin and Insulin-Related Peptides: Implications for the Central Nervous System, held January 19–20, 1987, in Gainesville, Florida

A Division of Plenum Publishing Corporation
233 Spring Street, New York, N.Y. 10013

Insulin, Insulin-like Growth Factors, and Their Receptors in the Central Nervous System

Edited by

Mohan K. Raizada
and M. Ian Phillips
University of Florida
Gainesville, Florida

and
Derek LeRoith
Diabetes Branch, NIDDK, NIH
Bethesda, Maryland

Plenum Press • New York and London

CONTENTS

INTERNALIZATION OF INSULIN AND ITS RECEPTOR: ROLE IN SIGNALING

Barry I. Posner, Masood N. Khan and John J. M. Bergeron*

Departments of Medicine and *Anatomy
McGill University
Montreal
Canada, H3A 1A1

INTRODUCTION

Tissue resistance to the action of insulin plays a role in the pathogenesis of Diabetes Mellitus, especially the Type II variety.[1] This has given clinical relevance to investigation of the mechanism of insulin action on target tissues. One approach to studying insulin action is to examine the nature of its interaction with target cells. In this article we shall briefly outline the fate of insulin following interaction with its receptor, and the role that subsequent cellular handling of insulin-receptor complexes might play in hormone signal transmission.

INSULIN CELL INTERACTIONS: STRUCTURES INVOLVED

The initial site of interaction between insulin and its target tissues is the cell surface receptor. This is followed by aggregation[2] and then internalization of insulin in a receptor-dependent manner.[3] The structures into which internalized hormone is rapidly concentrated have been studied in considerable detail.[4,5] In rat liver these entities are initially small vesicles and then lipoprotein-containing vesicles (LPVs). The latter are not lysosomes since they are not enriched in acid phosphatase.[6] Furthermore the low uptake of ^{125}I-insulin into purified lysosomes can be accounted for exclusively by uptake into LPVs contaminating the lysosomal fractions.[7]

Based on morphologic considerations and the enrichment in galactosyltransferase (GT) of cell fractions containing a preponderance of LPVs we initially suggested these LPVs were Golgi vesicular elements.[3] However, it was soon apparent that the lipoprotein-containing vesicles in Golgi fractions were heterogeneous and could be resolved by Percoll gradient centrifugation into two receptor-rich vesicle populations - lighter density structures cosedimenting with GT, and heavier density vesicles containing no GT but low levels of acid phosphatase.[8] Insulin was rapidly internalized into the lower density structures and only later appeared in the higher density components. These studies thus showed that the structures involved in endocytosis were heterogeneous and were, at least partially, resolvable from Golgi elements as defined by marker enzyme (i.e. GT) content.

The next question addressed the degree of uniformity of lower density lipoprotein-containing vesicles. Perhaps one pool reflected a biogenetic route and a

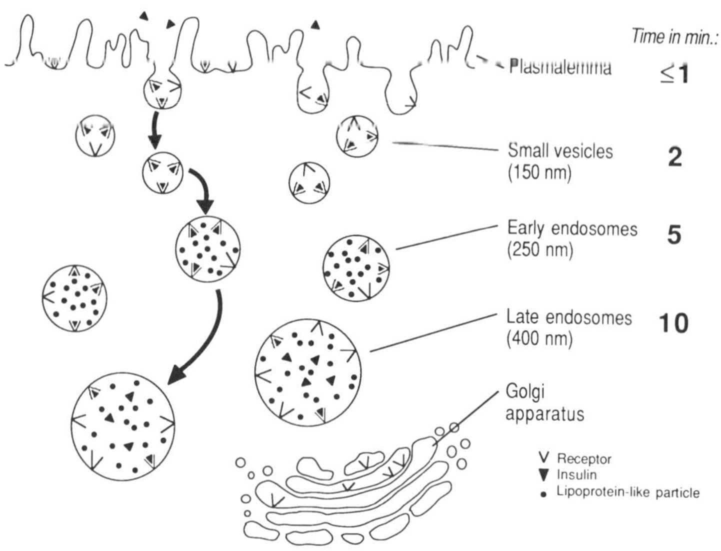

Figure 1. Receptor mediated endocytosis of insulin. The hormone is seen attaching to receptors at the cell surface. Following this hormone-receptor complexes appear sequentially in small vesicles, early endosomes and then late endosomes. In the latter the low intravesicular pH effects dissociation of hormone-receptor complexes. The estimated average size of the depicted structures is noted in parentheses.

second endocytosis and catabolism. This latter possibility was supported by the appreciation that the liver in most animals probably accounts for the bulk of low density lipoprotein catabolism.[9] The advent of a new and powerful method by Courtoy et al.[10] for resolving endocytic structures permitted us to examine more critically the extent to which internalized ^{125}I-insulin cosediments with GT. This technique is based upon the polymerization of diaminobenzidine (DAB) to a dense complex by horse-radish peroxidase (HRP) in the presence of H_2O_2. HRP, coupled to galactosylated bovine serum albumin, is internalized via the asialoglycoprotein receptor into rat liver endocytic vesicles. Following preparation of cell fractions the addition of DAB and H_2O_2 shifted endocytic structures to a higher density on subsequent centrifugation.[10] When we applied this procedure and coinjected ^{125}I-insulin it became clear that the bulk of low density endocytic elements containing ^{125}I-insulin shifted to a higher density and were devoid of GT.[11]

THE ENDOSOMAL APPARATUS

The structures involved in concentrating internalized ligands within the cell have been referred to in various ways (viz. lysosomes, ligandosomes, receptosomes, etc.). It is now clear that they can be distinguished from plasma membrane[3] and lysosomes[7] and, in large part, from Golgi elements as well.[11] The term now commonly used to designate this apparently distinctive intracellular system is the endosomal apparatus or endosomes.[5,12]

The prior discussion has noted that endosomes are heterogeneous and consist of several different components which can be separated kinetically and by fractionation procedures.[4,5] We have resolved by cell fractionation 3 distinctive components which participate sequentially in endocytosis as depicted in Fig. 1. Data from our laboratories have indicated that early endosomes are at near-neutral pH whereas late endosomes have acidic interiors and can concentrate the acidotropic substance chloroquine.[13] The extent to which this system consists of tubular elements which vesiculate on cell homogenization as suggested by Geuze et al.[14] remains to be ascertained.

ENDOSOME FUNCTIONS

A. Recycling of Receptors

Insulin is internalized in the form of insulin-receptor complexes. This is indicated by the fact that: (a) ligand uptake is receptor-mediated[15]; (b) photolabeled receptors become sequestered from receptor-modifying agents; (i.e. protease) with time[16]; (c) ligand administration accumulates receptors intracellularly[17]; and (d) antibodies to receptor and ligand colocalize at the cell surface and in intracellular vesicles.[14] It is also evident that most ligand-receptor complexes are dissociated within the endosomal system and that receptors recycle to the cell surface for repetitive utilization in effecting ligand internalization. Thus, whereas insulin is metabolized rapidly ($t_{\frac{1}{2}} \approx 10$ min) its receptor is metabolized slowly ($t_{\frac{1}{2}} \approx 10$ hr) by target cells.[17] Cell surface receptors (photolabeled) first lose and then regain sensitivity to protease.[18] Acidotropic agents accumulate both ligand and receptors intracellularly.[13,19,20] Finally, using antibodies to both asialoglycoprotein and its receptor Geuze et al. demonstrated the separation of the internalized complex in tubulovesicular elements within the hepatocyte.[21]

Though for many ligand receptor complexes there is intracellular degradation of ligand and receptor recycling (viz. LDL, peptide hormones, transcobalamin II, asialoglycoprotein) for others the ligand largely recycles with its receptor (e.g., transferrin[22]). Receptor-mediated endocytosis has also been documented to function as a mechanism for transporting ligand from one compartment to another. Thus, placental IgG receptors transport maternal IgG to the fetus[23]; hepatic IgA receptors transport circulating IgA to bile[24]; and choroid plexus prolactin receptors transport systemic prolactin into the CSF.[25] Thus the endosomal system plays a key role in directing the flow of ligand-receptor complexes between different cell compartments.

B. Ligand Processing

Since the original observations of Terris and Steiner identifying insulin degradation by hepatocytes as a receptor-mediated phenomenon[26] it has become ever clearer that an important consequence of the internalization of peptide hormones is their degradation within target cells. As noted above the dissociation of hormone from receptor within the endosomal apparatus might be an essential prior step. This could explain why the administration of chloroquine, an acidotropic agent, led to insulin accumulation in endosomes[7] whereas prolactin accumulation was unaffected by chloroquine.[27] Correspondingly prolactin binding to its receptor was far less sensitive to acid pH than was that of insulin binding.[28] The more rapid clearance of internalized insulin than internalized prolactin from the liver[29,30] is consistent with the processing of insulin within endosomes. Several groups have identified cathepsin D in endosomes[31,32] and Diment and Stahl have proposed that selective ligand processing is regulated by pH in macrophage endosomes.[31] In contrast Pease et al. have concluded that liver endosomes are a locus for insulin processing but by specific protease whose pH optimum is 6 to 7.[33] The independence of insulin processing from its dissociation from receptor by low pH has recently received strong support from the work of Hamel et al.[34] showing the onset of insulin degradation in early endosomes, a near-neutral pH vesicular compartment.

C. Hormonal Signaling

An interesting possibility is that internalized insulin-receptor complexes may play a key role in insulin action via several possibilities. Thus, insulin degradation

(continued after Figure 4)

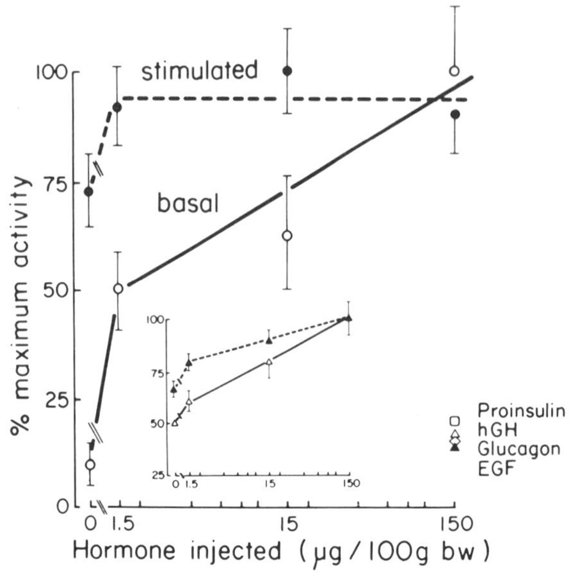

Figure 2. Autophosphorylation of solubilized insulin receptors from rat liver microsomes prepared 15 min after insulin injection at noted doses. Microsomes (20 mg protein/ml) were solubilized in 50 mM Hepes buffer (pH 7.6) - 1.0% Triton X-100 containing $MgCl_2$ (20 mM), sodium fluoride (1 mM), sodium vanadate (2 mM), sodium molybdate (20 mM), aprotinin (1000 KIU/ml), benzamidine (1 mM) and p-methylsulfonylfluoride (PMSF, 1 mM). After shaking for 1 hr at 4°C the suspension was centrifuged (100,000 g_{av} x 60 min) and the supernatant assayed for protein, insulin binding and insulin content as previously described.[19] Solubilized receptor (300-400 μg) was incubated for 1 hr at 4°C in 50 mM Hepes (pH 7.6) - 0.08% Triton X-100 and other additions as previously outlined[39] with or without 0.1 μM insulin in a final volume of 120 μl. Phosphorylation was initiated by adding 30 μl of γ-^{32}P-ATP at a final concentration of 50 μM (70 μCi/tube). The reaction was terminated after 25 min by adding 50 μl of 50 mM Hepes (pH 7.6) - 0.2% Triton X-100 containing ATP (100 mM), EDTA (40 mM) and PMSF (2 mM). Samples containing identical amounts of receptor (19 fmol specific binding) were immunoprecipitated by incubating with 10 μl (140 μg) anti-insulin receptor antibody for 4 hr at 4°C, followed by 40 μl of protein A-Sepharose for one hr. The immunoprecipitate was recovered by centrifugation (10,000 x g, 5 min), washed, solubilized and subjected to SDS-PAGE and radioautography as described previously.[39] The results are the mean ± SEM of 3 experiments. Identical studies were performed on rats injected with 150 μg of proinsulin (□), human growth hormone (△), glucagon (◇) and EGF (▲). Inset: Equivalent experiments where phosphorylation of synthetic substrate poly glu:tyr (4:1) was evaluated. Solubilized microsomal membrane receptors from control and insulin-injected rats were incubated with (▲) or without (△) insulin (0.1 μM). Phosphorylation was initiated with ^{32}P-ATP (50 μM final) for 10 min at room temp, and terminated by spotting 80 μl on Whatman filter papers (No. 3, 2 x 2 cm squares) which were immersed in TCA (10%) - sodium pyrophosphate (10 mM) for 18 hr at 4°C. After two washes at 4°C and two at room temp. (30 min each) the squares were dipped in anhydrous ethanol for 10 min and air dried at room temp. Radioactivity, determined in a Tri-Carb scintillation spectrometer (Packard, model 3003) using Aquasol-2, was normalized to the same amount of receptor (19 fmol specific binding) for each assay sample. Results are mean ± SEM of 3 experiments.

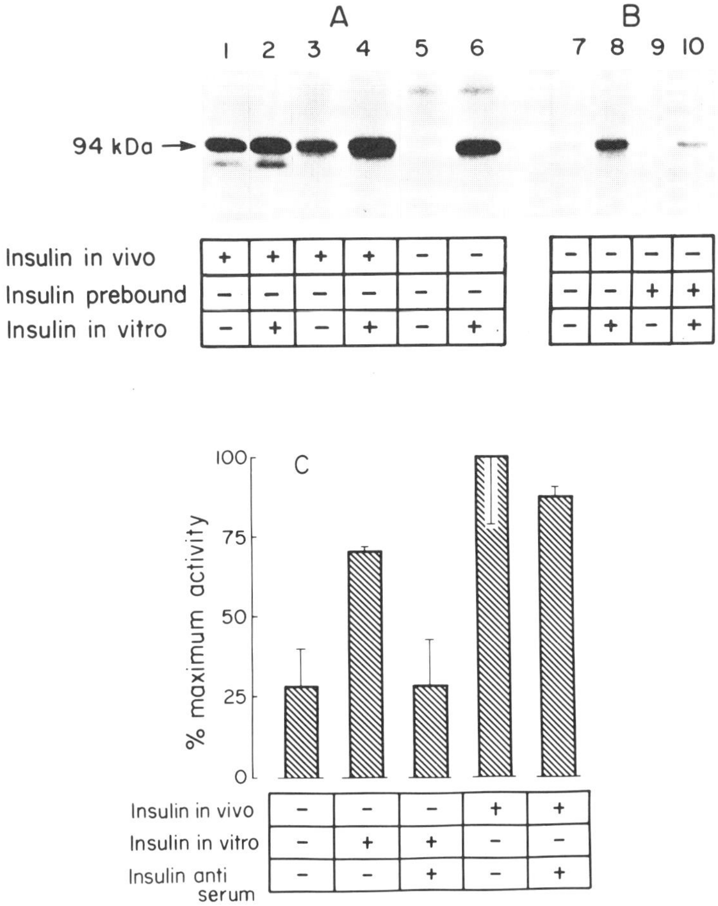

Figure 3. In vivo activation of the insulin receptor kinase activity in microsomes cannot be due to the carry over of associated ligand. (A) Comparison of receptor phosphorylation in solubilized microsomes from insulin injected rats [15 min, 150 μg/100 g body weight (lanes 1 and 2)] with that of lectin-purified (WGA-Sepharose) receptor from the same microsomes (lanes 3 and 4) or non-injected control rats (lanes 5 and 6). Receptor phosphorylation was carried out in the absence (lanes 1, 3 and 5) or presence (lanes 2, 4 and 6) of insulin then followed by immunoprecipitation as described in the legend to Fig. 1. (B) Autophosphorylation of lectin-purified (WGA-Sepharose) receptors from control microsomes (lanes 7 and 8) and from microsomes which had previously bound insulin in vitro (lanes 9 and 10). The microsomes (frozen and thawed 4 times) were incubated without (lanes 7 and 8) or with (lanes 9 and 10) insulin (100 ng/mg protein) in 25 mM Tris HCl, pH 7.4, 10 mM $MgCl_2$, 0.1% BSA for 20 hr at 4°C and then pelleted by centrifugation at 200,000g x 30 min. Specific insulin binding was 29.6 ng/mg protein as observed in separate experiments using ^{125}I-insulin. After binding membranes were solubilized and insulin receptors partially purified by WGA-Sepharose chromatography. Autophosphorylation was performed in the absence (lanes 7 and 9) or presence (lanes 8 and 10) of 0.1 μM insulin. Equivalent amounts of receptor (9.3 fmols of insulin binding activity) were loaded onto each lane. (C) Histogram: Effect of antiserum to insulin on insulin-stimulated autophosphorylation. Lectin-purified receptors (8 fmol insulin binding activity) from livers of control or insulin-injected rats (as above) were incubated with or without guinea pig anti-insulin antiserum (final titer 1:120) in the presence or absence of in vitro insulin (0.1 μM) for 30 min at 22°C followed by incubation for 60 min at 4°C. Phosphorylation was initiated by the addition of γ-^{32}P-ATP and terminated after 15 min at 4°C as described in Fig. 1. The results are mean ± SEM of three assays.

products may augment insulin action.[35] Other investigations suggest that small, membrane-derived molecules, released by insulin, may mediate its action as second messengers.[36] More recently it has been found that the β-subunit of the insulin receptor is a protein kinase[37] which is markedly activated on contact with insulin.[38] It has been suggested that this kinase may effect action by phosphorylating key intracellular proteins. All three of these possible modes of insulin action may occur during and following internalization of insulin-receptor complexes.

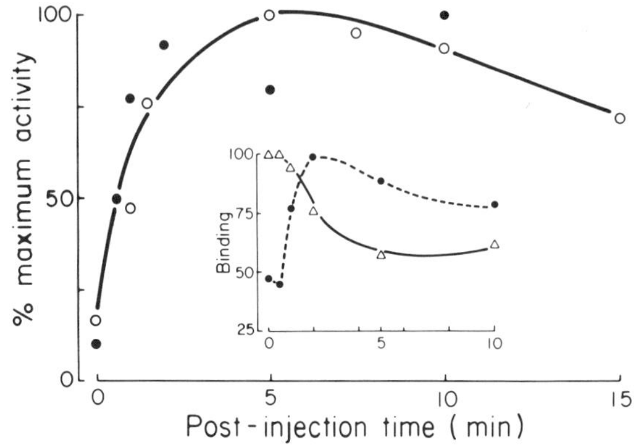

Figure 4. Time course of receptor activation and translocation. At various times after the injection of insulin (150 μg/100 g body weight) microsomes and derived endosomes[39] were isolated from liver homogenates. Autophosphorylation of solubilized microsomal receptors was carried out as described for Fig. 1 with 19 fmol insulin binding activity in each assay before immunoprecipitation (o---o). Endosome fractions were partially purified from parent microsomes by discontinuous sucrose gradient centrifugation and harvested at the 0.60/0.86 M sucrose interface. Detailed characterization of this fraction has shown no significant contamination by plasmalemma constituents.[39] Insulin receptors were lectin-purified (WGA-Sepharose) from solubilized endosome fractions and subjected to autophosphorylation in the absence of in vitro insulin (9.5 fmol insulin binding activity) as described in Figs. 1 and 2 (o——o). Inset: Kinetics of receptor change in PM (△——△) and endosomes (●---●). Plasmalemma (method of Hubbard et al.),[45] and endosome fractions were isolated as described by Khan et al.,[39] and specific binding determined as previously described.[39]

In initial studies we showed that injection of insulin in vivo augmented both β-subunit autophosphorylation (Fig. 2) as well as tyrosine kinase activity against the exogenous substrate poly glu:tyr, (4:1) (Fig. 2, inset). A dose-dependent augmentation of both insulin receptor kinase activities in rat liver microsomes can be seen. The specificity of in vivo activation was evaluated by the parallel injection of pro-insulin, human growth hormone, glucagon or epidermal growth factor, none of which altered basal autophosphorylation activity of the insulin receptor.

Studies were designed to determine whether the apparent activation seen in Fig. 2 was simply due to the continued association of insulin with the receptor preparations during their partial purification and assay. Following the binding of ^{125}I-insulin to microsomes the receptors were solubilized and partially purified by wheat germ agglutinin-Agarose (WGA)-chromatography. This procedure resulted in the dissociation of around 95% of the microsome-associated ^{125}I-insulin. Nevertheless, as seen in Fig. 3A the autophosphorylating activity of lectin-purified receptors from rats receiving in vivo insulin (lanes 3 and 4) was comparable to that of the solubilized parent microsomes (lanes 1 and 2), and much greater than that from uninjected controls (lane 5). Furthermore, the in vitro binding of insulin, at high concentration, to microsomes from control rats did not augment basal autophosphorylation of the subsequently lectin-purified insulin receptors (Fig. 3B). Finally, antiserum to insulin, added at a concentration sufficient to block the stimulatory effect of 100 nM insulin on autophosphorylation, did not inhibit the augmented level of basal autophosphorylation of receptors from insulin-treated rats (Fig. 3C). Thus in vivo insulin administration produced activation of its receptor kinase.

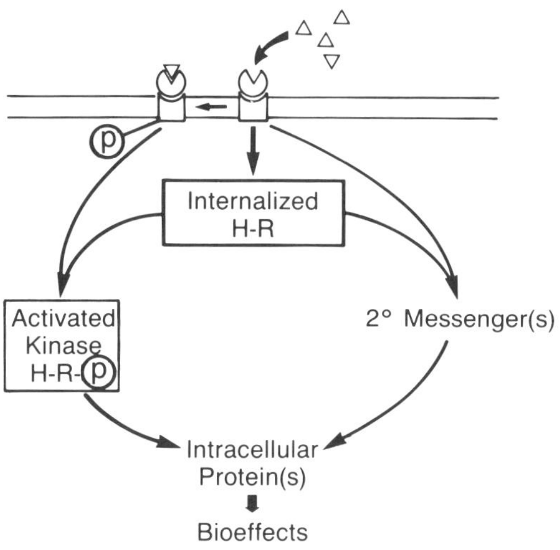

Figure 5. Internalization and activation of insulin-receptor complexes. Receptor is depicted as accumulating intracellularly in the form of hormone-receptor (H-R) complexes and activated receptor kinase (H-R-P). The possibilities that activation, through autophosphorylation, both precedes and follows internalization of H-R, are considered. The realization of hormone action through the release of second (2°) messenger(s) at the plasma membrane and/or intracellularly is also noted.

The time course of receptor activation following in vivo insulin was maximal by 5 min and extended for at least 15 min after insulin injection for receptors from microsomes and endosomes derived therefrom (Fig. 4). Comparison of the time course of kinase activation with receptor internalization (Fig. 4, inset) showed the latter may be even faster with a peak time of ca 2.5 min for receptor internalization into endosomes. The kinetics of receptor translocation shown here confirm and extend the previous work of Khan et al.[39] and Desbuquois et al.[19] and suggest that activation occurs following and/or during internalization to peripheral (early) endosomes.

In more recent studies the detailed time course of insulin receptor kinase activation has been studied following the injection of different doses of insulin.[40]

Activation of the plasma membrane (PM) receptor kinase was maximal at 30 sec after insulin injection whereas activation of the endosomal (EN) kinase reached maximal levels at 2 to 5 min postinjection. The PM and EN kinases were augmented by insulin doses as low as 15 ng/100 g body weight, attesting to the physiologic relevance of this process. The pattern of activation was the same for autophosphorylation and exogenous kinase activity. Activated receptors were solubilized and treated with phosphatase prior to assaying for kinase activity. The treatment with phosphatase yielded a marked reduction in the augmented activity seen after in vivo insulin administration. This decrease was prevented by phosphatase inhibitors. A model summarizing the essential features supported by the above data is depicted in Fig. 5.

The rapid internalization and concentration within endosomes of activated insulin receptor kinase is consistent with a role for the endosomal system in facilitating transmembrane signaling. Thus insulin dissociation from its receptor, which likely occurs in endosomes, need not limit the biological response to insulin. This view is supported by mounting evidence which points to a critical role for the insulin receptor tyrosine kinase in effecting insulin action. Thus, some patients with insulin resistance have normal receptor levels but decreased receptor kinase activity.[41] The injection into Xenopus Laevis oocytes of antibody to the kinase region of the insulin receptor β-subunit blocked insulin-induced meiosis.[42] Mutagenesis of receptor cDNA at tyr 1162 and 1163 (tyrosine replaced by phenylalanine) of the proreceptor sequence produced a kinase with greatly reduced ability to be stimulated by insulin and a parallel decrease in insulin-stimulable glucose uptake.[43] Finally, studies with insulin, vanadate and hydrogen peroxide have revealed a correlation between the extent of kinase activation and insulin-like growth factor receptor translocation to the cell surface of rat adipocytes.[44]

In summary, the endosomal system is a complex cellular organelle for which three functions are beginning to be discerned. First, considerable data point to a role for endosomes in regulating the cellular traffic of ligand-receptor complexes. Second, selective ligand processing seems to occur within endosomes. Finally, a role for this system in transducing the hormonal signal appears likely.

ACKNOWLEDGEMENTS

The work summarized in this article has been supported by grants from the U.S.P.H.S., the M.R.C. of Canada and the Canadian Diabetes Association.

REFERENCES

1. G. M. Reaven, Insulin resistance in noninsulin-dependent diabetes mellitus. Does it exist and can it be measured? Amer. J.Med. 74 (No.lA): 3 (1983).
2. Y. Schecter, J. Schlessinger, S. Jacobs, K.-J. Chang, and P. Cuatrecasas, Fluorescent labeling of hormone receptors in viable cells: Preparation and properties of highly fluorescent derivatives of epidermal growth factor and insulin, Proc. Natl. Acad. Sci. USA 75:2135 (1978).
3. B. I. Posner, J. J. M. Bergeron, Z. Josefsberg, M. N. Khan, R. J. Khan, B. A. Patel, R. A. Sikstrom, and A. K. Verma, Polypeptide Hormones: Intracellular receptors and internalization, Recent Prog. Horm. Res. 37:539 (1981).
4. B. I. Posner, M. N. Khan, and J. J. M. Bergeron, Endocytosis of peptide hormones and other ligands, Endocr. Revs. 3: 280 (1982).
5. J. J. M. Bergeron, J. Cruz, M. N. Khan, and B. I. Posner, Uptake of insulin and other ligands into receptor-rich endocytic components of target cells. The endosomal apparatus, Annual Rev. of Physiol. 47: 383(1985).
6. J. J. M. Bergeron, R. Sikstrom, A. R. Hand and B. I. Posner, Binding and uptake of ^{125}I-insulin into rat liver hepatocytes and endothelium: An in vivo radioautographic study, J. Cell Biol. 80: 427 (1979).

7. B. I. Posner, B. Patel, M. N. Khan, and J. J. M. Bergeron, Effect of chloroquine on the internalization of ^{125}I-insulin into subcellular fractions of rat liver: Evidence for an effect of chloroquine on Golgi elements, J. Biol. Chem. 257:5789 (1982).
8. M. N. Khan, B. I. Posner, R. J. Khan, and J. J. M. Bergeron, Internalization of insulin into rat liver Golgi elements: Evidence for vesicle heterogeneity and the path of intracellular processing, J. Biol. Chem. 257:5969 (1982).
9. A. D. Attie, R. C. Pittman, and D. Steinberg, Hepatic catabolism of low density lipoprotein: Mechanisms and metabolic consequences, Hepatology 2:269 (1982).
10. P. J. Courtoy, J. Quintart, and P. Baudhuin, Shift of equilibrium density induced by 3, 3-diaminobenzidine cytochemistry: A new procedure for the analysis and purification of peroxidase-containing organelles, J. Cell Biol. 98:870 (1984).
11. D. G. Kay, M. N. Khan, B. I. Posner, and J. J. M. Bergeron, ^{125}I-insulin in hepatic Golgi fractions: Application of the diaminobenzidine (DAB)-shift protocol, Biochem. Biophys Res. Commun. 123:1144 (1984).
12. A. Helenius, J. Mellman, D. Wall, and A. Hubbard, Endosomes, Trends Biochem. Sci. 7:245 (1983).
13. M. N. Khan, S. Savoie, J. J. M. Bergeron, and B. I. Posner, Insulin and insulin receptor uptake into Golgi fractions: Effect and possible site of chloroquine action, Diabetes 34:1025 (1985).
14. H. J. Geuze, J. W. Slot, G. J. A. M. Strous, H. F. Lodish, and A. L. Schwartz, Intracellular site of asialoglycoprotein receptor-mediated endocytosis, Cell 32:277 (1983).
15. Z. Josefsberg, B. I. Posner, B. Patel, and J. J. M. Bergeron, Uptake of prolactin into female rat liver: Concentration of intact hormone in the Golgi apparatus, J. Biol. Chem. 254:209 (1979).
16. M. Fehlmann, J.-L. Carpentier, A. Le Cam, P. Thamm, D. Saunders, D. Brandenburg, L. Orci, and P. Freychet, Biochemical and morphological evidence that the insulin receptor is internalized with insulin in hepatocytes, J. Cell Biol. 93:82 (1982).
17. M. Krupp and M. D. Lane, On the mechanism of ligand-induced down-regulation of insulin receptor level in the liver cell, J. Biol. Chem. 256:1689 (1981).
18. M. Fehlmann, J.-L. Carpentier, E. Van Obberghen, P. Freychet, P. Thamm, D. Saunders, D. Brandenburg, and L. Orci, Internalized insulin receptors are recycled to the cell surface in rat hepatocytes, Proc. Natl. Acad. Sci. USA 79:5921 (1982).
19. B. Desbuquois, S. Lopez, and H. Burlet, Ligand-induced translocation of insulin receptors in intact rat liver, J. Biol. Chem. 257:10852 (1982).
20. V. Pezzino, R. Vigneri, N. B. Pliam, and I. D. Goldfine, Rapid regulation of plasma membrane insulin receptors, Diabetologia 29:211 (1980).
21. H. J. Geuze, J. W. Slot, G. J. A. M. Strous, J. Peppard, K. von Figura, A. Hasilik, and A. L. Schwartz, Intracellular receptor sorting during endocytosis: Comparative immunoelectron microscopy of multiple receptors in rat liver, Cell, 37:195 (1984).
22. W. S. May, Jr. and P. Cuatrecasas, Transferrin receptor: Its biological significance, J. Membr. Biol. 88:205 (1985).
23. D. R. Abrahamson and R. Rodewald, Evidence for the sorting of endocytic vesicle contents during the receptor-mediated transport of IgG across the newborn rat intestine, J. Cell Biol. 91:270 (1981).
24. L. C. Kuhn and J. P. Kraehenbuhl, The sacrificial receptor-translocation of polymeric IgA across epithelia, Trends Biochem.Sci. 7:299 (1982).
25. R. Walsh, F. J. Slaku and B. I. Posner, Prolactin transport from blood to CSF: A specific receptor-mediated mechanism, Endocrinology (in press).
26. S. Terris, and D. F. Steiner, Binding and degradation of ^{125}I-insulin by rat hepatocytes, J.Biol. Chem. 250:8389 (1975).
27. R. J. Khan, M. N. Khan, J. J. M. Bergeron, and B. I. Posner, Prolactin uptake into liver endocytic components: Reduced sensitivity to chloroquine, Biochim. Biophys. Acta 838:77 (1985).

28. B. I. Posner, Z. Josefsberg, and J. J. M. Bergeron, Intracellular polypeptide hormone receptors: Characterization and induction of prolactin receptors in the Golgi apparatus of rat liver, J. Biol. Chem. 254:12494 (1979).
29. J. J. M. Bergeron, N. Searle, M. N. Khan, and B. I. Posner, Differential and analytical subfractionation of rat liver components internalizing insulin and prolactin, Biochemistry 25: 1756 (1986).
30. M. N. Khan, S. Savoie, J. J. M. Bergeron, and B. I. Posner, Differential kinetics and sensitivity to chloroquine for receptor-mediated insulin and prolactin endocytosis in liver parenchymal cells, Biochim. Biophys. Acta 888:100 (1986).
31. S. Diment and P. Stahl, Macrophage endosomes contain protease which degrade endocytosed protein ligands, J. Biol. Chem. 260:15311 (1985).
32. H. J. Geuze, J. W. Slot, G. J. A. M. Strous, A. Hasilik, and K. von Figura, Possible pathways for lysosomal enzyme delivery, J. Cell Biol. 101:2253 (1985).
33. R. J. Pease, G. D. Smith, and T. J. Peters, Degradation of endocytosed insulin in rat liver is mediated by low-density vesicles, Biochem. J. 228:137 (1985).
34. F. G. Hamel, B. I. Posner, M. Vanderwel, J. J. M. Bergeron, and W. C. Duckworth, Insulin degradation by endosomes in intact liver, Abstract, Forty seventh Annual Meeting of the American Diabetes Association, Diabetes (submitted).
35. K. Kikuchi, J. Larner, R. J. Freer, and A. R. Day, Effect of insulin fragments on biological activity of insulin and desoctapeptide insulin, I. Potentiation of biological activities, J. Biol. Chem. 256:9441 (1981).
36. A. R. Saltiel, J. A. Fox, P. Sherline, and P. Cuatrecasas, Insulin-stimulated hydrolysis of a novel glycolipid generates modulators of cAMP phosphodiesterase, Science 233:967 (1986).
37. M. Kasuga, Y. Fujita-Yamaguchi, D. L. Blithe, M. F. White, and C. R. Kahn, Characterization of the insulin receptor kinase purified from human placental membranes, J. Biol. Chem. 258:10973 (1983).
38. O. M. Rosen, R. Herrera, Y. Olowe, L. M. Petruzzelli, and M. H. Cobb, Phosphorylation activates the insulin receptor tyrosine protein kinase, Proc. Natl. Acad. Sci. USA 80:3237 (1983).
39. M. N. Khan, S. Savoie, J. J. M. Bergeron, and B. I. Posner, Characterization of rat liver endosomal fractions: in vivo activation of insulin-stimulable kinase in these structures, J. Biol. Chem. 261:8462 (1986).
40. M. N. Khan, J. J. M. Bergeron, and B. I. Posner, Internalization of the activated insulin receptor kinase in rat liver endosomes, J. Cell. Biol. 103 (No.5, Part 2): 450a (1986). [Abstr. No. 1679].
41. G. Grunberger, Y. Zick, and P. Gorden, Defect in phosphorylation of insulin receptors in cells from an insulin-resistant patient with normal insulin binding, Science 223: 932 (1984).
42. D. O. Morgan, L. Ho, L. J. Korn, and R. A. Roth, Insulin action is blocked by a monoclonal antibody that inhibits the insulin-receptor kinase, Proc. Natl. Acad. Sci. USA 83:328 (1986).
43. L. Ellis, E. Clauser, D. O. Morgan, M. Edery, R. A. Roth, and W. J. Rutter, Replacement of insulin receptor tyrosine residues 1162 and 1163 compromises insulin-stimulated kinase activity and uptake of 2-deoxyglucose, Cell 45:721 (1986).
44. S. Kadota, I. G. Fantus, H. Guyda, and B. Posner, Vanadate augments adipocyte IGF-2 binding in a manner similar but not identical to insulin, Diabetes 35 (Suppl. 1): 53A (1986) [Abstr. No. 211].
45. A. L. Hubbard, D. A. Wall, and A. Ma, Isolation of rat hepatocyte plasma membranes. 1. Presence of the three major domains, J. Cell Biol. 96:217 (1983).

INSULIN-ACTIVATED PHOSPHORYLATION ON TYROSINE OF A 15 KILODALTON CYTOSOLIC PROTEIN IN 3T3-L1 ADIPOCYTES*

Michel Bernier[1], Susan C. Frost[2], Don M. Laird[2], Ronald A.Kohanski[2], M. Daniel Lane

Department of Biological Chemistry
The Johns Hopkins University School of Medicine
Baltimore, Maryland 21205

I. INTRODUCTION

The action of insulin is initiated by its interaction with the insulin receptor located on the surface of target cells (1). This interaction generates a signal, which when transmitted across the plasma membrane, is propagated and distributed to pleitropic control points of cellular metabolism. Modulation by insulin of flux through these controlled reactions is responsible for regulation of the major energy storage pathways in many cell types. In the adipocyte, glucose uptake, glycogenesis and lipogenesis are accelerated by insulin.

The insulin receptor is a transmembrane allosteric enzyme which has an $\alpha_2\beta_2$ oligomeric structure (1). Insulin binds to a specific site on the α-subunit which is located at the face of the plasma membrane and is covalently attached (through disulfide bonds) to the membrane-spanning β-subunit. This binding interaction apparently induces a conformational change which is transmitted through the receptor across the plasma membrane to the β-subunit's cytoplasmic tyrosine kinase catalytic site. This action first activates autophosphorylation of the β-subunit which, in turn, activates catalysis of phosphorylation of protein substrates (1).

The fundamental question to be addressed in this paper is, "How is the insulin signal transmitted from its receptor in the plasma membrane to the enzymes (or other proteins) that regulate energy metabolism?". The regulated metabolic process that we have focused on in the studies to be described is the activation of glucose uptake by insulin in the 3T3-L1 adipocyte. In these studies we discovered a 15 kDa phosphotyrosyl protein that we believe is an intermediate in the signal transmission pathway from the insulin receptor to the glucose transport system (2).

We have employed the fully-differentiated 3T3-L1 adipocyte in culture as a model insulin-sensitive cell system. The 3T3-L1 preadipocyte, a cell line established more than ten years ago in Howard Green's laboratory (3,4), undergoes differentiation when stimulated appropriately into a cell type which possesses the morphological (5) and biochemical (6-13) characteristics of an adipocyte. During differentiation

3T3-L1 cells acquire the capacity to elicit insulin-stimulated hexose uptake (12). This increased sensitivity to insulin is due in part to a 20-fold increase in the number of insulin receptors the differentiated adipocyte acquires (10).

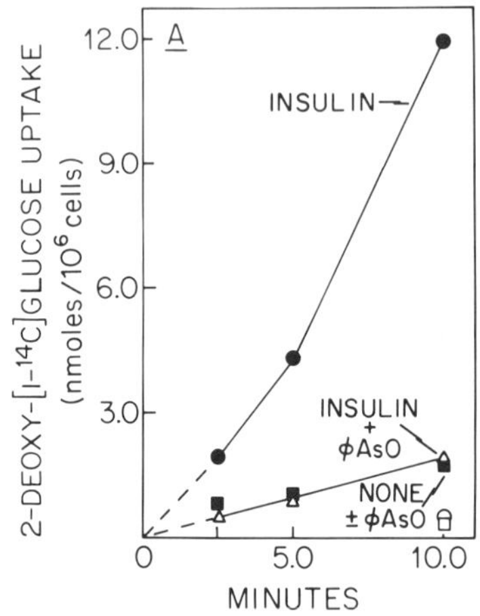

Figure 1. Inhibition by phenylarsine oxide of insulin-activated 2-deoxyglucose uptake in 3T3-L1 adipocytes. 2-deoxy[1-^{14}C]glucose (0.2 mM) uptake was measured over a 10 minute period in the presence or absence of 1 μM insulin in cells pretreated or not with 35 μM phenylarsine oxide. Some monolayers were pretreated for 10 minutes with cytochalasin B (20 μM) and then assayed for hexose uptake with (●) or without (■) insulin as above. Half-maximal transport activation is achieved at 7 nM insulin. The results are from Frost and Lane (12).

II. INHIBITION BY PHENYLARSINE OXIDE OF SIGNAL TRANSMISSION FROM THE INSULIN RECEPTOR TO THE GLUCOSE TRANSPORT SYSTEM

The rate of 2-deoxyglucose uptake by 3T3-L1 adipocytes is markedly stimulated by insulin (12, 14). Figure 1 shows that after a short lag period hexose uptake rate is increased approximately 10-fold by insulin relative to that by control cells not treated with insulin. Several years ago we observed (12) that phenylarsine oxide blocks the activation of hexose uptake by insulin, but does not alter hexose uptake *per se* (Figure 1).

This observation suggested that signal transmission from the insulin receptor to the glucose transport system is blocked by the inhibitor. Trivalent arsenicals, such as phenylarsine oxide, form stable ring complexes with vicinal dithiols as illustrated in Figure 2. While trivalent arsenicals are known to inhibit several different enzymes which contain functional vicinal dithiols, these inhibitors are chemically quite specific. Although the reaction of phenylarsine oxide with neighboring sulfhydryl groups gives rise to stable ring complexes (15), this reaction can be reversed by dithiol competitors, such as 2,3-dimercaptopropanol (Figure 2).

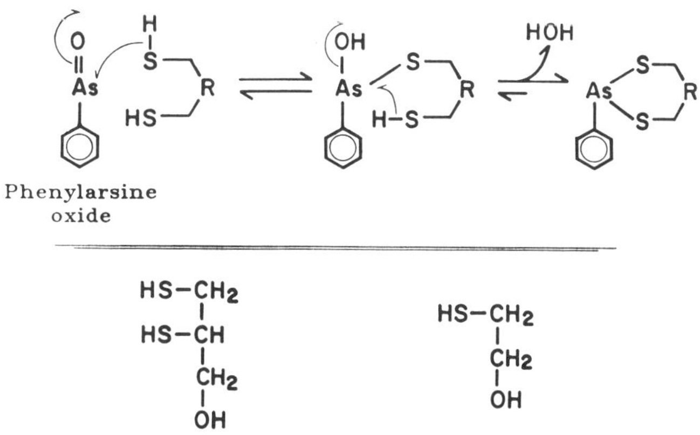

Figure 2. Reaction of vicinal dithiols with phenylarsine oxide: structures of 2,3-dimercaptopropanol and 2-mercaptoethanol.

Importantly, this reversibility can be demonstrated in the intact cell. For example, the inhibition of the activation of hexose uptake by phenylarsine oxide can be fully reversed by the use of 2,3-dimercaptopropanol in the 3T3-L1 adipocyte (12).

The fact that phenylarsine oxide inhibits the activation of hexose uptake by insulin, but not hexose transport *per se*, indicates that the inhibitor interrupts the signal transmission process itself. Furthermore, the mechanism by which trivalent arsenicals act suggests involvement in the signalling process of a protein with functional vicinal sulfhydryl groups.

III. KINETICS OF INSULIN-ACTIVATED INSULIN RECEPTOR β-SUBUNIT PHOSPHORYLATION AND HEXOSE UPTAKE

To assess the temporal relationship between insulin-activated phosphorylation of the insulin receptor's β-subunit and of hexose uptake, the rates of activation of these two processes by insulin were compared (14). In order to determine the rate of β-subunit phosphorylation upon stimulation by insulin, it was necessary to label the cellular ATP pool with ^{32}P. This was accomplished with a 2-hour preliminary incubation of 3T3-L1 adipocytes with $^{32}P_i$. It was determined that this time period was sufficient to achieve constant specific activity in the α, β, and γ phosphate groups of ATP (14). Then, at various times after the addition of insulin, further phosphorylation and/or dephosphorylation were prevented by the addition of sodium dodecylsulfate (SDS). The detergent extract was diluted by addition of Triton X-100, a non-ionic detergent, to trap SDS in Triton micelles. Following centrifugation the insulin receptor-containing extract was subjected to wheat germ lectin Sepharose affinity chromatography after which the eluted glycoprotein fraction (containing the insulin receptor) was subjected to 2-dimensional non-reducing/reducing SDS polyacrylamide gel electrophoresis. This process readily resolves the α and the β subunits of the receptor from each other and all other proteins in the extracts by virtue of the unique S-S covalent $\alpha_2\beta_2$ structure of the receptor in the non-reduced state and its dissociation into free α and β subunits in the reduced state (14, 17).

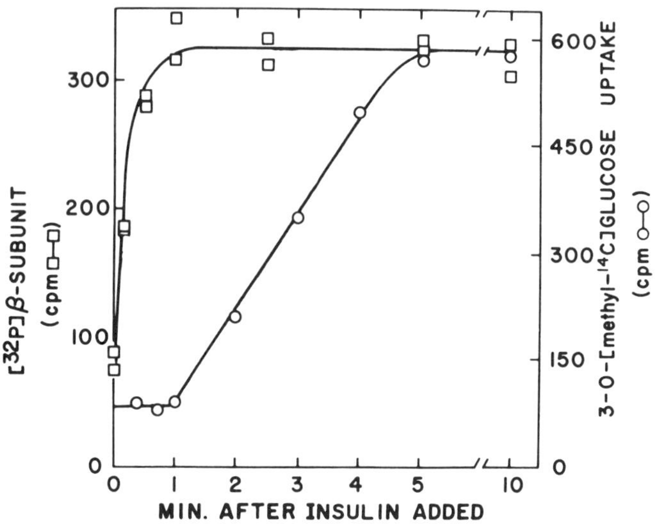

Figure 3. Kinetics of activation by insulin of insulin receptor β-subunit phosphorylation and of 3-O-methylglucose uptake. 3T3-L1 adipocytes were exposed to 1 μM insulin for time periods indicated. The uptake of 3-O-[methyl-^{14}C]glucose (average from 4 cell monolayers) was measured for a 20-sec period after the indicated periods of time following the addition of insulin. Thus, each point shown on the plot represents the rate of hexose uptake. To determine the extent of phosphorylation of the insulin receptor β-subunit, cells were first exposed to medium containing $^{32}P_i$ for 2 hours to label the ATP pool to constant ^{32}P specific activity (14). At various times after exposing the cells to insulin further phosphorylation or dephosphorylation was quenched by the addition of 0.1% SDS. This was followed by dilution with 1% Triton X-100 and adsorbing the receptor quantitatively to wheat-germ lectin Sepharose and elution with N-acetylglucosamine. ^{32}P-labeled β-subunit was then isolated by 2-dimensional SDS polyacrylamide gel electrophoresis. Radioactivity associated with the β-subunit was quantitated by cutting out the gel spot and counting. The results shown in this figure and the methods employed are described in Kohanski _et. al._ (14).

Cells treated similarly (but without $^{32}P_i$ or detergent treatment) were subjected to 30-second 3-O-methylglucose uptake assays following the addition of insulin (14). These results are illustrated in Figure 3.

It is shown that the receptor was phosphorylated to a significant extent prior to the addition of insulin; this phosphorylation is primarily on phosphoserine with a trace on phosphotyrosine (14). Upon addition of insulin there is a rapid rise (about 4-5-fold) in the extent of β-subunit phosphorylation after which the new steady-state level of phosphorylation is maintained for at least 10 minutes. Phosphoamino acid analysis showed that the insulin-stimulated rise in β-subunit phosphorylation is due exclusively to a 7-8-fold increase in tyrosine phosphorylation with no change in the initial basal level of serine phosphorylation (14). The rise in tyrosine phosphorylation is extremely rapid exhibiting a $t_{1/2}$ of approximately 10 seconds.

Correlated with this change in tyrosine phosphorylation is a change in the rate of hexose uptake. The rate of uptake of 3-O-methylglucose following insulin addition exhibits a 60-second lag and then rises for an additional 4 minutes at which point a steady-state uptake rate is achieved (Figure 3). From these results it may be concluded that any intermediary events in signal transmission must occur between the time of incipient β-subunit phosphorylation and the rise in the rate of hexose uptake (Figure 3).

In other studies (14) it was determined that half-maximal stimulation β-subunit phosphorylation and 3-O-methylglucose occurs at an insulin concentration of 3-6 nM and that maximal hexose uptake occurs when 70-80% of the insulin receptor is phosphorylated. Both IGF-I and IGF-II (insulin-like growth factors I and II) stimulate hexose uptake at comparable concentrations (K_a = 5 nM); however, neither IGF-I nor IGF-II activated phosphorylation of the β-subunit of the insulin receptor (14). These results indicate that neither IGF-I nor IGF-II activate hexose uptake by a mechanism involving phosphorylation of the insulin receptor *per se*.

IV. INSULIN AND PHENYLARSINE OXIDE-DEPENDENT ACCUMULATION OF A 15 KILODALTON PROTEIN PHOSPHORYLATED ON TYROSINE

Based on the results cited above, we set out to search for a cellular intermediate in the signal transmission pathway that is phosphorylated by the insulin receptor's tyrosine kinase catalytic site. The strategy employed in our search for a protein target of the receptor in intact 3T3-L1 adipocytes was based on the use of phenylarsine oxide. As demonstrated above, this inhibitor interrupts signal transmission between the receptor and the glucose transport system. It was anticipated that a blockade by this inhibitor might cause accumulation of a phosphorylated intermediate(s) proximal to the receptor and upstream from the site of inhibition (see Figure 4A). Importantly, earlier work had established that phenylarsine oxide does not significantly alter cellular ATP levels in 3T3-L1 adipocytes using the protocol described below (12).

Fully-differentiated 3T3-L1 adipocytes, incubated with $^{32}P_i$ for 2 hours to achieve steady-state labeling of cellular ATP (14), were incubated for 10 minutes with or without phenylarsine oxide and then were stimulated or not for 10 minutes with insulin. The cells were quickly lysed with urea-containing buffer and the phosphorylated proteins in the extract were analyzed by 2-dimensional gel electrophoresis using non-equilibrium isoelectric focusing and then SDS polyacrylamide gel electrophoresis. As shown in Figure 5D, addition of insulin and phenylarsine oxide to 3T3-L1 adipocytes led to the appearance of several phosphorylated polypeptides. The most striking change was the marked accumulation of a 15 kDa ^{32}P-labeled protein (pp15) (2). In the absence of insulin and phenylarsine oxide or with insulin added alone or with phenylarsine oxide added alone, virtually no ^{32}P-labeled pp15 was detected. In other experiments using equilibrium isoelectric focusing pp15 was found to have a pI of 6.3 (2).

2-Dimensional phosphoamino acid analysis of partial acid hydrolysates of ^{32}P-labeled pp15 revealed that phosphorylation occurred exclusively on tyrosyl residues with no evident phosphorylation on serine or threonine (Figure 6). Although changes in the phosphorylation states of other cellular polypeptides occur upon treatment with insulin and/or phenylarsine oxide (Figure 5), all of those examined (with the exception of the insulin receptors β-subunit itself) were found to be phosphorylated on serine or threonine rather than on tyrosine (results not shown). These results and those described below are consistent with the putative intermediate, X-Tyr-P shown in Figure 4A, as being pp15 (Figure 4B).

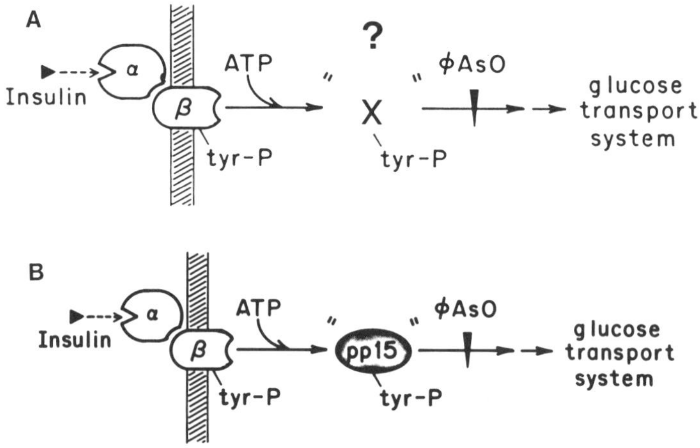

Figure 4. Possible effect of phenylarsine oxide on the insulin-activated signal transmission pathway. A) Pathway showing X-tyr-P as an hypothetical intermediate. B) Pathway showing pp15-tyr-P as an intermediate.

To ascertain the temporal relationship between insulin-activated phosphorylation of the β-subunit of the receptor and of pp15 and the activation of hexose uptake, the kinetics of these three processes were followed after the addition of insulin to phenylarsine oxide-treated 3T3-L1 adipocytes (Figure 7). The inhibitor had no effect on the kinetics of phosphorylation of the β-subunit which, as previously reported (14), reached a steady-state level of phosphorylation rapidly ($t_{1/2}$ = 10 sec) following insulin addition. The rate of phosphorylation of pp15, which followed immediately, is compatible with its involvement as an intermediate in the signal transmission pathway to the glucose transport system, since the insulin-stimulated phosphorylation of pp15 preceded activation of hexose transport (Figure 7). Moreover, the insulin concentration dependency and the K_a of insulin for the activation of β-subunit and pp15 phosphorylation and the activation of hexose uptake are identical (results not shown; see reference 2). These findings support the concept that p15 (or its precursor) is a cellular substrate of the tyrosine-specific receptor kinase and is on the signal transmission pathway to the glucose transport system (see Figure 4B).

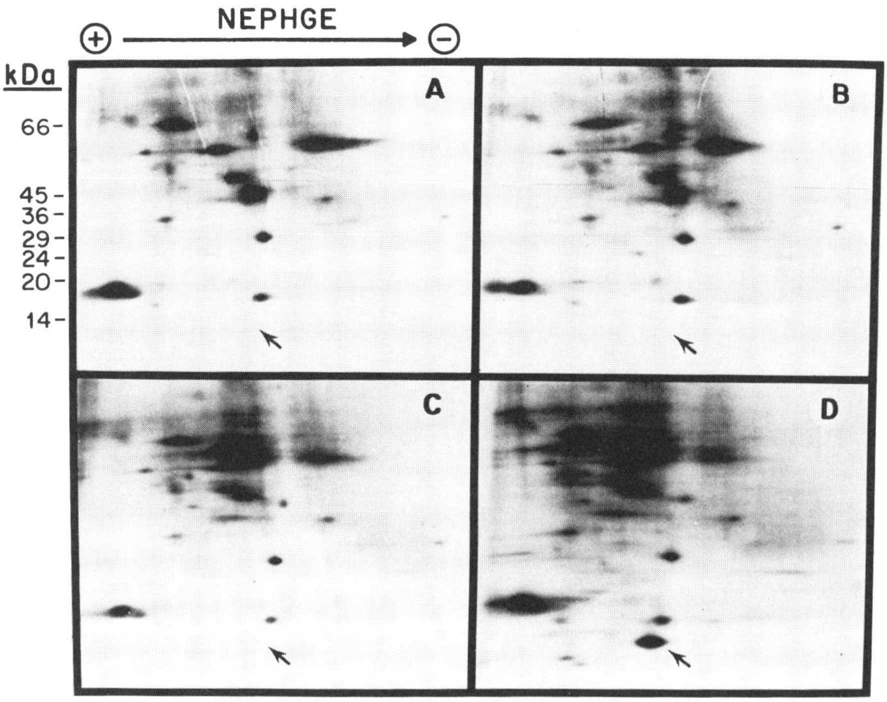

Figure 5. Insulin- and phenylarsine oxide-dependent accumulation of a phosphorylated 15 kDa polypeptide in 3T3-L1 adipocytes. Cell monolayers were first labeled for 2 hours with $^{32}P_i$-containing medium. This was followed by a 10-min preincubation without (A, B) or with (C, D) phenylarsine oxide (35 μM) and then a 10-min incubation without (A, C) or with (B, D) insulin (1 μM). Cells were lysed in urea-containing sample buffer and phosphorylated proteins were analyzed by 2-dimensional gel electrophoresis with non-equilibrium isoelectric focusing (NEPHGE) in the first dimension and SDS/polyacrylamide gel electrophoresis in the second dimension. Equal amounts (equivalent to 250,000 cells) of cell extract were loaded onto gels. ^{32}P-labeled proteins were detected by autoradiography. The results shown in this figure are from Bernier *et.* al. (2).

Phenylarsine oxide has no effect on the insulin concentration dependence (results not shown) or on the kinetics of β-subunit phosphorylation (Figure 7) indicating that the inhibitor acts downstream from the insulin receptor. In previous studies (Frost, Kohanski and Lane, manuscript submitted) it was observed that insulin receptor isolated from phenylarsine oxide-treated and untreated 3T3-L1 adipocytes exhibited identical insulin binding, autophosphorylation, and model substrate phosphorylation activities. Thus, it does not seem likely that phenylarsine oxide has any effect on the functions of the insulin receptor, but rather acts downstream from the receptor.

The specificity of the insulin-induced accumulation of pp15 (in the presence of phenylarsine oxide) was examined by comparing the effects of

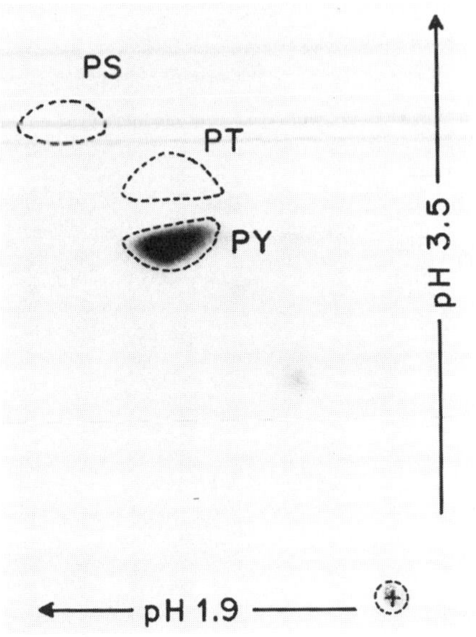

Figure 6. Phosphoamino acid analysis of ^{32}P-labeled pp15. 3T3-L1 adipocytes labeled with $^{32}P_i$, as described in Figure 5, were incubated with 35 μM phenylarsine oxide followed by 1 μM insulin. The phosphorylation reaction was terminated by extraction of the cells with urea sample buffer (as in Figure 5). ^{32}P-labeled proteins were resolved by 2-dimensional polyacrylamide gel electrophoresis (see Figure 5). The gel segment corresponding to ^{32}P-phospho-p15 was cut out and subjected to partial acid hydrolysis with 6 N HCl *in vacuo* for 2 hours. ^{32}P-phosphoamino acids were then analyzed by 2-dimensional thin-layer high-voltage electrophoresis in the presence of unlabeled phosphoamino acid markers. PY refers to phosphotyrosine, PT to phosphothreonine, and PS to phosphoserine. The ^{32}P-labeled phosphoamino acids were detected by autoradiography. Results shown in this figure were obtained from Bernier *et. al.* (2).

IGF-I, IGF-II, EGF and PDGF with that of insulin (Table 1). In other studies (results not shown) we have established that 3T3-L1 adipocytes possess cell-surface receptors for all of these growth factors. The receptors for IGF-I (18), EGF (19), and PDGF (20), like the insulin receptor, are ligand-activated tyrosine-specific protein kinases. As illustrated in Table 1 these peptide growth factors differ considerably in their ability to activate hexose uptake in 3T3-L1 adipocytes, with insulin and IGF-I being equally active and EGF and PDGF exhibiting little, if any, activity. On the other hand, only insulin was active in stimulating the phosphorylation of pp15 (Table 1). These results indicate that activation by insulin of the phosphorylation of pp15 is highly specific and moreover, that IGF-I and IGF-II, which also activate hexose uptake, enter the signal transmission pathway at points beyond, or parallel to, pp15.

Further support for the proposed role of pp15 in the signalling pathway leading to the activation of hexose uptake and of the involvement of the insulin receptor in the phosphorylation of pp15 (Figure 4B), is derived from experiments with vanadate. Vanadate, which is known to inhibit phosphotyrosine protein phosphatases, activates hexose uptake (Table 2). Like the activation of hexose uptake by insulin, activation by vanadate is blocked by phenylarsine oxide. Furthermore as illustrated in Table 2, vanadate in the presence of phenylarsine oxide, but not vanadate alone, causes the accumulation of pp15. This is directly analogous to the accumulation of pp15 induced by insulin and phenylarsine oxide (Table 2). The fact that both insulin and vanadate cause an increase in insulin receptor β-subunit phosphorylation (Table 2), which is virtually unaffected by phenylarsine oxide, further implicates

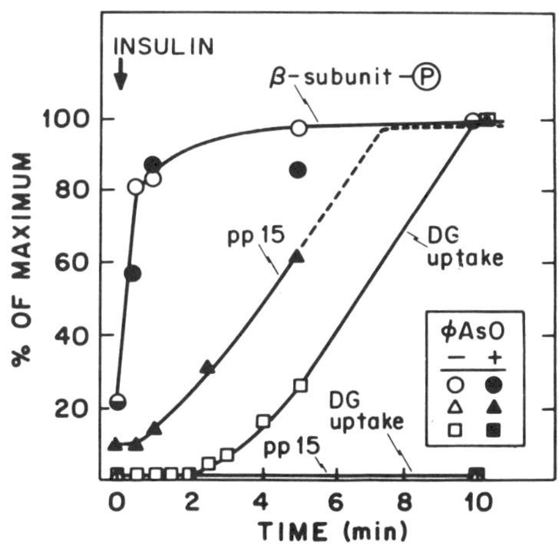

Figure 7. Comparison of the kinetics of insulin-stimulated insulin receptor β-subunit phosphorylation, pp15 phosphorylation and 2-deoxy-[1-^{14}C]glucose uptake in 3T3-L1 adipocytes. To follow the kinetics of phosphorylation of the insulin receptor's β-subunit and of pp15, cells were first labeled with medium containing $^{32}P_i$ as described in Figure 5. The cells were then treated (●, ▲) or not (o, Δ) with phenylarsine oxide for 10 minutes followed by insulin addition. The kinetics of 2-deoxy-[1-^{14}C]glucose uptake were determined in cells previously treated (■) or not (□) with 35 μM phenylarsine oxide and stimulated with 1 μM insulin. The maximal level of [^{32}P]labeled β-subunit in the insulin-stimulated steady-state was 542 c.p.m. per 10^6 cells and the maximal level of [^{32}P]-pp15 was 601 c.p.m. per 10^6 cells. [^{14}C]2-Deoxyglucose uptake is expressed as insulin-stimulated uptake, corrected for basal uptake, at each time point. Maximal uptake at 10 min was 11.5 nmoles per 10^6 cells. β-Subunit-P refers to [^{32}P]labeled insulin receptor β-subunit and DG refers to [^{14}C] 2-deoxyglucose. The results shown in this figure are from Bernier et. al. (2).

the insulin receptor's tyrosine-specific protein kinase in the phosphorylation of pp15.

Table 1. Specificity of Polypeptide pp15 Phosphorylation and Hexose Uptake. For phosphorylation studies, cells were preincubated for 2 hours with $^{32}P_i$-containing medium, then were incubated for 10 minutes with 35 μM phenylarsine oxide followed by 100 nM peptide. For hexose uptake studies, cells were treated with 100 nM of the appropriate peptide for 10 minutes prior to measurement of 2-deoxy-[1-^{14}C]glucose uptake. The results are from Bernier et. al. (2).

Treatment	^{32}P-pp15*	Hexose uptake
	c.p.m./10^6 cells	nmoles/min/10^6 cells
none	0	0.22
insulin	1203	1.26
IGF-I	0	1.14
IGF-II	0	0.82
EGF	0	0.41
PDGF	157	0.44

*in the presence of phenylarsine oxide

Table 2. Comparison of the Effects of Insulin and Vanadate. Treatment with insulin and phenylarsine oxide for hexose uptake and ^{32}P-pp15 phosphorylation were as described in Table 1. Cells were treated with 1 mM vanadate 15 hours prior to the addition of phenylarsine oxide. The results are from Laird et. al. (22). ØAsO refers to phenylarsine oxide.

Additions	^{32}P-Insulin receptor (β-subunit)	^{32}P-pp15	Hexose uptake
	c.p.m./10^6 cells	c.p.m./10^6 cells	nmoles/min/10^6 cells
none	220	0	0.3
insulin	1200	0	2.4
ØAsO	150	0	0.4
insulin + ØAsO	1000	1200	0.6
vanadate	900	0	2.2
vanadate + ØAsO	740	1000	0.6

V. ROLE OF pp15 IN THE ACTIVATION OF GLUCOSE UPTAKE

Two additional findings link insulin-stimulated phosphorylation of pp15 to the activation of hexose uptake. First, phenylarsine oxide affects both processes reciprocally and reversibly (Figure 7), inhibiting insulin-activated hexose uptake and causing the accumulation of pp15 in the presence of insulin; both of these effects are specifically reversed by the vicinal dithiol reagent, 2,3-dimercaptopropanol, but not by a monothiol, 2-mercaptoethanol (see Figure 2). The results in Table 3 show that the complete recovery of insulin-activated hexose uptake by

2,3-dimercaptopropanol was accompanied by a decreased accumulation of phospho-p15. Moreover, 2-mercaptoethanol was neither capable of reversing the inhibition of insulin-activated deoxyglucose uptake by phenylarsine oxide, nor the dependence of pp15 accumulation upon phenylarsine oxide. These results strongly suggest the involvement of a cellular dithiol in the signal transmission pathway between the insulin receptor and the glucose transport system, downstream from pp15.

Table 3. Reversal of the Effects of Phenylarsine Oxide on Insulin-Activated pp15 Phosphorylation and 2-Deoxy-glucose Uptake in 3T3-L1 Adipocytes. 3T3-L1 adipocytes were treated with 35 μM phenylarsine oxide (ØAsO) for 5 minutes where indicated, then 75 μM 2,3-dimercapto-propanol (DMP) or 150 μM 2-mercaptoethanol (ME) was added or not for an additional 5 minutes. The cells were then incubated in the absence or presence of 1 μM insulin for 10 minutes, after which 2-deoxy-[1-^{14}C]-glucose uptake or the incorporation of $^{32}P_i$ into pp15 was determined. The results are from Bernier et. al. (2).

Treatment	^{32}P-pp15	Hexose uptake
	c.p.m./10^6 cells	nmoles/min/10^6cells
none	0	0.19
insulin	0	1.48
ØAsO	55	0.18
ØAsO, then insulin	533	0.17
ØAsO, then DMP, then insulin	75	1.33
ØAsO, then ME, then insulin	501	0.13

Second, we have obtained kinetic evidence (Figure 8) that the formation of phospho-p15 is the rate-limiting step in signal transmission to the glucose transport system and is responsible for the long lag (about 5 min) in achieving maximal hexose uptake rate following insulin addition (see Fig. 7). As shown in Figure 8, by allowing cellular phospho-p15 to accumulate for 5 min in the presence of insulin and phenylarsine oxide, and then quickly releasing the phenylarsine oxide-induced blockade with 2,3 dimercaptopropanol, in effect by-passing the rate limiting step, eliminates the lag in achieving maximal hexose uptake rate. This result is consistent with the proposed sequence of events shown in Figure 4B and provides an explanation of why pp15 fails to accummulate when 3T3-L1 adipocytes are treated with insulin alone (see Figure 5B versus 5D). Taken together these results suggest that the rate of turnover of the phosphoryl moiety of pp15 is much faster than its rate of formation and further that dephosphorylation of pp15 is tightly coupled to signal transmission to the glucose transport system.

VI. DISCUSSION

There is now abundant evidence that the pleiotropic actions of insulin are mediated through the protein kinase activity of the β-subunit of the insulin receptor. The insulin receptor kinase is capable of phosphorylating only tyrosine residues (1, 16, 17), while most of the proteins whose phosphorylation states are altered by insulin in intact cells (eg. glycogen synthase, pyruvate dehydrogenase, acetyl-CoA carboxylase and ribosomal protein S_6) involve phosphoserine residues. Thus, it is necessary to implicate a switch from tyrosine phosphorylation, proximal to the receptor, to serine phosphorylation at the distal multiple termini of the insulin-initiated regulatory cascade. Such a cascade, although complex, would have the potential for signal amplification.

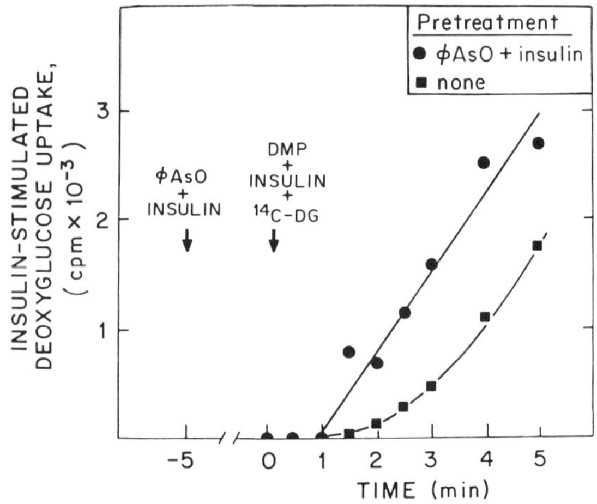

Figure 8. Effect of prior pp15 accumulation on the lag in hexose uptake. 3T3-L1 adipocytes were treated or not for 5 minutes with phenylarsine oxide and insulin prior to initiating hexose uptake by the addition of 2,3-dimercaptopropanol (which reverses inhibition by phenylarsine oxide), insulin and [^{14}C]-2-deoxyglucose. ^{14}C-Hexose uptake was then followed as described in Figure 1. The results are from Bernier et. al. (21).

The objective of the present study was to characterize events proximal to the insulin receptor when cells are stimulated by insulin. In intact 3T3-L1 adipocytes, insulin-stimulated phosphorylation of the receptor's β-subunit (14; Figures 3 and 7). This stimulation of β-subunit phosphorylation was due entirely to an increased level of

[^{32}P]phosphotyrosine without a change in the level of [^{32}P]phosphoserine in the receptor (14). To determine whether there are kinetic grounds for a connection between insulin-stimulated β-subunit phosphorylation and the acceleration of hexose transport rate, the time dependencies of both processes were measured. It is a requiremnt of any functional association that the presumed regulatory event occur before, or coincident with, the process under its control. Results satisfying this requirement are presented here (Figures 3 and 7), and also in studies published elsewhere (14), for the stimulation and relaxation of both processes following the addition and removal, respectively, of insulin. Under both circumstances, the change in β-subunit phosphorylation state coincided with the addition or removal of insulin; this change in phosphorylation state was followed by a lag after which hexose uptake increased or decreased, respectively.

The question, still unanswered, however, was how the receptor tyrosine kinase transmits its signal to the ultimate targets of insulin action, including the glucose transport system? As shown in this paper and elsewhere (2, 21-23), we have employed phenylarsine oxide which inhibits insulin-activated hexose uptake by producing an apparent post-receptor blockade of signal transmission to the hexose transport system (Figure 4). In 3T3-L1 adipocytes labeled with $^{32}P_i$, this blockade appears to cause the insulin-stimulated accumulation of [^{32}P]pp15 (Figure 5), a 15 kDa polypeptide which is phosphorylated exclusively on tyrosine (Figure 6). In results not shown (2) we have determined that phospho-p15 is localized in the cytosolic fraction of 3T3-L1 cells. Thus, pp15 (or its precursor) would be expected to be mobile and capable of translocating from its site of phosphorylation at the cytoplasmic face of the plasma membrane (by the cytoplasmic tyrosine kinase domain of the β-subunit) to the intracellular membrane site of the glucose transporter. The cytosolic localization of phospho-p15 raises the possibility that this agent may act pleiotropically to mediate other insulin-activated processes.

Phospho-p15 has the expected characteristics of a cytosolic intermediate in the insulin signal transmission pathway. First, activation of the accumulation of ^{32}P-pp15 in 3T3-L1 adipocytes is specific. IGF-I, IGF-II, EGF, and PDGF do not induce ^{32}P-pp15 accumulation (Table 1) despite the presence on 3T3-L1 cells of receptors for all four of these growth factors. Since IGF-I and IGF-II, like insulin, activate hexose uptake in 3T3-L1 adipocytes (2, 14 and Table 1), the mediators generated by these factors must enter the signaling pathway downstream from, or parallel to, pp15. Also in support of the role of both the insulin receptor and pp15 in the same signalling pathway is the finding that phosphorylation of both tyrosyl residues, i.e. of the receptor's β-subunit and of pp15, exhibit identical insulin concentration dependencies (2). Since phenylarsine oxide does not affect insulin-dependent β-subunit phosphorylation (2, 23 and Figure 7), but is required for the accumulation of ^{32}P-pp15, pp15 must lie proximal to the receptor, and upstream from the site of phenylarsine oxide action as depicted in Figure 4B. Finally, the kinetics of phosphorylation of the insulin receptor's β-subunit and pp15 are consistent with a role for pp15 in mediating insulin-activated hexose uptake (Figure 7). Insulin rapidly activates the apparent autophosphorylation of the receptor's β-subunit (on tyrosine, see Figure 7 and Reference 17) which is followed in succession by the initial appearance of phospho-p15 and then an increased rate of hexose uptake.

The role of tyrosine phosphorylation in signal transmission from the insulin receptor is further supported by studies with vanadate (22 and Table 2). Vanadate, a potent inhibitor of certain phosphotyrosine protein phosphatases, increased phosphorylation of the insulin receptor's β-subunit on tyrosine in rat adipocytes (24). Vanadate, which mimics the action of insulin in activating hexose uptake by isolated rat (25) and 3T3-L1 adipocytes (Table 2), also causes insulin receptor β-subunit phosphorylation in both cell types. Furthermore, phenylarsine oxide blocks vanadate-stimulated hexose transport in 3T3-L1 adipocytes and, like the combined action of insulin and phenylarsine oxide, vanadate and phenylarsine oxide together cause the accumulation of pp15 (Table 2).

Finally, two observations link insulin-stimulated phosphorylation of pp15 to the activation of hexose uptake. First, phenylarsine oxide affects both processes in an inverse manner (Figure 7 and Table 3) and these effects are specifically reversed by the vicinal dithiol reagent, 2,3-dimercaptopropanol, but not by a monothiol, 2-mercaptoethanol (Table 3). This result implicates an essential dithiol intermediate in the signal transmission pathway which interacts with, or downstream from, pp15. Second, kinetic evidence (Figure 8) suggests that the formation of phospho-p15 in response to insulin is the rate-limiting step in signal transmission to the glucose transport system and is responsible for the long (5 min) lag in achieving maximal hexose uptake following insulin addition (Figure 7). Thus, by allowing cellular phospho-p15 to accumulate for 5 min in the presence of insulin and phenylarsine oxide and then quickly releasing the phenylarsine oxide-induced blockade with 2,3-dimercaptopropanol, thereby by-passing the rate-limiting step, eliminates the lag in achieving maximal hexose uptake rate (Figure 8). This result, predicted by the proposed sequence of events shown in Figure 4B, further suggests that dephosphorylation of (or transphosphorylation from) pp15 is coupled to signal transmission to the glucose transport system.

VII. SUMMARY

Insulin activates hexose (2-deoxyglucose or 3-O-methylglucose) uptake by approximately 10-fold in the mature 3T3-L1 adipocyte. Following insulin addition there is a 4-5 minute lag period before maximal hexose uptake rate is achieved. Phenylarsine oxide, a trivalent arsenical that forms stable ring complexes with vicinal dithiols, prevents the activation of hexose uptake by insulin in a concentration-dependent manner (K_i = 7 μM), but has no inhibitory effect on basal hexose uptake. 2,3-Dimercaptopropanol at a level nearly stoichiometric to that of phenylarsine oxide prevents, or rapidly reverses, the inhibition of hexose uptake, while 2-mercaptoethanol does not reverse inhibition of hexose uptake. These results suggest that phenylarsine oxide inhibits signal transmission from the receptor to the glucose transport system.

Upon addition of insulin to 3T3-L1 adipocytes, ^{32}P-orthophosphate incorporation into the β-subunit of the insulin receptor on tyrosyl residues is increased 7-fold and is complete within 1 minute ($t_{1/2}$ = 10 seconds). Kinetic experiments with the intact 3T3-L1 adipocyte support the hypothesis that β-subunit phosphorylation is an intermediate step connecting insulin binding to increased hexose transport rate.

Insulin activates the phosphorylation of a tyrosyl residue(s) on a 15 kilodalton cytosolic protein (pp15) which accumulates when 3T3-L1 adipocytes are treated with phenylarsine oxide. Several lines of evidence implicate pp15 in insulin receptor-induced signal transduction to the glucose transport system. The reciprocal effects of phenylarsine oxide on the insulin-stimulated accumulation of phospho-p15 and on insulin-stimulated hexose uptake are both reversed by the vicinal dithiol, 2,3-dimercaptopropanol, but not by the monothiol, 2-mercaptoethanol. Thus, a cellular dithiol appears to function in the signal transmission pathway downstream from pp15. Furthermore, both hexose uptake and phenylarsine oxide-dependent pp15 accumulation exhibit identical insulin concentration dependencies. Like insulin-activated autophosphorylation of the receptors' β-subunit (on tyrosine), activation of the phosphorylation of pp15 is specific, with IGF-I and II, EGF and PDGF being inactive. Vanadate, which activates hexose uptake and insulin receptor β-subunit phosphorylation, also causes the accumulation of pp15 in the presence of phenylarsine oxide. The temporal kinetic relationship of insulin-activated receptor β-subunit phosphorylation, followed by the phosphorylation of pp15 and then increased hexose uptake rate is consistent with an intermediary signalling role for pp15 in the insulin-stimulated glucose uptake.

VIII. REFERENCES

1. Lane, M.D., Life-Cycle and Regulation of the Insulin Receptor, in: "Insulin: Its Receptor and Diabetes," M.D. Hollenberg, ed., Marcel Dekker, Inc., New York, pp. 237-264 (1985).
2. Bernier, M., Laird, D. and Lane, M.D., Proc. Natl. Acad. Sci., USA, In Press (1986).
3. Green, H. and Kehinde, O., Cell 1:113-116 (1974).
4. Green, H. and Meuth, M., Cell, 3:127-133 (1974).
5. Novikoff, A., Novikoff, P., Rosen, O., and Rubin, C., J. Cell Biol. 87:180-196 (1980).
6. Mackall, J.C., Student, A.K., Polakis, S.E. and Lane, M.D., J. Biol. Chem. 251:6462-6464 (1976).
7. Mackall, J.C. and Lane, M.D. Biochem. Biophys. Res. Communs. 79:720-725 (1977).
8. Coleman, R.A., Reed, B.C., Mackall, J.C., Student, A.K., Lane, M.D. and Bell, R.M., J. Biol. Chem. 253:7256-7261 (1978).
9. Student, A.K., Hsu, R.Y., and Lane, M.D., J. Biol. Chem. 255: 4745-4750 (1980).
10. Reed, B.C., Ronnett, G.V., Clements, P.R. and Lane, M.D. J. Biol. Chem. 256:3917-3925 (1981).
11. Bernlohr, D.A., Angus, C.W., Lane, M.D., Bolanowski, M.A., and Kelly, Jr., T.J., Proc. Natl. Acad. Sci., USA 81:5468-5472 (1984).
12. Frost, S.C. and Lane, M.D., J. Biol. Chem. 260:2646-2652 (1985).
13. Bernlohr, D.A., Bowlanowski, M.A., Kelly, Jr., T.J. and Lane, M.D., J. Biol. Chem. 260:5563-5567 (1985).
14. Kohanski, R.A., Frost, S.C., and Lane, M.D., J. Biol. Chem., 261, 12272-12281 (1986).
15. Webb, J.L., Enzyme and Metabolic Inhibitors, Vol. III, pp. 595-793, Academic Press, New York,1966.
16. Kohanski, R.A. and Lane, M.D., Biochem. Biophys. Res. Communs. 134: 1312-1318 (1986).
17. Kohanski, R.A. and Lane, M.D., J. Biol. Chem. 260:5014-5025 (1985).
18. Jacobs, S., Kull, F.C.,Jr. Earp, H.S., Svoboda,M.E., Van Wyck, J.J. and Cuatrecasas, P., J. Biol. Chem. 258:9581-9584 (1983).
19. Cohen, S., Carpenter, G., and King, L.E., Jr., J. Biol. Chem. 255:4834-4841 (1980).
20. Bishayee, S., Ross, A.H., Womer, R., and Scher, C.D. Proc. Natl.Acad. Sci, USA 83:6756-6760 (1986).
21. Bernier, M., Laird, D.M., and Lane, M.D. (1987) submitted for publication.
22. Laird, D.M., Bernier, M., and Lane, M.D. (1987) submitted for publication.
23. Frost, S.C., Kohanski, R.A. and Lane, M.D. (1987) submitted for publication.

24. Tamura, S., Brown, T.A., Whipple, J.H., Fujita-Yamaguchi, Y., Dublers, R.E., Cheng, K. and Larner, J., J. Biol. Chem. 259: 6650-6658 (1984).
25. Dubyak, G.R. and Kleinzeller, A. J. Biol. Chem. 255:5306-5312 (1980).

---

[*] This work was supported by research grants from the National Institute of Health and the Juvenile Diabetes Foundation.
[1] Supported by a postdoctoral fellowship from the Medical Research Council of Canada.
[2] Supported by a postdoctoral fellowship from the National Institutes of Health, USPHS.

ROLE OF PROTEIN PHOSPHORYLATION IN GROWTH FACTOR SIGNAL TRANSDUCTION

S. L. Pelech, D. A. Tinker, C. P. Chan and E. G. Krebs

Howard Hughes Medical Institute, University of Washington
Mail Stop SL-15, Seattle, WA 98195

The molecular basis for the actions of insulin and other growth factors remains an outstanding problem in biology today. Delineation of the early steps of the mitogenic response is important for a proper understanding of the processes of both normal and abnormal cell proliferation, and other pathological conditions including diabetes. In this paper, which consists primarily of a review of work carried out here and elsewhere, a role for protein phosphorylation in the mediation of many of the metabolic responses of cells to growth factors is examined.

PROTEIN-TYROSINE PHOSPHORYLATION

Although our knowledge is incomplete, major insights into the intracellular mechanisms of growth factor action have been realized over the last decade. The cell surface receptors for insulin, insulin-like growth factor 1 (IGF-1), epidermal growth factor (EGF), platelet-derived growth factor (PDGF), fibroblast growth factor (FGF) (also referred to as bovine brain-derived growth factor) and macrophage colony stimulating factor 1 have been identified as ligand-stimulatable protein-tyrosine kinases[1,2] (reviewed in ref. 3). Sequencing studies have revealed that many of the known oncogenes implicated in neoplastic cell proliferation encode either the aforementioned growth factors (e.g. *sis*[4,5]), their receptors (e.g. *erb-B*[6], *fms*[7]) or related proteins (e.g. *neu*[8,9], *ros*[10], *trk*[11], *kit*[12], *met*[13], *sea*[14]). Furthermore, many of the products of other oncogenes (e.g. *src*[15,16], *lck*[17,18], *fps*(*fes*)[19], *abl*[20], *fgr*[21], *rel*[22,23], *syn*[24], *yes*[25]) are also protein-tyrosine kinases, some of which may also be associated with the plasma membrane. Although a role for protein-tyrosine phosphorylation has been strongly implicated in the regulation of cell proliferation, complementary processes such as polyphosphoinositol turnover and cAMP production may also participate (reviewed in ref. 26).

Various mouse 3T3 culture cell lines have been particularly useful in the study of growth factor action. For example, when deprived of exogenous growth factors, Swiss 3T3 cells exit from the cell cycle and enter the G_0 or stationary phase. Upon addition of defined growth factors, the quiescent cultures can be prompted to resume the cell cycle leading to DNA synthesis and cell division. These cells express receptors for a wide range of mitogens that can be subclassified as of the "competence" or "progression" type. Competence factors such as PDGF, FGF and bombesin can

Table 1. Targets for growth factor-stimulated protein phosphorylation.

System[1]	Apparent M_r by SDS polyacrylamide gel electrophoreses[2,3]	References
INSULIN-STIMULATED		
m 3T3-L1	22K[A,B], 31K[B]	A=35, B=36
r adipocytes	23K[A], 40K[B], 62K[C]	A=37, B=38, C=39
l adipocytes	110K[A]	A=40
r hepatocytes	22K[A], 34K[A,B], 46K[A,B], 110K[C], 120K[D]	A=41, B=42, C=40, D=43
r hepatoma	185K[A]	A=44
EGF-STIMULATED		
h fibroblasts	21K[A,B], 22K[A,B], 26K[A], 30K[C], 35K[A,B], 36K[C], 41K[C], 43K[C], 45K[A], 56K[C], 60K[C], 85K[C]	A=45, B=46, C=47
m 3T3	21K[A], 42K[A,B], 43K[B], 45K[B]	A=48, B=49
m 3T3-L1	22K[A]	A=35
h A431	35K[A], 200K[B], 250K[B], 300K[B], 330K[B], 360K[B]	A=50, B=51
m hepatocytes	120K[A]	A=52
r hepatocytes	21K[A], 25K[A], 35K[A], 36K[A], 38K[A], 42K[A], 67K[A]	A=53
PDGF-STIMULATED		
h fibroblasts	30K[A], 35K[B], 36K[A], 41K[A], 43K[A], 45K[B], 54K[B], 56K[A], 60K[A], 72K[B], 85K[A], 115K[B], 200K-300K[B]	A=47, B=54
h osteosarcoma	115K[A]	A=55
m 3T3	33K[A], 36K[B], 40K-45K[C,D], 60K[B], 62K[C], 74K[C], 80K[E], 92K[C], 116K[C], 140K[C]	A=56, B=57, C=58, D=49, E=59
m 3T3-L1	22K[A], 31K[A], 80K[A]	A=36
FGF-STIMULATED		
h fibroblasts	30K[A], 36K[A], 41K[A], 43K[A], 56K[A], 60K[A], 85K[A]	A=47
m 3T3	80K[A]	A=59
m 3T3-L1	22K[A], 31K[A], 80K[A]	A=36
r adipocytes	22K[A], 31K[A], 80K[A]	A=36

SRC KINASE-STIMULATED		
c embryo fibroblasts	14K[A], 19K[A], 20K-200K[B], 28K[A,C,D], 34K-36K[A,D,E,F,G], 39K[C,D], 44K-46K[A,C,D], 50K[D,H,I], 55K[A], 70K[J], 75K[J], 125K[J], 130K[A,D], 135K[J]	A=60, B=61, C=62, D=63, E=64, F=65, G=66, H=67, I=68, J=69
PHORBOL ESTER- OR PROTEIN KINASE C-STIMULATED		
h fibroblasts	41K-43K[A]	A=47
c embryo fibroblasts	40K-43K[A,B], 60K[C], 80K[C], 93K[C]	A=70, B=71, C=72
m 3T3	20K[A], 36K[A], 42K[A], 58K[A], 66K[A], 80K[B], 180K[A]	A=48, B=73
m 3T3-L1	22K[A], 31K[A], 80K[A]	A=36
h A431	180K[A]	A=74
r adipocytes	40K[A]	A=38
h erythrocytes	46K[A], 80K[A], 100K[A]	A=75
h platelets	180K[A]	A=76
h B lymphocytes	28K[A], 35K[A], 40K[A], 43K[A], 56K[A], 61K[A], 66K[A], 75K[A], 94K[A], 98K[A], 116K[A], 130K[A], 140K[A], 155K[A], 180K[A], 205K[A], 220K[A], 245K[A], 280K[A]	A=77
h U-937	45K[A], 61K[A], 67K[A], 116K[A], 140K[A]	A=78
l neutrophils	40K[A], 50K[A], 55K[A], 64K[A], 70K[A], 90K[A]	A=79
r Leydig	17K[A], 33K[A]	A=80
m pancreatic islets	17K[A], 19K[A], 20K[A], 28K[A], 30K[A], 38K[A], 43K[A], 48K[A], 66K[A], 75K[A], 120K[A], 155K[A], 170K[A], 190K[A]	A=81
c heart	27K[A], 42K[A], 51K[A], 85K[A]	A=82

[1] c=chicken, h=human, l=rabbit, m=mouse, r=rat.

[2] Proteins that undergo autophosphorylation are not listed.

[3] Proteins that have been shown to be phosphorylated on tyrosine residues are underlined.

singly elicit a full mitogenic response when added to quiescent Swiss 3T3 cells. By contrast, progression factors like insulin, IGF-1, and prostaglandins E_1 and $F_{2\alpha}$ augment the action of suboptimal amounts of competence factors or cooperate in specific combinations with other progression factors to stimulate DNA synthesis and cell division. EGF cannot readily be classified as either a competence or progression factor for Swiss 3T3 cells since long but not short-term treatment can induce about half of the quiescent cells to reenter the cell cycle and synthesize DNA. The ability of PDGF, FGF and bombesin to facilitate the full mitogenic response may arise from the potential of these hormones to stimulate protein-tyrosine phosphorylation, polyphosphoinositol turnover and elevate cAMP levels. Progression factors appear to activate only one or two of these parameters[26].

Just how protein-tyrosine phosphorylation mediates the mitogenic response is an enigma. The most prominent and earliest targets for growth factor-stimulated protein-tyrosine phosphorylation are the receptors for these hormones. With the insulin[27-30], IGF-1[31,32] and EGF[33,34] receptors, autophosphorylation has been correlated with an enhanced ability to phosphorylate exogenous proteins on tyrosine residues. It is possible that growth factor-induced autophosphorylation of the receptors represents the first amplification step of a cascade involved in the transduction of the growth factor signal. The nature of the next step of the mitogenic pathway is controversial, but is likely to involve the phosphorylation of one or more as yet undefined regulatory proteins on tyrosine residues.

Many studies have focused on the identification of possible substrates for growth factor receptor protein-tyrosine kinases. One commonly adopted approach has been to preincubate cultured cells with ^{32}P-labelled orthophosphate and monitor the incorporation of the label into cellular proteins in the absence and presence of mitogens. Another method involves phosphorylation of endogenous proteins in cell-free extracts reconstituted with growth factors and/or purified receptors in the presence of [γ-^{32}P]ATP. Subsequent resolution of the ^{32}P-labelled proteins has revealed that numerous proteins undergo growth factor-induced phosphorylation not only on tyrosine residues, but also on serine and threonine residues (see Table 1). However, with the exception of the EGF receptor-catalyzed phosphorylation of the 35 kDa protein lipocortin I (calpactin II)[83,84], few of these phosphotyrosine-containing proteins have been identified with respect to function, nor has it been demonstrated that they are directly phosphorylated by the receptor kinases. Furthermore, the patterns of protein phosphorylations induced by insulin, EGF, FGF and PDGF, though partly overlapping, appear to be distinct (Table 1).

It should be appreciated that part of the difference between insulin- and EGF-induced protein phosphorylation as compared to that evoked by PDGF and FGF in murine 3T3 cell lines may stem from the ability of the latter two hormones, but not the former, to promote polyphosphoinositol turnover (reviewed in ref. 26). In particular, an 80 kDa protein has been identified as a major substrate for serine phosphorylation by protein kinase C. This kinase is activated as a consequence of polyphosphoinositol breakdown or following treatment with the phorbol ester tumor promoter, 12-O-tetradecanoyl-phorbol acetate (TPA)[36,85-87].

The results of in vitro substrate specificity studies on purified growth factor receptors and the src-encoded kinase (summarized in Table 2) further demonstrate that these kinases exhibit divergent preferences. Moreover, these kinases may phosphorylate unique sites on the same proteins. For example, the insulin and EGF receptors phosphorylate microtubule-associated protein 2 at similar sites, but the src kinase phosphorylates different tyrosine residues on this protein[91].

Table 2. Substrate preferences of protein-tyrosine kinases.

Substrate	Preference[1,2,3]	Reference
angiotensin II	EGF-R >> insulin-R	88
band 3 (erythrocyte)	src kinase ≃ EGF-R	89
α-casein	insulin-R > EGF-R	88
ß-casein	EGF-R > insulin-R	88, 90
fodrin α-subunit	src kinase > EGF-R	91
ß-subunit	EGF-R > src kinase	91
histone H1	insulin-R ≃ EGF-R	90
histone H2B	insulin-R >> EGF-R	88
histone H2B	insulin-R ≃ EGF-R	90, 92
myosin light chains (smooth muscle)	EGF-R > insulin-R	90
poly(E,A,Y) (1:1:10)	EGF-R > insulin-R	92
poly(E,A,Y) (6:3:1)	EGF-R > insulin-R, IGF-1-R	93
poly(E,Y) (4:1)	insulin-R, IGF-1-R > EGF-R	88, 92, 93
progesterone receptor	insulin-R, EGF-R >> PDGF-R	94
src peptide (RRLIEDAEYAARG)	insulin-R ≃ EGF-R ≃ PDGF-R	88, 90, 95
troponin I	insulin-R ≃ EGF-R	90
tubulin α-subunit	src kinase > EGF-R	91
ß-subunit	src kinase ≃ EGF-R	91

1 These comparisons are based on Vmax/Km ratio values obtained with the growth factor receptors and src kinase whenever possible.
2 "Receptor" is abbreviated as "R".
3 "≃" corresponded to no greater than a 2-fold difference; ">" corresponded to no greater than a 5-fold difference; ">>" corresponded to greater than a 5-fold difference.

Early studies on the specificities of various protein-tyrosine kinases failed to reveal substantial differences[90,96]. Sequence analysis of the sites phosphorylated by the insulin and EGF receptors and the src kinase implies that each kinase may recognize some of the same positive determinants for phosphorylation. As shown in Table 3, acidic residues at the first, third and fourth residues N-terminal to the phosphorylated tyrosine residue are commonly featured. However, most of these substrates were originally selected for examination because of their preponderance of acidic residues near a tyrosine residue. Proteins such as lipocortin II, enolase and lactate dehydrogenase, which are substrates for the src kinase in intact cells, do not display appreciable homology in the region of the tyrosine phosphorylation site. The apparent homology between autophosphorylation sites of various protein-tyrosine kinases may simply reflect their common ancestry. The ability of these phosphorylation sites to adopt a ß-turn conformation may be a positive determinant for phosphorylation[115].

It may be that the various growth factor receptors and src kinase phosphorylate a common subset of regulatory proteins that are components of a cascade that mediates many of the events typically associated with

Table 3. Phosphorylation sites for protein-tyrosine kinases.

Substrate[1]	Amino acid sequence[2]	Reference
A. AUTOPHOSPHORYLATION SITES		
h insulin receptor - Tyr-960 (minor)	SSNPEYLSARR	97
- Tyr-1150 (major)	DIYETDYYRK	97
- Tyr-1316 (minor)	YEEHIPYTHMNG	97
h EGF receptor - Tyr-1068 (minor)	FLPVPEYINQSVP	98, 99
- Tyr-1148 (minor)	SLDNPDYQQDFFP	98, 99
- Tyr-1173 (major)	TAENAEYLRVAPQ	98, 99
c src kinase - Tyr-416	RLIEDNEYTARQGAK	100-103
m lck kinase	LIEDNEYTAREG	18, 104
c yes kinase	RLIEDNEYTARQGAK	25
c fps kinase	RQEEDGVYASTGGMK	19
f fes kinase	REEADGVYAASGGLR	105
f fes kinase	REAADGIYAASGGLR	105
c abl kinase	RLMTGDTYTAHAGAG	20
B. INSULIN RECEPTOR CATALYZED PHOSPHORYLATION		
c src kinase peptide patterned after Tyr-416	LIEDAEYAARG	90,96,97
h angiotensin II - Tyr-4	DRVYIHPF	96

C.	EGF RECEPTOR CATALYZED PHOSPHORYLATION		
h	angiotensin I - Tyr-4	DRVYIHPFHL	106
h	angiotensin II - Tyr-4	DRVYIHPF	107
h	band 3 (erythrocyte) - Tyr-8	EELEDDYEDD	89
b	cAMP-dependent protein kinase R_{II} peptide patterned after Tyr-95	RFDRRVYVAAE	106
h	gastrin peptide patterned after Tyr-29	LEEEEEAYG	108
h	growth hormone - Tyr-35	QEFEEAYIPK	109
p	lipocortin I (calpactin II) - Tyr-9	DNEEQEYIKTVK	84
h	lipocortin I (calpactin II) - Tyr-20	ENEEQEYVQTV	110
b	myosin light chains (smooth muscle) - Tyr-142	DEEVDEMYREAPID	111
	- Tyr-155	GNFNYVEFTR	111
	polyoma middle T	LEEEEEEYMPM	109
m	Ha-ras peptide patterned after Tyr-63	DTTGQEEYSA	108
c	src kinase peptide patterned after Tyr-416	LIEDAEYAARG	90
c	src kinase peptide patterned after Tyr-416	LIEDNEYTARQG	98, 108
D.	SRC KINASE CATALYZED PHOSPHORYLATION		
h	angiotensin II - Tyr-4	DRVYIHPF	107
h	band 3 (erythrocyte) - Tyr-8	EELEDDYEDD	89
l	enolase (muscle) - Tyr-43?	GASTGIYEALEL	112
c	lactate dehydrogenase (muscle) - Tyr-238	QVVDSAYEVIKLK	112
b	lipocortin II (calpactin I) - Tyr-23	STPPSAYGSVKAY	113
h	c-myc peptide patterned after N-terminus	RRGDEEENFYQQQQQQG	114

---

[1] b=bovine, c=chicken, f=cat, h=human, l=rabbit, m=mouse, p=pig.

[2] Phosphorylated residue is underlined.

the mitogenic response (Table 4)*. If these phosphoproteins are near the top of such a putative cascade, it is possible that they are not present in quantities sufficient in the cell for detection by the methods employed for Table 1. Moreover, even if these phosphoproteins could be isolated, without some additional insights into their action, their precise functions would be extremely arduous to establish. An alternative strategy towards elucidation of the mitogenic cascade is to exploit the tendency of various growth factors to induce a subset of common responses.

PROTEIN-SERINE/THREONINE PHOSPHORYLATION

Although elevated protein-tyrosine phosphorylation may represent one of the earliest events subsequent to growth factor binding to cells, a majority of the phosphoproteins represented in Table 1 undergo serine/threonine phosphorylation, including most of those that are also substrates for protein-tyrosine kinases. Furthermore, some oncogene products that appear to facilitate tumorigenic cell transformation are protein-serine/threonine kinases (e.g. mos[150], raf (mil)[151], pim-1[152] and pks[153]), as is the tumor promoter-activated enzyme protein kinase C[154]. Therefore, a role for protein-serine/threonine phosphorylation in the mitogenic response can be anticipated. Indeed, certain proteins that are known to modulate the processes that are affected by growth factors are subject to regulation by reversible serine/threonine phosphorylation (see Table 5).

Insulin promotes the dephosphorylation of glycogen synthase, pyruvate dehydrogenase and pyruvate kinase (Table 5), and this can account for the increased catalytic activity of each of these enzymes. These changes are consistent with the effects of insulin on the anabolic processes that these enzymes govern (Table 4). EGF and PDGF also stimulate the glycogen synthase activity ratio (activity in the absence of glucose 6-phosphate/activity in the presence of glucose 6-phosphate) in Swiss 3T3 cells (Figure 1A). Maximal stimulation by these mitogens is observed within 30 min, and the synthase activity ratio returns to basal levels by 100 min. With acetyl-CoA carboxylase, activation induced by insulin and EGF is correlated with increased serine phosphorylation of the protein (Table 5). The mitogen-triggered phosphorylation is apparently at a different site(s) on the carboxylase from that phosphorylated by cAMP-dependent protein kinase which is inactivating[136,170,173]. The relative activation of acetyl-CoA carboxylase does not persist after purification, despite preservation of the mitogen-induced phosphorylation[136]. It may be that the insulin-dependent phosphorylation regulates the ability of carboxylase to respond to a modulator. A stimulated cAMP-independent protein kinase that phosphorylates carboxylase has been reported in cytosolic extracts from insulin-treated rat adipose tissue[171]. Casein kinases 1 and 2 have been shown to phosphorylate carboxylase at or near the insulin-modulated phosphorylation site[173]. In this regard, it is intriguing that insulin-treatment of mouse 3T3-L1 preadipocytes results in activation of a casein kinase 1-like protein kinase that also phosphorylates ribosomal subunit S6[204].

Phosphorylation of subunit S6 on at least five serine residues in the C-terminus of the protein (Table 5) may mediate the increase in protein synthesis induced by growth factors (Table 4). A variety of studies imply

---

* Expression of the src kinase activity can supplant the growth factor requirement for proliferation of cells[144-147] and induce at least some of the responses listed in Table 4 (e.g. increased hexose uptake and glycolysis[148]). The src kinase has been shown to catalyze the phosphorylation and activation of the insulin receptor kinase[149] and has been implicated in the mitogenic response to PDGF[57].

Table 4. Some common metabolic responses to growth factors.

1. Increased Na^+/H^+ exchange leading to cell alkalinization: insulin[116,117]; EGF[116-118]; PDGF[119,120]; TPA[118,120].
2. Increased amino acid uptake: insulin[121,122]; IGF-1[123,124]; PDGF[125]; not EGF[126].
3. Increased hexose uptake: insulin[127,128]; IGF-1[123,124]; EGF[129]; PDGF[130,131]; TPA[127,128].
4. Increased glycolysis: insulin[127,132]; EGF[132]; TPA[127].
5. Increased glycogen synthesis: insulin[133,134]; IGF-1[135]; EGF[134].
6. Increased fatty acid synthesis: insulin[136-138]; EGF[136-138].
7. Increased protein synthesis: insulin[139]; IGF-1[135]; EGF[140]; PDGF[125].
8. Induction of ornithine decarboxylase: insulin[141 but not 142]; EGF[141 but not 142]; PDGF[141,142]; TPA[141,143].

Table 5. Growth factor-induced changes in the serine/threonine phosphorylation states of proteins

A. INCREASED PHOSPHORYLATION
1. insulin receptor: insulin[155-160]; TPA[155,,161,162].
2. IGF-1 receptor: IGF-1[32,155]; TPA[155,162].
3. EGF receptor: EGF[34,163-165]; PDGF[166]; TPA[34,164,165,167-169].
4. PDGF receptor: PDGF[54].
5. acetyl-CoA carboxylase: insulin[136,170-173]; EGF[136].
6. ATP-citrate lyase: insulin[136,171,174-176]; EGF[136].
7. ribosomal subunit S6: insulin[177-180]; IGF-1[180]; EGF[140,179,181]; PDGF[182,183]; TPA[184,185].

B. DECREASED PHOSPHORYLATION
1. glycogen synthase: insulin[186-188].
2. pyruvate dehydrogenase: insulin[189-191].
3. pyruvate kinase: insulin[192].

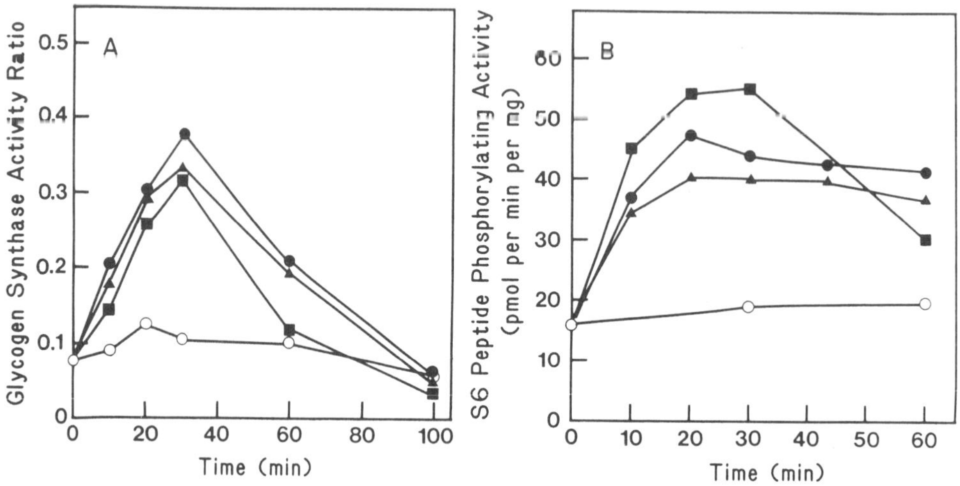

Figure 1. Time courses of activations of glycogen synthase and S6 kinase by mitogens. Confluent quiescent cultures of 3T3 cells were incubated in the absence (○) or presence of 100 ng insulin/ml (▲), 100 ng EGF/ml (■) and 5 ng PDGF/ml (●). The glycogen synthase activity ratio data (panel A) was previously presented in ref. 194, and the S6 kinase activity towards a synthetic peptide (arg-arg-leu-ser-ser-leu-arg-ala) patterned after a phosphorylation site in ribosomal protein S6 (panel B) was determined for ref. 197.

that the rates of polysome formation and protein synthesis initiation become stimulated when S6 is phosphorylated (see ref. 209 and 210 for summary of evidence). Table 6 lists a number of model systems where an enhanced S6 kinase activity is detectable in soluble extracts from cells exposed to mitogens or TPA. In addition, src kinase expression in chick embryo fibroblasts results in elevated S6 phosphorylation[181,184], apparently due to activation of the same S6 kinase[202,207].

Treatment of 3T3 cells with various combinations of insulin, EGF and PDGF yields no further stimulation of the S6 kinase activity than a saturating dose of any of these mitogens alone[197]. This observation, which also holds true for mitogenic stimulation of the glycogen synthase activity ratio[194], is consistent with the notion of a common activation pathway. This is further supported by the very similar time courses of glycogen synthase and S6 kinase activations by insulin, EGF and PDGF (Figure 1).

A number of observations point to a phosphorylation reaction directly involved in the activation of the S6 kinase. The stimulated state of the S6 kinase is maintained in crude cell extracts only in the presence of phosphatase inhibitors such as EGTA, ß-glycerophosphate, p-nitrophenyl-phosphate, phosphotyrosine and vanadate (ref. 199,203 and 206; S. Pelech and E. Krebs, unpublished observations). In the absence of phosphatase inhibitors, the S6 kinase activity declines in a time-dependent fashion, which is consistent with a catalytic inactivation mechanism (ref. 199; S. Pelech and E. Krebs, unpublished observations). The stimulated form of the S6 kinase retains activity after various types of column fractionation, which is indicative of a covalent-modification[197,202,206]. Moreover, fractionated S6 kinase can be apparently phosphorylated and activated upon incubation with purified protein kinase C (K. Meier and E. Krebs, preliminary studies).

Table 6. Growth factor-induced activations of glycogen synthase, acetyl-CoA carboxylase and S6 kinase.

1. Increased glycogen synthase activity (-glucose-6-phosphate/+glucose-6-phosphate activity ratio).
   i. m[1] Swiss 3T3 cells: insulin[193,194]; EGF[193,194]; PDGF[194].
   ii. r hepatocytes: insulin[134]; EGF[134].
   iii. r adipocytes: insulin[187].
   iv. h fibroblasts: insulin[195].
   v. h A431 cells: EGF[193].
   vi. l skeletal muscle: insulin[188].

2. Increased acetyl-CoA carboxylase activity.
   i. r mammary gland: insulin[189].
   ii. r adipocytes: insulin[138,170,171,196]; EGF[138].

3. Increased ribosomal subunit S6 kinase activity.
   i. m Swiss 3T3 cells: insulin[197]; IGF-1[197]; EGF[197-199]; FGF[200]; TPA[197,200].
   ii. r kidney fibroblasts: insulin[201]; EGF[201].
   iii. c embryo fibroblasts: TPA[202].
   iv. r H4 hepatoma: insulin[203].
   v. m 3T3-L1 adipocytes: insulin[204-207]; TPA[205].
   vi. m BC3H-1 myocytes: insulin[208]; TPA[208].

[1] c=chicken, h=human, l=rabbit, m=mouse, r=rat.

The mitogen-activated S6 kinase may be the mammalian equivalent of the amphibian S6 kinase that becomes activated when Xenopus oocytes are induced to mature with insulin or progesterone[211-214]. Activation of an S6 kinase and phosphorylation of S6 in frog oocytes can be triggered following microinjection of the human placenta insulin receptor[212-215] or the abl kinase[216] into the oocytes. A similar S6 kinase is also activated when sea star oocytes are stimulated to mature with 1-methyladenine[217]. Studies with the Xenopus S6 kinase imply that it is an 80-90 kDa protein which undergoes autophosphorylation[211,214].

Although it was reported[211] that the purified Xenopus S6 kinase is highly specific for phosphorylation of S6, partially purified preparations of this kinase from extracts of progesterone-treated frog oocytes also exhibit enhanced phosphorylating activity toward Sigma histone-IIIS, myelin basic protein, glycogen synthase and acetyl-CoA carboxylase[214]. This could implicate the mitogen-activated S6 kinase in adipocytes in the insulin-induced phosphorylation of acetyl-CoA carboxylase. Since the S6 kinase is activated by phorbol ester tumor promoters, it is plausible that this kinase may participate along with protein kinase C in TPA-induced phosphorylation and inhibition of glycogen synthase[218-220].

Another well documented action of TPA is its ability to stimulate serine/threonine phosphorylation of the receptors for insulin, IGF-1 and EGF (Table 5). Phorbol ester-induced phosphorylation of these receptors has been correlated with decreased ligand binding and autophosphorylation activity[155,166,221-228]. By contrast, TPA exposure does not appreciably affect the ability of PDGF to stimulate autophosphorylation of its receptor or polyphosphoinositol breakdown[228], although PDGF activation of Na^+/H^+ exchange can be blocked by TPA[229]. The src kinase also undergoes increased serine phosphorylation as a consequence of TPA or PDGF treatment[230,231], and protein kinase C has been shown to phosphorylate Ser-12 of the cellular src kinase in vitro, although without any apparent effect on the catalytic activity[232].

It has been proposed that PDGF-reduced binding of EGF and autophosphorylation of the EGF-receptor may be mediated through activation of protein kinase C[166] (see Figure 2). This is most likely since protein

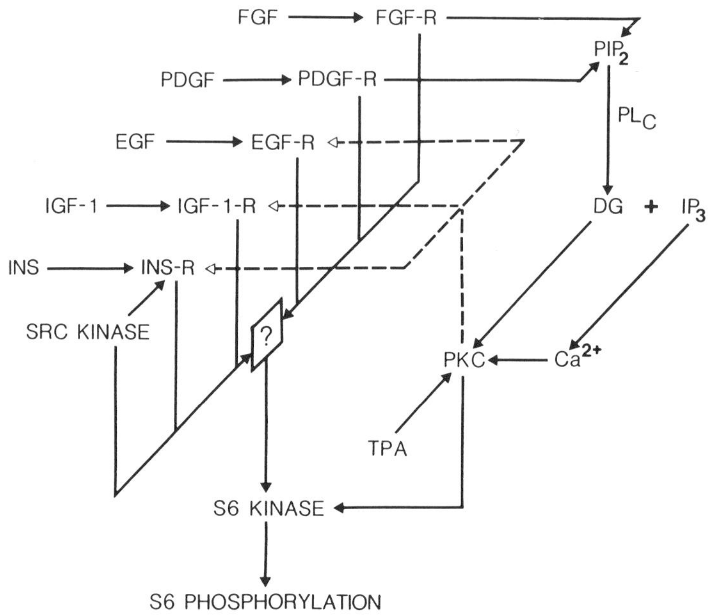

Figure 2. Pathways for growth factor-stimulation of 40S ribosomal protein S6 phosphorylation. Activating pathways are indicated with solid arrows and inhibiting pathways with broken arrows. Abbreviations: DG, diacylglycerol; EGF, epidermal growth factor; FGF, fibroblast growth factor; IGF-1, insulin-like growth factor 1; INS, insulin; IP_3, inositol-1,4,5-trisphosphate; PDGF, platelet-derived growth factor; PIP_2, phosphatidyl-4,5-bisphosphate; PKC, protein kinase C; PL_C, phospholipase C; R, receptor; TPA, 12-O-tetradecanoyl-phorbol acetate.

kinase C has been demonstrated to phosphorylate the EGF receptor at Thr-654 and other sites, and decrease EGF binding and autophosphorylation of the receptor[233,234]. However, it is possible to deplete protein kinase C in 3T3 cell lines by preincubation with TPA[235], and PDGF still effectively reduces EGF binding in cells refractory to TPA[236]. This implies that PDGF is capable of stimulating phosphorylation of Thr-654 and other sites in the EGF receptor by another protein kinase that is distinct from protein kinase C.

The S6 kinase appears to be activated via protein kinase C-dependent and independent mechanisms (Figure 2). Although, the stimulation of the S6 kinase activity by TPA and agents that induce polyphosphoinositol turnover such as vasopressin and prostaglandin $F_{2\alpha}$ is lost in cells in which protein kinase C has been down-regulated by phorbol ester pretreatment, activation via the src kinase[237] and the growth factor receptor kinases[197,200,208] is preserved. Hence, feedback phosphorylation of the EGF and other growth factor receptors by the S6 kinase is an attractive possibility that merits closer scrutiny in the future.

How increased protein-tyrosine phosphorylation is translated into stimulation of the S6 kinase remains to be determined. A simple working hypothesis is that the S6 kinase is phosphorylated on a serine/threonine residue and activated by an intermediate S6 kinase kinase, which is phosphorylated on a tyrosine residue and activated by another kinase (presumably a growth factor receptor or src kinase). Thus far, attempts to activate partially purified S6 kinase with insulin and EGF receptor preparations have failed. Potential candidates for the S6 kinase kinase included the kinases specified by the oncogenes mos, raf(mil), pim-1 and pks, and stimulated kinase activities in extracts from insulin-treated cells that have been shown to phosphorylate actin[238], casein[204], microtubule-associated protein 2[239] and histone H2B[240]. Solution of this problem will bring us one step closer towards establishing the mechanism of insulin action.

1. S. S. Huang and J. S. Huang, J. Biol. Chem. 261:9568 (1986).
2. C. W. Rettenmier, J. H. Chen, M. F. Roussel and C. J. Sherr, Science 228:320 (1985).
3. M. F. White and C. R. Kahn, The Enzymes 17:247 (1986).
4. R. F. Doolittle, M. W. Hunkapiller, L. E. Hood, S. G. Devare, K. C. Robbins, S. A. Aaronson and H. N. Antoniades, Science 221:275 (1983).
5. M. D. Waterfield, G. T. Scrace, N. Whittle, P. Stroobant, A. Johnsson, A. Wasteson, B. Westermark, C. H. Heldin, J. S. Huang and T. F. Deuel, Nature 304:35 (1983).
6. J. Downward, Y. Yarden, E. Mayes, G. Scrace, N. Totty, P. Stockwell, A. Ullrich, J. Schlessinger and M. Waterfield, Nature 307:521 (1984).
7. A. Hampe, M. Gobet, C. J. Sherr and F. Galibert, Proc. Natl. Acad. Sci. USA 81:85 (1984).
8. C. I. Bargmann, M. C. Hung and R. A. Weinberg, Nature 319:226 (1986).
9. L. Coussens, T. L. Yang-Feng, Y.C. Liao, E. Chen, A. Gray, J. McGrath, P. H. Seeburg, T. A. Libermann, J. Schlessinger, U. Francke, A. Levinson and A. Ullrich, Science 230:1132 (1985).
10. T. Hunter, Nature 313:740 (1985).
11. D. Martin-Zanca, S. H. Hughes and M. Barbacid, Nature 319:743 (1986).
12. P. Besmer, J. E. Murphy, P. C. George, F. Qiu, P. J. Bergold, L. Lederman, H. W. Snyder, D. Brodeur, E. E. Zuckerman and W. D. Hardy, Nature 320:415 (1986).
13. M. Dean, M. Park, M. Le Beau, T. S. Robins, M. O. Diaz, J. D. Rowley, D. G. Blair and G. F. Van de Woude, Nature 318:385 (1985).
14. M. J. Hayman, G. Kitchener, P. K. Vogt and H. Beug, Proc. Natl. Acad. Sci. USA 82:8237 (1985).
15. D. E. Schwartz, R. Tizard and W. Gilbert, Cell 32:853 (1983).
16. A. P. Czernilofsky, A. D. Levinson, H. E. Varmus, J. M. Bishop, E. Tischer and H. Goodman, Nature 301:736 (1983).

17. J. D. Marth, R. Peet, E. G. Krebs and R. M. Perlmutter, Cell 43:393 (1985).
18. A. F. Voronova and B. M. Sefton, Nature 319:682 (1986).
19. M. Shibuya and H. Hanafusa, Cell 30:787 (1982).
20. E. P. Reddy, M. J. Smith and A. Srinivasan, Proc. Natl. Acad. Sci. USA 80:3623 (1983).
21. G. Naharro, K. C. Robbins and E. P. Reddy, Science 223:63 (1984).
22. R. Stephens, N. Rice, R. Hiebsch, H. Bose and R. Gilden, Proc. Natl. Acad. Sci. USA 80:6229 (1983).
23. K. Wilhelmsen, K. Eggleton and H. Temin, J. Virol. 52:172 (1984).
24. K. Semba, M. Nishizawa, N. Miyajima, M. C. Yoshida, J. Sukegawa, Y. Yamanashi, M. Sasaki, T. Yamamoto and K. Toyoshima, Proc. Natl. Acad. Sci. USA 83:5459 (1986).
25. N. Kitamura, A. Kitamura, K. Toyoshima, Y. Hirayama and M. Yoshida, Nature 297:205 (1982).
26. E. Rozengurt, Science 234:161 (1986).
27. O. M. Rosen, R. Herrera, Y. Olowe, L. M. Petruzzelli and M. H. Cobb, Proc. Natl. Acad. Sci. USA 80:3237 (1983).
28. K. T. Yu and M. P. Czech, J. Biol. Chem. 261:4715 (1986).
29. R. A. Kohanski and M. D. Lane, Biochem. Biophys. Res. Commun. 134:1312 (1986).
30. H. H. Klein, G. R. Freidenberg, M. Kladde and J. M. Olefsky, J. Biol. Chem. 261:4691 (1986).
31. N. Sasaki, R. W. Rees-Jones, Y. Zick, S. P. Nissley and M. M. Rechler, J. Biol. Chem. 260:9793 (1985).
32. K. T. Yu, M. A. Peters and M. P. Czech, J. Biol. Chem. 261:11341 (1986).
33. P. J. Bertics and G. N. Gill, J. Biol. Chem. 260:14642 (1985).
34. C. S. King and J. A. Cooper, J. Biol. Chem. 261:10073 (1986).
35. P. J. Blackshear, R. A. Nemenoff and J. Avruch, Biochem. J. 214: 11 (1983).
36. P. J. Blackshear, L. A. Witters, P. R. Girard, J. F. Kuo and S. N. Quamo, J. Biol. Chem. 260:13304 (1985).
37. S. Ramakrishna and W. B. Benjamin, Biochem. Biophys. Res. Commun. 117:758 (1983).
38. C. B. Graves and J. M. McDonald, J. Biol. Chem. 260:11286 (1985).
39. J. C. Lawrence, J. F. Hiken, M. Inkster, C. W. Scott and M. C. Mumby, Proc. Natl. Acad. Sci. USA 83:3649 (1986).
40. J. L. Sadoul, J. F. Peyron, R. Ballotti, A. Debant, M. Fehlmann and E. V. Obberghen, Biochem. J. 227:887 (1985).
41. A. Le Cam, P. Auberger and M. Samson, Biochem. Biophys. Res. Commun. 106:1062 (1982).
42. A. Le Cam, J. Biol. Chem. 257:8376 (1982).
43. R. W. Rees-Jones and S. I. Taylor, J. Biol. Chem. 260:4461 (1985).
44. M. F. White, R. Maron and C. R. Kahn, Nature 318:183 (1985).
45. T. D. Giugni, L. C. James and H. T. Haigler, J. Biol. Chem. 260: 15081 (1985).
46. B. Ek and C. H. Heldin, J. Biol. Chem. 257:10486 (1982).
47. M. Kohno, J. Biol. Chem. 260:1771 (1985).
48. R. Bishop, R. Martinez, M. J. Weber, P. J. Blackshear, S. Beatty, R. Lim and H. R. Herschman, Mol. Cell. Biol. 5:2231 (1985).
49. J. A. Cooper, D. F. Bowen-Pope, E. Raines, R. Ross and T. Hunter, Cell 31:263 (1982).
50. S. T. Sawyer and S. Cohen, J. Biol. Chem. 260:8233 (1985).
51. G. E. Landreth, L. K. Williams and G. D. Rieser, J. Cell. Biol. 101:1341 (1985).
52. J. C. Ehrhart, C. Creuzet, E. Rollet and J. Loeb, Biochem. Biophys. Res. Commun. 102:602 (1981).
53. R. M. Johnson, P. A. Connelly, R. B. Sisk, B. F. Pobiner, E. L. Hewlett and J. C. Garrison, Proc. Natl. Acad. Sci. USA 83:2032 (1986).

54. B. Ek and C. H. Heldin, J. Biol. Chem. 259:11145 (1984).
55. C. Betsholtz, B. Westermark, B. Ek and C. H. Heldin, Cell 39:447 (1984).
56. J. Nishimura and T. F. Deuel, Biochem. Biophys. Res. Commun. 103: 355 (1981).
57. R. Ralston and J. M. Bishop, Proc. Natl. Acad. Sci. USA 82:7845 (1985).
58. A. R. Frackelton, P. M. Tremble and L. T. Williams, J. Biol. Chem. 259:7909 (1984).
59. T. Tsuda, K. Kaibuchi, Y. Kawahara, H. Fukuzaki and Y. Takai, FEBS Lett. 191:205 (1985).
60. E. V. Maytin, P. C. Balduzzi, M. F. D. Notter and D. A. Young, J. Biol. Chem. 259:12135 (1984).
61. K. Beemon, T. Ryden and E. A. McNelly, J. Virol. 42:742 (1982).
62. J. A. Cooper and T. Hunter, J. Biol. Chem. 258:1108 (1983).
63. T. Hunter, Cell 22:647 (1980).
64. E. Erikson and R. L. Erikson, Cell 21:829 (1980).
65. K. Radke, T. Gilmore and G. S. Martin, Cell 21:821 (1980).
66. R. Martinez, K. D. Nakamura and M. J. Weber, Mol. Cell. Biol. 2: 653 (1982).
67. J. S. Brugge and D. Darrow, Nature 295:250 (1982).
68. T. D. Gilmore, K. Radke and G. S. Martin, Mol. Cell. Biol. 2:199 (1982).
69. G. Gacon, S. Gisselbretch, J. P. Piau, M. Y. Fiszman and S. Fischer, Eur. J. Biochem. 125:453 (1982).
70. R. Bishop, R. Martinez, K. D. Nakamura and M. J. Weber, Biochem. Biophys. Res. Commun. 115:536 (1983).
71. T. Gilmore and G. S. Martin, Nature 306:487 (1983).
72. A. Laszlo, K. Radke, S. Chin and M.J. Bissell, Proc. Natl. Acad. Sci. USA 78:6241 (1981).
73. E. Rozengurt, M. Rodriguez-Pena and K. A. Smith, Proc. Natl. Acad. Sci. USA 80:7244 (1983).
74. S. O. Moon, H. C. Palfrey and A. C. King, Proc. Natl. Acad. Sci. USA 81:2298 (1984).
75. P. J. Raval and D. Allan, Biochem. J. 232:43 (1985).
76. L. Y. W. Bourguignon, G. Walker and G. J. Bourguignon, J. Biol. Chem. 260:11775 (1985).
77. A. E. Nel, M. Navailles, D. F. Rosberger, G. E. Landreth, P. J. Goldschmidt-Clermont, G. J. Baldwin and R. M. Galbraith, J. Immunol. 135:3448 (1985).
78. G. Grunberger, Y. Zick, S. I. Taylor and P. Gorden, Proc. Natl. Acad. Sci. USA 81:2762 (1984).
79. J. R. White, C. K. Huang, J. M. Hill, P. H. Naccache, E. L. Becker and R. I. Sha'afi, J. Biol. Chem. 259:8605 (1984).
80. A. P. N. Themmen, J. W. Hoogerbrugge, F. F. G. Rommerts and H. J. Van der Molen, FEBS Lett. 203:116 (1986).
81. P. Thams, K. Capito and C. J. Hedeskov, Biochem. J. 221:247 (1984).
82. Y. Iwasa and M. M. Hosey, J. Biol. Chem. 259:534 (1984).
83. R. B. Pepinsky and L. K. Sinclair, Nature 321:81 (1986).
84. B. K. De, K. S. Misono, T. J. Lukas, B. Mroczkowski and S. Cohen, J. Biol. Chem. 261:13784 (1986).
85. A. Rodriguez-Pena and E. Rozengurt, EMBO. J. 4:71 (1985).
86. A. Rodriguez-Pena and E. Rozengurt, EMBO. J. 5:77 (1986).
87. P. J. Blackshear, L. Wen, B. P. Glynn and L. A. Witters, J. Biol. Chem. 261:1459 (1986).
88. H. H. Klein, G. R. Freidenberg, R. Cordera and J. M. Olefsky, Biochem. Biophys. Res. Commun. 127:254 (1985).
89. T. Shiba, T. Akiyama, T. Kadowaki, Y. Fukami, T. Tsuji, T. Osawa, M. Kasuga and F. Takaku, Biochem. Biophys. Res. Commun. 135:720 (1986).

90. L. J. Pike, E. A. Kuenzel, J. E. Casnellie and E. G. Krebs, J. Biol. Chem. 259:9913 (1984).
91. T. Akiyama, T. Kadowaki, E. Nishida, T. Kadooka, H. Ogawara, Y. Fukami, H. Sakai, F. Takaku and M. Kasuga, J. Biol. Chem. 261: 14797 (1986).
92. S. Braun, W. E. Raymond and E. Racker, J. Biol. Chem. 259:2051 (1984).
93. Y. Zick, G. Grunberger, R. W. Rees-Jones and R. J. Comi, Eur. J. Biochem. 148:177 (1985).
94. D. D. L. Woo, S. P. Fay, R. Griest, W. Coty, I. Goldfine and F. C. Fox, J. Biol. Chem. 261:460 (1986).
95. L. J. Pike, D. F. Bowen-Pope, R. Ross and E. G. Krebs, J. Biol. Chem. 258:9383 (1983).
96. L. A. Stadtmauer and O. M. Rosen, J. Biol. Chem. 258:6682 (1983).
97. L. Stadtmauer and O. M. Rosen, J. Biol. Chem. 261:10000 (1986).
98. J. Downward, P. Parker and M. D. Waterfield, Nature 311:483 (1984).
99. J. Downward, M. D. Waterfield and P. J. Parker, J. Biol. Chem. 260: 14538 (1985).
100. A. P. Czernilofsky, A. D. Levinson, H. E. Varmus, J. M. Bishop, E. Tischler and H. M. Goodman, Nature 287:193 (1980).
101. T. Takeya, R. A. Feldman and H. Hanafusa, J. Virol. 44:1 (1982).
102. T. Patschinsky, T. Hunter, F. S. Esch, J. A. Cooper and B. M. Sefton, Proc. Natl. Acad. Sci. USA 79:973 (1982).
103. D. E. Schwartz, R. Tizard and W. Gilbert, Cell 32:853 (1983).
104. J. E. Casnellie, M. L. Harrison, K. E. Hellstrom and E. G. Krebs, J. Biol. Chem. 257:13877 (1982).
105. A. Hampe, I. Laprevotte, F. Galibert, L. A. Fedele and C. Scherr, Cell 30:775 (1982).
106. C. P. Chan, B. Gallis, D. K. Blumenthal, C. J. Pallen, J. H. Wang and E. G. Krebs, J. Biol. Chem. 261:9890 (1986).
107. T. W. Wong and A. R. Goldberg, J. Biol. Chem. 258:1022 (1983).
108. G. S. Baldwin, I. J. Stanley and E. C. Nice, FEBS Lett. 153:257 (1983).
109. G. S. Baldwin, B. Grego, M. T. W. Hearn, J. A. Knesel, F. J. Morgan and R. J. Simpson, Proc. Natl. Acad. Sci. USA 80:5276 (1983).
110. B. P. Wallner, R. J. Mattaliano, C. Hession, R. L. Cate, R. Tizard, L. K. Sinclair, C. Foeller, P. E. Chow, J. L. Browning, K. L. Ramachandran and R. B. Pepinsky, Nature 320:77 (1986).
111. B. Gallis, A. M. Edelman, J. E. Casnellie and E. G. Krebs, J. Biol. Chem. 258:13089 (1983).
112. J. A. Cooper, F. S. Esch, S. S. Taylor and T. Hunter, J. Biol. Chem. 259:7835 (1984).
113. T. Kristensen, C. J. M. Saris, T. Hunter, L. J. Hicks, D. J. Noonan, J. R. Glenney and B. F. Tack, Biochemistry 25:4497 (1986).
114. J. M. Trevillyan, A. Nordstrom and T. J. Linna, Biochim. Biophys. Acta 845:1 (1985).
115. D. A. Tinker, E. G. Krebs, I. Feltham, S. K. Attah-Poku and V. S. Ananthanarayanan, Fed. Proc. 45:1799 (1986).
116. S. Talha and L. Harel, Biochem. Biophys. Res. Commun. 133:265 (1985).
117. F. Vara and E. Rozengurt, Biochem. Biophys. Res. Commun. 130:646 (1985).
118. J. Pouyssegur, J. C. Chambard, A. Franchi, G. L'Allemain, S. Paris and E. Van Obberghen-Schilling, Cancer Cells 3:409 (1985).
119. A. Lopez-Rivas, P. Stroobant, M. D. Waterfield and E. Rozengurt, EMBO J. 3:939 (1984).
120. W. H. Moolenaar, L. G. J. Tertoolen and S. W. de Laat, Nature 312:371 (1984).
121. A. Zorzano, T. W. Balon, M. N. Goodman and N. B. Ruderman, Biochem. Biophys. Res. Commun. 134:1342 (1986).

122. I. Yuli, S. Incerpi, P. Luli and M. Shinitzky, Experientia 38:1114 (1982).
123. K. T. Yu and M. P. Czech, J. Biol. Chem. 259:3090 (1984).
124. F. Beguinot, C. R. Kahn, A. C. Moses and R. J. Smith, J. Biol. Chem. 260:15892 (1985).
125. A. J. Owen, R. P. Geyer and H. N. Antoniades, Proc. Natl. Acad. Sci. USA 79:3203 (1982).
126. O. Morin, C. Forest and M. Fehlmann, FEBS Lett. 127:109 (1981).
127. L. Bosca, G. G. Rousseau and L. Hue, Proc. Natl. Acad. Sci. USA 82:6440 (1982).
128. D. H. Nelson and D. K. Murray, Biochem. Biophys. Res. Commun. 138:463 (1986).
129. K. Yamanishi, H. Nishino and A. Iwashima, Biochem. Biophys. Res. Commun. 117:637 (1983).
130. P. Davies and R. Ross, J. Cell Biol. 79:663 (1978).
131. C. W. Castor, J. C. Ritchie, M. E. Scott and S. L. Whitney, Arthritis Rheum. 20:859 (1977).
132. I. Diamond, A. Legg, J. A. Schneider and E. Rozengurt, J. Biol. Chem. 253:866 (1978).
133. T. B. Miller, A. K. Garnache, J. Cruz, R. K. McPherson and C. Wollenben, J. Biol. Chem. 261:785 (1986).
134. F. Bosch, B. Bouscarel, J. Slaton, P. F. Blackmore and J. H. Exton, Biochem. J. 239:523 (1986).
135. J. L. Parkes, R. R. Cardell and G. Grieninger, Biochem. Biophys. Res. Commun. 134:427 (1986).
136. R. Holland and D. G. Hardie, FEBS Lett. 181:308 (1985).
137. W. J. Vaartjes, C. G. M. de Haas and S. G. Van den Bergh, Biochem. Biophys. Res. Commun. 131:449 (1985).
138. T. A. J. Haystead and D. G. Hardie, Biochem. J. 234:279 (1986).
139. S. J. Fuller and P. H. Sugden, FEBS Lett. 201:246 (1986).
140. G. Thomas, I. Novak-Hofer, J. Martin-Perez, G. Thomas and M. Siegmann, Cancer Cells 3:33 (1985).
141. C. A. Rinehart and E. S. Canellakis, Proc. Natl. Acad. Sci. USA 82:4365 (1985).
142. J. G. Hovis, D. J. Stumpo, D. L. Halsey and P. J. Blackshear, J. Biol. Chem. 261:10380 (1986).
143. E. Tragni, A. Corsini, R. Fumagalli, L. Flaminio and C. L. Galli, Biochem. Biophys. Res. Commun. 139:186 (1986).
144. J. P. Durkin and J. F. Whitfield, Biochem. Biophys. Res. Commun. 123:411 (1984).
145. S. D. Balk, P. I. Polimeni, B. S. Hoon, Le Stourgeon and R. S. Mitchell, Proc. Natl. Acad. Sci. USA 76:3913 (1979).
146. A. F. Chambers and S. Wilson, Mol. Cell. Biol. 5:728 (1985).
147. B. Weissman and S. A. Aaronson, Mol. Cell. Biol. 5:3386 (1985).
148. J. Cooper, K. Nakamura, T. Hunter and M. J. Weber, J. Viol. 46: 15 (1983).
149. K. T. Yu, D. K. Werth, I. H. Pastan and M. P. Czech, J. Biol. Chem. 260:5838 (1985).
150. W. S. Kloetzer, S. A. Maxwell and R. B. Arlinghaus, Proc. Natl. Acad. Sci. USA 80:412 (1980).
151. K. Moelling, B. Heimann, P. Beimling, U. R. Rapp and T. Sander Nature 312:558 (1984).
152. G. Selten, H. T. Cuypers, W. Boelens, E. Robanus-Maandag, J. Verbeek, J. Domen, C. Van Beveren and A. Berns, Cell 46: 603 (1986).
153. G. E. Mark, T. W. Seely, T. B. Shows and J. D. Mountz, Proc. Natl. Acad. Sci. USA 83:6312 (1986).
154. Y. Nishizuka, Science 233:305 (1986).
155. S. Jacobs and P. Cuatrecasas, J. Biol. Chem. 261:934 (1986).
156. D. T. Pang, B. R. Sharma, J. A. Shafer, M. F. White and C. R. Kahn, J. Biol. Chem. 260:7131 (1985).

157. L. Stadtmauer and O. M. Rosen, J. Biol. Chem. 261:3402 (1986).
158. M. Kasuga, Y. Zick, D. L. Blith, F. A. Karlsson, H. U. Haring and C. R. Kahn, J. Biol. Chem. 257:9891 (1982).
159. H. Gazzano, A. Kowalski, M. Fehlmann and E. Van Obberghen, Biochem. J. 210:575 (1983).
160. Y. Zick, G. Grunberger, J. M. Podskalny, U. Moncada, S. I. Taylor, P. Gorden and J. Roth, Biochem. Biophys. Res. Commun. 116:1129 (1983).
161. S. Takayama, M. F. White, V. Lauris and C. R. Kahn, Proc. Natl. Acad. Sci. USA 81:7797 (1984).
162. S. Jacobs, S. May, S. Watson, E. Lapetina and P. Cuatrecasas, Cancer Cells 3:139 (1985).
163. R. J. Davis and M. P. Czech, J. Biol. Chem. 260:2543 (1985).
164. M. Chinkers and D. L. Garbers, Biochem. Biophys. Res. Commun. 123: 618 (1984).
165. S. J. Decker, Mol. Cell. Biol. 4:1718 (1984).
166. R. J. Davis and M. P. Czech, Proc. Natl. Acad. Sci. USA 82:4080 (1985).
167. R. J. Davis and M. P. Czech, Biochem. J. 233:435 (1986).
168. S. Iwashita and C. F. Fox, J. Biol. Chem. 259:2559 (1984).
169. P. G. McCaffrey, B. A. Friedman and M. R. Rosner, J. Biol. Chem. 259:12502 (1984).
170. R. W. Brownsey and R. M. Denton, Biochem. J. 202:77 (1982).
171. R. W. Brownsey, N. J. Edgell, T. J. Hopkirk and R. M. Denton, Biochem. J. 218:733 (1984).
172. L. A. Witters, Biochem. Biophys. Res. Commun. 100:872 (1981).
173. L. A. Witters, J. P. Tipper and G. W. Bacon, J. Biol. Chem. 258: 5643 (1983).
174. G. J. Belsham, R. W. Brownsey and R. M. Denton, Biochem. J. 204: 345 (1982).
175. M. W. Pierce, J. L. Palmer, H. T. Keutmann, T. A. Hall and J. Avruch, J. Biol. Chem. 257:10681 (1982).
176. G. D. Swergold, O. M. Rosen and C. J. Rubin, J. Biol. Chem. 257: 4207 (1982).
177. C. J. Smith, P. J. Wejksnora, J. R. Warner, C. J. Rubin and O. M. Rosen, Proc. Natl. Acad. Sci. USA 76:2725 (1979).
178. S. M. Lastik and E. H. McConkey, J. Biol. Chem. 256:583 (1981).
179. J. Martin-Perez, M. Siegmann and G. Thomas, Cell 36:287 (1984).
180. G. K. Haselbacher, R. E. Humbel and G. Thomas, FEBS Lett. 100:185 (1979).
181. S. Decker, Proc. Natl. Acad. Sci. USA 78:4112 (1981).
182. R. E. H. Wettenhall, C. N. Chesterman, T. Walker and F. J. Morgan, FEBS Lett. 162:171 (1983).
183. J. Nishimura and T. F. Deuel, FEBS Lett. 156:130 (1983).
184. J. Blenis, J. G. Spivack and R. L. Erikson, Proc. Natl. Acad. Sci. 81:6408 (1984).
185. J. M. Trevillyan, R. K. Kulkarni and C. V. Byus, J. Biol. Chem. 259:897 (1984).
186. V. S. Sheorain, H. Juhl, M. Bass and T. R. Soderling, J. Biol. Chem. 259:7024 (1984).
187. J. C. Lawrence, C. James and J. F. Hiken, J. Biol. Chem. 261:669 (1986).
188. P. J. Parker, F. B. Caudwell and P. Cohen, Eur. J. Biochem. 130: 227 (1983).
189. K. Cheng and J. Larner, J. Biol. Chem. 260:5279 (1985).
190. W. A. Hughes, R. W. Brownsey and R. M. Denton, Biochem. J. 192: 469 (1980).
191. A. P. Thomas and R. M. Denton, Biochem. J. 238:93 (1986).
192. L. Lopez-Alarcon, M. Mojena, L. Monge and J. E. Feliu, Biochem. Biophys. Res. Commun. 134:292 (1986).

193. C. P. Chan and E. G. Krebs, Proc. Natl. Acad. Sci. USA 82:4563 (1985).
194. C. P. Chan, D. F. Bowen-Pope, R. Ross and E. G. Krebs, J. Biol. Chem. (in press) (1987).
195. J. M. Podskalny and C. R. Kahn, Diabetes 29:724 (1980).
196. R. W. Brownsey, G. J. Belsham and R. M. Denton, FEBS Lett. 124: 145 (1981).
197. S. L. Pelech and E. G. Krebs, J. Biol. Chem. (submitted) (1987).
198. I. Novak-Hofer and G. Thomas, J. Biol. Chem. 259:5995 (1984).
199. I. Novak-Hofer and G. Thomas, J. Biol. Chem. 260:10314 (1985).
200. S. L. Pelech, B. B. Olwin and E. G. Krebs, Proc. Natl. Acad. Sci. USA 83:5968 (1986).
201. B. Like and J. Massague, J. Biol. Chem. 261:13426 (1986).
202. J. Blenis and R. L. Erikson, Proc. Natl. Acad. Sci. USA 82:7621 (1985).
203. R. A. Nemenoff, J. R. Gunsalus and J. Avruch, Arch. Biochem. Biophys. 245:196 (1986).
204. M. H. Cobb and O. M. Rosen, J. Biol. Chem. 258:12472 (1983).
205. D. Tabarini, J. Heinrich and O. M. Rosen, Proc. Natl. Acad. Sci. USA 82:4369 (1985).
206. M. H. Cobb, J. Biol. Chem. 261:12994 (1986).
207. M. H. Cobb, J. G. Burr, M. E. Linder, T. B. Gray and J. S. Gregory, Biochem. Biophys. Res. Commun. 137:702 (1986).
208. D. H. Spach, R. A. Nemenoff and P. J. Blackshear, J. Biol. Chem. 261:12750 (1986).
209. S. J. Burkhard and J. A. Traugh, J. Biol. Chem. 258:14003 (1983).
210. A. Hansson and M. Ingelman-Sundberg, Eur. J. Biochem. 151:97 (1985).
211. E. Erikson and J. L. Maller, Proc. Natl. Acad. Sci. USA 82:742 (1985).
212. D. Stefanovic, E. Erikson, L. J. Pike and J. L. Maller, EMBO J. 5: 157 (1986).
213. J. Martin-Perez, B. B. Rudkin, M. Siegmann and G. Thomas, EMBO J. 5:725 (1986).
214. M. Cicirelli, S. L. Pelech and E. G. Krebs, (manuscript in preparation) (1987).
215. J. L. Maller, L. J. Pike, G. R. Freidenberg, R. Cordera, B. J. Stith, J. M. Olefsky and E. G. Krebs, Nature 320:459 (1986).
216. J. L. Maller, J. G. Foulkes, E. Erikson and D. Baltimore, Proc. Natl. Acad. Sci. USA 82:272 (1985).
217. S. L. Pelech, L. Meijer and E. G. Krebs, J. Biol. Chem. (submitted) (1987).
218. P. J. Roach and M. Goldman, Proc. Natl. Acad. Sci. USA 80:7170 (1983).
219. J. Arino and J. J. Guinovart, Biochem. Biophys. Res. Commun. 134: 113 (1986).
220. P. F. Blackmore, W. G. Strickland, S. B. Bocckino and J. H. Exton, Biochem. J. 237:235 (1986).
221. S. Takayama, M. F. White, V. Lauris and C. R. Kahn, Proc. Natl. Acad. Sci. USA 81:7797 (1984).
222. M. Rouis, P. Thomopoulos, C. Cherier and U. Testa, Biochem. Biophys. Res. Commun. 130:9 (1985).
223. H. Haring, D. Kirsch, B. Obermaier, B. Ermel and F. Machicao, J. Biol. Chem. 261:3869 (1986).
224. R. J. Davis and M. P. Czech, J. Biol. Chem. 259:8545 (1984).
225. R. J. Davis, B. R. Ganong, R. M. Bell and M. P. Czech, J. Biol. Chem. 260:5315 (1985).
226. L. Beguinot, J. A. Hanover, S. Ito, N. D. Richert, M. C. Willingham and I. Pastan, Proc. Natl. Acad. Sci. USA 82:2774 (1985).
227. S. Jacobs, N. E. Sahyoun, A. R. Saltiel and P. Cuatrecasas, Proc. Natl. Acad. Sci. USA 80:6211 (1983).

228. E. Sturani, L. M. Vicentini, R. Zippel, L. Toschi, A. Pandiella-Alonso, P. M. Comoglio and J. Meldolesi, Biochem. Biophys. Res. Commun. 137:343 (1986)
229. B. Whitely, T. Deuel and L. Glaser, Biochem. Biophys. Res. Commun. 129:854 (1985).
230. T. Tamura, R. R. Friis and H. Bauer, FEBS Lett. 177:151 (1984).
231. A. F. Purchio, M. Shoyab and L. E. Gentry, Science 229:1393 (1985).
232. K. L. Gould, J. R. Woodgett, J. A. Cooper, J. E. Buss, D. Shalloway and T. Hunter, Cell 42:849 (1985).
233. C. Cochet, G. N. Gill, J. Meisenhelder, J. A. Cooper and T. Hunter, J. Biol. Chem. 259:2553 (1984).
234. J. Downward, M. D. Waterfield and P. J. Parker, J. Biol. Chem. 260:14538 (1985).
235. A. Rodriguez-Pena and E. Rozengurt, Biochem. Biophys. Res. Commun. 120:1053 (1984).
236. N. E. Olashaw, E. J. O'Keefe and W. J. Pledger, Proc. Natl. Acad. Sci. USA 83:3834 (1986).
237. J. Blenis and R. L. Erikson, Proc. Natl. Acad. Sci. USA 83:1733 (1986).
238. J. M. Carrascosa and O. H. Wieland, FEBS Lett. 201:81 (1986).
239. T. W. Sturgill and L. B. Ray, Biochem. Biophys. Res. Commun. 134:565 (1986).
240. R. Ballotti, A. Kowalski, Y. Le Marchand-Brustel and E. Obberghen, Biochem. Biophys. Res. Commun. 139:179 (1986).

THE PROCESSING AND TRANSPORT OF PEPTIDE HORMONES ACROSS ENDOTHELIAL CELL BARRIERS

Donald P. Bottaro and George L. King

Research Division, Joslin Diabetes Center, Department of Medicine, Brigham and Women's Hospital, Harvard Medical School, Boston, MA

INTRODUCTION

Transcytosis is the transcellular transport of substances from one side of the cell to the other side within vesicles. Transported substances are taken up by endocytosis at one plasma membrane surface and are released via exocytosis at a different surface, which allows these substances to bypass intercellular junctions. The term was originally proposed for vesicular transport across endothelial cells (1), where the transcellular route is the main route of vesicle traffic, especially in capillaries with a continuous endothelium like those of skeletal and cardiac muscle, and brain. Transcytosis is also observed in many other types of cells, such as the transport of IgG from the lumen of the intestine to the perivascular space in the newborn rat (2), and the transport of IgA from the vascular front to the bile capillary front by hepatocytes (3,4).

The ultrastructure of endothelial cells suggests that vesicular traffic to the lysosomes and Golgi apparatus is minimal, whereas the transcellular route appears to be highly amplified. The attenuated cytoplasm of endothelial cells brings the lumenal and ablumenal surfaces into close apposition and thus facilitates transcytosis by shortening the transit pathway. Endothelial vesicles can occupy up to 35% of the cytoplasmic volume, at densities estimated from 228 (5) to 800 (6) per square micrometer of endothelial cell surface, as estimated by transmission electron microscopy. Using electron-dense tracers, a shuttle mechanism whereby vesicles pick up material from the lumenal surface and release it on the adventitial surface, has been demonstrated (7). More recently, the receptor-mediated transport of LDL (8), insulin (9) and albumin (10) across endothelia have been reported.

At least five distinct steps can be observed in all examples of transcytosis: 1) the association of the substance to be transported with a particular region of the plasma membrane; 2) endocytosis; 3) vesicular movement across the cytoplasm; 4) exocytosis; and 5) the dissociation of the transported substance from a second region of the plasma membrane. In this light, transcytosis appears to be an organized combination of several fundamental processes that occur separately otherwise. For example, the endocytosis of insulin by adipocytes involves receptor-binding, endocytosis, and eventual degradation of some of the insulin within lysosomes or other prelysosomal compartment (11). The secretion of insulin by the β-cells of the pancreatic islets occurs by fusion of storage granules with the plasma membrane (exocytosis), and the diffusion of released insulin away from the membrane (12). It is assumed that transcytosis occurs by (and perhaps during) a sequence of these more fundamental events, and that each additional pathway can transmit to the next the information required to identify the final destination of the transported substance.

The nature of the transported substance and its association with the plasma membrane may in part determine the signal(s) that specify the transport pathway. In receptor-mediated transcytosis, a signaling mechanism (ligand binding) already exists that could specify a particular pathway, while it is likely that absorptive phase or fluid phase transcytosis may occur by constitutive mechanisms. Association with the plasma membrane, through specific binding or non-specific adsorption, can also affect other aspects of transport. Binding moieties can diffuse laterally in the plane of the membrane, effectively concentrating the bound ligand before endocytosis. Once concentrated, the dissociation of bound material following exocytosis may also be enhanced by a local diffusion gradient. Receptor clustering has been documented in the receptor-mediated endocytosis of LDL, prior to its internalization in coated pits (13). Insulin is not preferentially endocytosed in coated pits by endothelial cells, nor is receptor clustering observed in this cell type (14). This may indicate that uptake in coated pits constitutes a degradative pathway for insulin, a more important pathway for this hormone within non-endothelial target cells.

Exploration of the mechanisms and regulation of transcytosis has been facilitated by the development of model systems *in vitro*. Insulin transport by vascular endothelial cells (9), and immunoglobulin (15) and viral protein (16,17) transport by epithelial cells have been studied using cultured cells grown on porous supports that separate two fluid compartments. Thyroglobulin transport has been studied in inside-out follicles isolated from pig thyroid glands (18,19). Several aspects of each particular event in transcytosis, namely uptake and endocytosis, sorting and targeting, and exocytosis and release, are now more clearly understood in these systems.

PEPTIDE HORMONE BINDING AND RECEPTOR STRUCTURE

The binding of insulin to surface receptors on vascular endothelial cells has been described (20,21,22). Binding studies using ^{125}I-iodinated insulin show that endothelial cells possess approximately 2 X 10^4 insulin receptors (22). Scatchard analysis of insulin binding to endothelial cells shows a curvilinear relationship characteristic of insulin binding in other cell types (22), suggesting that receptors with high and low affinity coexist on the endothelial cell surface. As in other cell types, the endothelial cell receptors can be down-regulated two- to three-fold with physiological concentrations of insulin.

Macro- and microvessel endothelial cells also possess IGF-I and IGF-II receptors similar to those reported found in other tissues with respect to affinity and number, though it appears that macrovessel endothelial cells bind more IGF-II than do microvessel endothelial cells (23,24). Scatchard analysis of IGF binding data shows that microvessel endothelial cells possess fewer receptors for IGF-II than do macrovessel endothelial cells, but with similar affinities (24). Scatchard plots for IGF-I and IGF-II binding data produce straight lines, suggesting homogeneous, non-interacting populations of receptors similar to those found in other cells and in contrast to the curvilinear plots characteristic of insulin binding (24). Although endothelial cells from micro- and macrovessels have IGF receptors with similar binding characteristics, IGF-I and -II exert differential effects on the rate of DNA synthesis as assessed by ^{3}H-thymidine incorporation. Retinal microvessel endothelial cells respond to insulin and the IGF's with increased DNA synthesis, but aortic endothelial cells are unaffected (24).

Cross-linking of ^{125}I-insulin to its receptor on aortic and retinal microvessel endothelial cells in the presence of 100 mM dithiotheitol (DTT) reveals three major bands at 310, 290, and 145 Kd (25; Figure 1). These bands are competed for by high concentrations of IGF-I, but not by IGF-II. Under non-reducing conditions three bands are also observed with molecular weights of 310, 250 and 145 Kd (25). These results suggest that the 145 Kd band represents the α-subunit of the insulin receptor, while the 250 Kd band represents an α-α dimer and the 310 Kd band represents the insulin receptor in its native form.

Microvascular endothelial cells also respond to insulin binding by autophosphorylation of the β-subunit of the insulin receptor <u>in vivo</u>, an event that activates the receptor as a kinase for other substrates and which has been implicated in the mediation of insulin action (25,26,27).

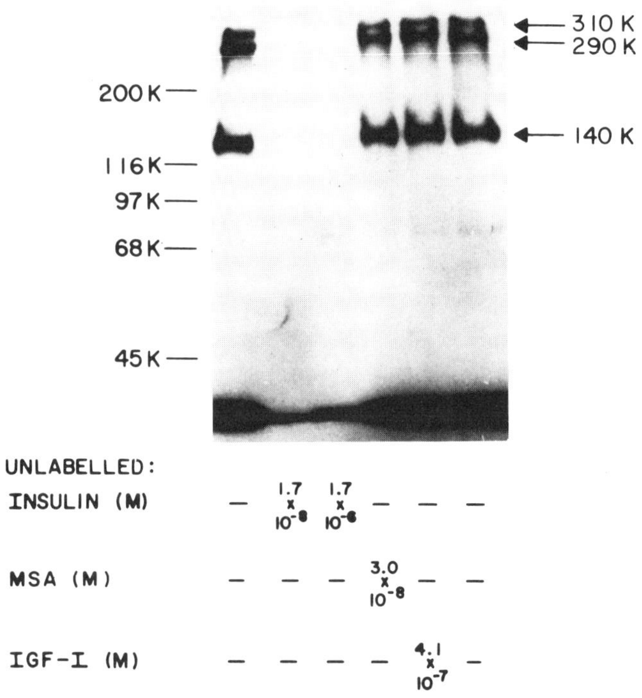

<u>Figure 1:</u> SDS-PAGE autoradiography of ^{125}I-insulin cross-linked to insulin receptors on bovine retinal capillary endothelial cells under reduced conditions. Competition studies with IGF-II (MSA) and IGF-I were performed as well (25).

Insulin does not appear to stimulate receptor autophosphorylation in intact bovine aortic endothelial cells, although if the receptor is partially purified from these cells on a wheat germ agglutinin-agarose affinity column, insulin-stimulated autophosphorylation can be observed using ^{32}P-ATP. Furthermore, none of the growth promoting effects of insulin are observed in this cell type (25).

IGF receptor structure has also been characterized via cross-linking (25). Macro- and microvessel endothelial cells show a single major band at 260 Kd when cross-linked to ^{125}I-IGF-II under reducing conditions. This band was displaced with cold IGF-II, but not with IGF-I or insulin. Under non-reducing conditions, the same molecular species migrates at approximately 230 Kd, suggesting that intrachain disulfide bonds are present in the IGF-II receptor. These results are similar to the characteristics of the IGF-II receptor described for other cells (28,29). Cross-linking using ^{125}I-IGF-I shows that under reducing conditions endothelial cells possess three major species with apparent molecular weights of 310, 290, and 145 Kd. The three bands are effectively displaced with unlabeled IGF-I, but much less by insulin (25). The two higher molecular weight forms are thought to result from cross-linking of the IGF-I receptor subunits to each other or to other membrane proteins, since these bands are minimized in the presence of less disuccinimidyl suberate (DSS). Under non-reducing conditions, two additional bands appear in aortic and retinal microvessel endothelial cells at 310 and 250 Kd. As with the insulin receptor, the 250 Kd band probably represents a complex of α- and β-subunits, whereas the 310 Kd band may represent an oligomer of α- and β-subunits.

PEPTIDE HORMONE PROCESSING AND TRANSPORT

The binding and processing of insulin and IGF-I are time- and temperature-dependent in macro- and microvessel endothelial cells (30,31; Figure 2). In the latter study, approximately 50% of the bound IGF-I and insulin were internalized in both microvessel and aortic endothelial cells after 30 min at 37°C. Internalization of both hormones was decreased to approximately 20% at 15°C, and to less than 20% at 4°C. Treatment with chloroquine or monensin, cellular inhibitors of hormone processing (32), enhanced cell-associated ^{125}I-insulin at 37°C approximately two-fold for aortic endothelial cells after 1 h (31). Accumulation of ^{125}I-IGF-I by aortic endothelial cells was also enhanced by these agents, but to a lesser extent. Microvessel endothelial cells treated with chloroquine or monensin displayed a similar accumulation of ^{125}I-insulin, but showed no change in the amount of cell-associated ^{125}I-IGF-I (31).

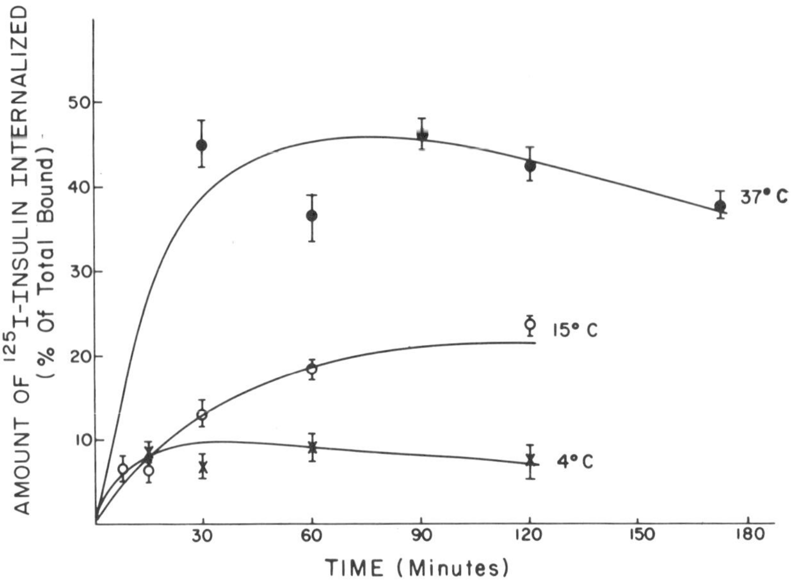

Figure 2: The time course and temperature dependence of internalization of bound insulin by rat capillary endothelial cells. Internalization was determined by acid washing the cells at 4°C after binding for various times and at various temperatures. The acid-resistant radioactivity was taken to represent the internalized portion of the bound hormone. Each point represents the mean ± SEM of samples from endothelial cells that were grown in three separate dishes and assayed independently (31).

Leupeptin, a lysosomal protease inhibitor, did not affect insulin or IGF-I processing by micro- or macrovessel endothelial cells (31). Once internalized, insulin and IGF-I were rapidly released, with approximately 80% of both hormones appearing in the medium after 2h. the released hormones were approximately 90% intact, as assessed by trichloroacetic acid (TCA) precipitability, gel filtration chromatography, and immunoprecipitation. Both insulin and IGF-I induced the down-regulation of their receptors, as shown by an approximate 60% decrease in hormone binding after 24h in aortic and microvessel endothelial cells (31). Taken together, these data indicate that macro- and microvessel endothelial cells specifically bind and process insulin and IGF-I by degradative and non-degradative pathways. Although dual pathways of insulin processing have been identified in adipocytes (33), the amplification of the non-degradative pathway for the processing of these hormones and the modulation of receptors by physiological hormone concentrations suggest a mechanism by which endothelial cells may regulate the access of insulin and IGF-I to target tissues.

Comparison of the processing of IGF-II and insulin by cultured bovine aortic endothelial cells revealed that 50-70% of the bound hormones were internalized within 60 min at $37^{o}C$ (34). Although most of both hormones were subsequently released intact, IGF-II degradation was two- to three-fold greater than insulin degradation, as measured by G-50 chromatography and TCA precipitability (34). These results suggest that aortic endothelial cells preferentially divert more IGF-II than insulin to a degradative pathway. The capacity of endothelial cells to differentially process polypeptide hormones of similar structure further suggests that the pathway(s) by which hormones are delivered to target tissues may be tightly regulated.

Direct measurement of the transport of ^{125}I-insulin by aortic endothelial cells <u>in vitro</u> using a two-compartment system confirms that insulin can be rapidly and unidirectionally transported by receptor-mediated transcytosis (9; Figure 3). The transport observed was inhibited by an excess of unlabeled insulin, and by specific antibodies to the insulin receptor, but not by an excess of unrelated polypeptide, such as nerve growth factor. ^{14}C-labeled inulin, a marker of comparable molecular weight to insulin, was transported at approximately 10% of the rate of ^{125}I-insulin, suggesting that a process of hormone sequestering enhanced its transport relative to a marker of bulk micropinocytosis. As expected, transport in this system was temperature-sensitive (approximately 3-fold greater at $37^{o}C$ than at $15^{o}C$), and more than 80% of the transported hormone was intact.

The kinetics of insulin receptor internalization and the regulation of this process have been studied in micro- and macrovessel endothelial cells (35). Specifically, the role of receptor phosphorylation in this process was examined using insulin and phorbol 12-myristate acetate (PMA). Phorbol esters produce a variety of effects on cellular metabolism, differentiation and growth, and have been shown to induce the internalization of receptors for transferrin, epidermal growth factor, and β-adrenergic agonists (36-41). In these systems it is likely that PMA acts as an analog of diacylglycerol and activates protein kinase C, which in turn phosphorylates the receptors mentioned above (40-41). The

β-subunit of the insulin receptor normally contains phosphoserine and phosphothreonine, and upon insulin binding, autophosphorylates tyrosine residues (26). In the presence of PMA, serine phosphorylation of the

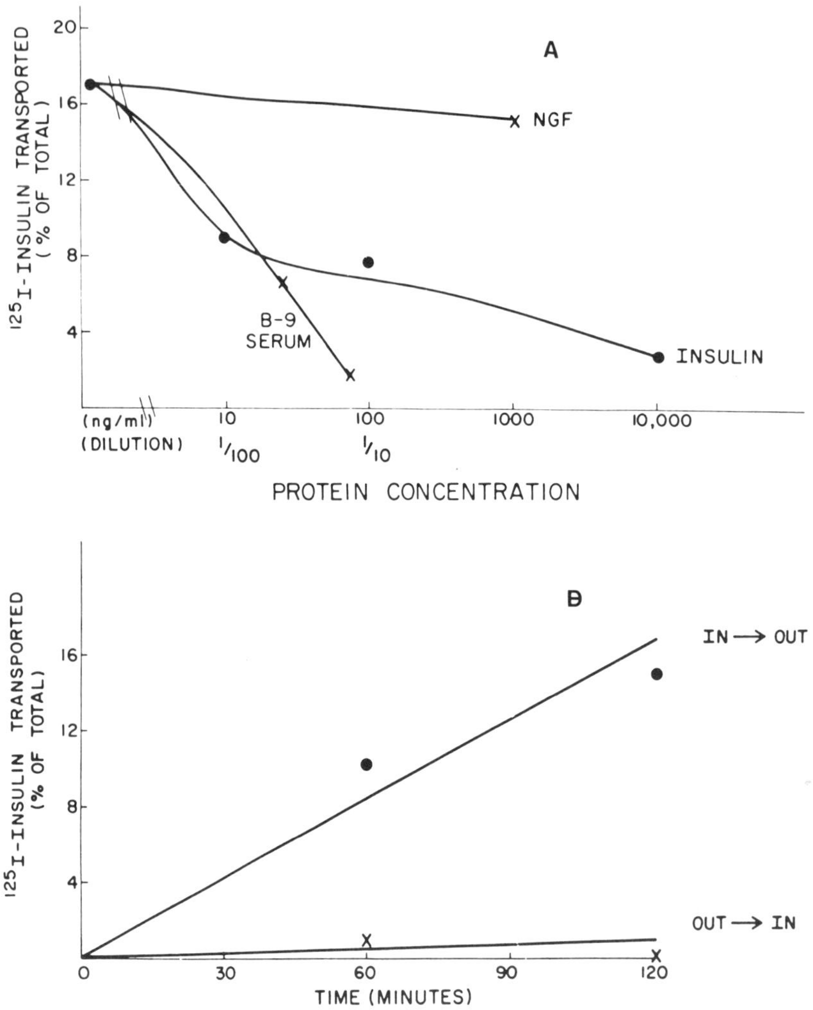

Figure 3: (A) Effects of insulin, nerve growth factor (NGF), and antiserum to the insulin receptor (B-9) on the inhibition of ^{125}I-labeled insulin transport after 2 hours (B) The directionality of ^{125}I-labeled insulin transport across bovine aortic endothelial cells. ^{125}I-labeled insulin was added to the upper chamber (lumenal surface; in→out) or lower chamber (out→in). At each time point, an aliquot of buffer from the upper or lower chamber was used to determine the counts of transported ^{125}I-labeled insulin (9).

receptor is approximately doubled (35). Insulin increases phosphorylation of the receptor almost 3-fold, and the combination of insulin and PMA increase phosphorylation almost 4-fold, suggesting an additive effect.

In the presence of PMA, endothelial cells accumulated between 1.5 and 2-times the amount of ^{125}I-insulin taken up by control cells after 1 h at 37°C (35). At 4°C, however, PMA had no effect on cell-associated ^{125}I-insulin, suggesting that PMA acts on energy-dependent processes, such as internalization of the hormone-receptor complex. This hypothesis was confirmed by further investigations to localize the ^{125}I-insulin associated with PMA-treated endothelial cells at 37°C. These studies revealed that the amount of labeled insulin removable by acid wash was comparable to that of control cells, and that the increase in cell-associated hormone was due to an increase in its intracellular accumulation (35). To determine whether the increased accumulation of hormone in PMA-treated cells was due to decreased degradation or release, these parameters were measured using ^{125}I-insulin-loaded endothelial cells. PMA had no effect on the level of hormone degradation, as assessed by TCA-precipitability after 1 h at 37°C, and a time course of insulin release showed that this process was also unaffected by PMA (35).

The internalization rate of the insulin receptors in endothelial cells was measured directly by observing the decrease in susceptibility of the ^{125}I-surface labeled receptor to tryptic digestion at 10°C (35; Figure 4). Steady-state for receptor internalization in the presence of 100 nM insulin was reduced within 15 min at 37°C. When surface-labeled endothelial cells were pre-incubated with PMA at 37°C, the initial rate of receptor internalization was increased 3-fold over controls. PMA did not appear to affect the internalization of unoccupied receptors, as determined by the absence of trypsin resistant receptor immediately following incubation with PMA (35). These results suggest that PMA acts at a site proximal to the divergence of the two hormone processing pathways already described for endothelial cells, specifically, at the level of insulin receptor internalization. Interestingly, PMA did not appear to affect the steady-state distribution of insulin receptors in endothelial cells. This suggests that PMA not only affects the rate of receptor internalization, but also the rate of receptor recycling, and that these two processes attain an equilibrium within the 30 min period required for internalization to plateau. Recent studies confirm this hypothesis: PMA enhances the insulin-stimulated insulin receptor recycling rate (42). these results further implicate the phosphorylation of the insulin receptor in the regulation of internalization and recycling.

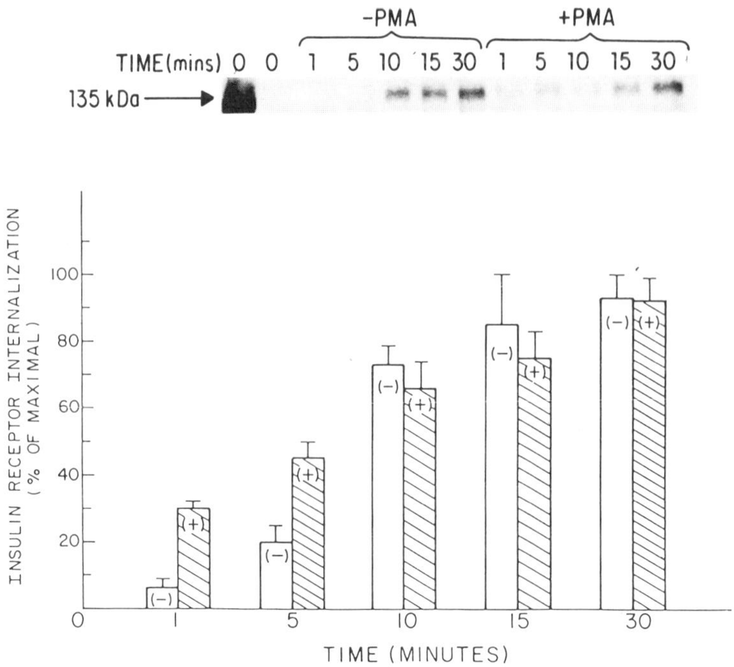

Figure 4: Effect of PMA on the time course of insulin-stimulated insulin receptor internalization. Insulin receptors on the surface of cells were labeled with ^{125}I and internalized by incubation with insulin (100 nM) for the indicated times at 37°C. Surface-labeled receptor was removed by trypsin. The cells were solubilized and the trypsin-resistant (internalized) receptors were quantitated by immunoprecipitation and SDS-PAGE autoradiography. Upper panel: Time course of insulin receptor α-subunit internalization in the presence and absence of PMA. Lower panel: Quantitation of internalized α-subunit by scanning densitometry, expressed as the percentage of maximum internalized at 30 min, in the absence (open bars) or presence (hatched bars) of PMA.

Collectively, these studies show that insulin receptors on endothelial cells may also function as transporters of insulin across the vascular barrier. In the continuously-lined capillaries of muscle and adipose tissue, where endothelial cells are the principal obstacle to the free diffusion of insulin from blood to tissue, receptor-mediated transcytosis most likely provides an efficient and highly regulated system of insulin delivery. In the special case of insulin transport across the blood-brain barrier, this scheme has been convincingly demonstrated *in vivo*. Both brain and retinal microvessel endothelial cells have insulin receptors with the same structural and functional properties as those found in non-neuronal tissues (21, 43-46). Peripheral intravenous infusion of insulin into human subjects raised plasma insulin levels from 12 $\pm$ 1.2 to 268 $\pm$ 35 mU/ml, and concommitantly raised cerebrospinal fluid insulin levels from 0.9 $\pm$ 0.1 to 2.8 $\pm$ 0.4 (47). The authors interpret these data as suggesting a potential mechanism by which peripheral insulin could provide a feedback signal to the central nervous system to regulate food intake.

SUMMARY

In summary, we are just beginning to understand the physiology of peptide hormone receptors in polarized cell types. The binding, processing, and transport of insulin and insulin-like growth factors by vascular endothelial cells suggest that a high degree of specificity may be involved in the delivery of peptide hormones from the circulation to target tissues. The regulation of hormone receptors on endothelial cells could affect the concentration of hormone in the extravascular space, and provide an additional site for the modulation of hormone action. The unraveling of transport and intracellular sorting processes will provide answers as to possible new roles of insulin receptors in mediating insulin action, and will improve our insight into the mechanisms of protein sorting and hormone processing in general.

REFERENCES

1. Simionescu, N. 1979. The microvascular endothelium: Segmental differentiations, transcytosis, selective distribution of anionic sites. Adv Inflammation Res **1**:64-70.
2. Rodewald, R. 1980. Distribution of immunoglobulin G receptors in the small intestine of the young rat. J Cell Biol **85**:18-32.
3. Renston, R.H., A.L. Jones, W.D. Christiansen, G. Hradeck, and B.J. Underdown. 1980. Evidence for a vesicular transport mechanism in hepatocytes for biliary secretion of immunoglobulin A. Science **208**:1276-1278.
4. Nagura, H., P.K. Nakame, and W.R. Brown. 1979. Translocation of dimeric IgA through neoplastic colon cells *in vitro*. J Immunol **123**:2359-2368.
5. Shea, S.M., M.J. Karnovsky, and W.H. Bossert. 1969. Vesicle transport across endothelium: Simulation of a diffusion model. J Theoret Biol **24**:30-42.

6. Casley-Smith, J.R. 1969. The dimensions and numbers of small vesicles in cells, endothelial and mesothelial and the significance of these for endothelial permeability. J Microsc **90**:251-269.
7. Palade, G.E., M. Simionescu, and N. Simionescu. 1979. Structural aspects of the permeability of the microvascular endothelium. Acta Physiol Scand Suppl **463**:11-32.
8. Vasile, E., M. Simionescu, and N. Simionescu. 1983. Visualization of the binding, endocytosis, and transcytosis of low-density lipoprotein in the arterial endothelium _in situ_. J Cell Biol **96**:1677-1689.
9. King, G.L., and S.M. Johnson. 1985. Receptor-mediated transport of insulin across endothelial cells. Science **227**:1583-1586.
10. Ghitescu, L., A. Fixman, M. Simionescu, and N. Simionescu. 1986. Specific binding sites for albumin restricted to plasma lemmal vesicles of continuous capillary endothelium: Receptor-mediated transcytosis. J Cell Biol **102**:1304-1311.
11. Marshall, S. 1985. Kinetics of insulin receptor internalization and recycling in adipocytes. Shunting of receptors to a degradative pathway by inhibitors of recycling. J Biol Chem **260**:4136-4144.
12. Malaisse, W.J. 1984. Stimulus-secretion coupling in the pancreatic B-cell. Experientia **40**:1025-1164.
13. Goldstein, J.L., R.G.W. Anderson, and M.S. Brown. 1979. Coated pits, coated vesicles, and receptor-mediated endocytosis. Nature (Lond) **5715**:679-685.
14. King, G.L. Unpublished observations.
15. Mostov, K.E., and D.L. Deitcher. 1986. Polymeric immunoglobulin receptor expressed in MDCK cells transcytoses IgA. Cell **46**:613-621.
16. Von Bondsdorff, C.H., S.D. Fuller, and K. Simons. 1985. Apical and basolateral endocytosis in Madin-Darby canine kidney (MDCK) cells grown on nitrocellulose filters. EMBO J **4**:2781-2792.
17. Pesonen, M., W. Ansorge, and K. Simons. 1984. Transcytosis of the G protein of vesicular stomatitis virus after implantation into the apical plasma membrane of Madin-Darby canine kidney cells. I Involvement of endosomes and lysosomes. J Cell Biol **99**:796-802.
18. Herzog, V. 1983. Preparation of inside-out thyroid follicles for studies on transcellular transport (transcytosis). Methods Enzymol **98**:447-458.
19. Herzog, V. 1983. Transcytosis in thyroid follicle cells. J Cell Biol **97**:607-617.
20. Bar, R.S., M.L. Peacock, R.G. Spanheimer, R. Veenstra and J.C. Hoak. 1980. Differential binding of insulin to human arterial and venous endothelial cells in primary culture. Diabetes **29**:991-995.
21. Frank, H.J.L., and W.M. Pardridge. 1981. A direct _in vitro_ demonstration of insulin binding to isolated brain microvessels. Diabetes **30**:757-761.
22. King, G.L., S.M. Buzney, C.R. Kahn, N. Hetu, S. Buchwald, S.G. MacDonald, and L.I. Rand. 1983. Differential responsiveness to insulin of endothelial and support cells from micro- and macrovessels. J Clin Invest **71**:974-979.
23. Bar, R.S., and M. Boes. 1984. Distinct receptors for IGF-I, IGF-II, and insulin are present on bovine capillary endothelial cells and large vessel endothelial cells. Biochem Biophys Res Commun **124**:203-209.
24. King, G.L., A.D. Goodman, S. Buzney, A. Moses, and C.R. Kahn. 1985. Receptors and growth-promoting effects of insulin and

insulin-like growth factors on cells from bovine retinal capillaries and aorta. J Clin Invest **75**:1028-1036.
25. Jialal, I., M. Crettaz, H.L. Hachiya, C.R. Kahn, A.C. Moses, S.M. Buzney, and G.L. King. 1985. Characterization of the receptors for insulin and the insulin-like growth factors on micro- and macrovascular tissues. Endocrinology **117**:1222-1229.
26. Kasuga, M., F.A. Karlsson, and C.R. Kahn. 1982. Insulin stimulates the phosphorylation of the 95,000-dalton subunit of its own receptor. Science **215**:185-187.
27. White, M.F., R. Maron, and C.R. Kahn. 1985. Insulin rapidly stimulates tyrosine phosphorylation of a Mr-185,000 protein in intact cells. Nature **318**:183-186.
28. Kasuga, M., E. Van Obberghen, S.P. Nissley, and M.M. Rechler. 1981. Demonstration of two subtypes of insulin-like growth factor receptors by affinity cross-linking. J Biol Chem **256**:5305-5308.
29. Massague, J., and M. Czech. 1982. The subunit structures of two distinct receptors for insulin-like growth factors I and II and their relationship to the insulin receptor. J Biol Chem **257**:5038-5045.
30. Bar, R.S., A. DeRose, A. Sandra, M.L. Peacock, and W.G. Owen. 1983. Insulin binding to microvascular endothelium: A kinetic and morphometric analysis. Am J Physiol **244**:E447-E452.
31. Banskota, N.K., J.L. Carpentier, and G.L. King. 1986. Processing and release of insulin and insulin-like growth factor I by macro- and microvascular endothelial cells. Endocrinology **119**:1904-1913.
32. Maxfield, F. 1982. Weak bases and ionophores rapidly and reversibly raise the pH of endocytic vesicles in cultured mouse fibroblasts. J Clin Biol **95**:676-681.
33. Marshall, S. 1985. Dual pathways for the intracellular processing of insulin. Relationship between retroendocytosis of intact hormone and the recycling of insulin receptors. J Biol Chem **260**:13524-13531.
34. Hachiya, H.L., J.L. Carpentier, and G.L. King. 1986. Comparative studies on insulin-like growth factor-II and insulin processing by vascular endothelial cells. Diabetes **35**:1065-1072.
35. Hachiya, H.L., S. Takayama, M.F. White, and G.L. King. 1987. Regulation of insulin receptor internalization in vascular endothelial cells by insulin and phorbol ester. J Biol Chem In press.
36. Klausner, R.D., J. Harford, and J. Van Renswoude. 1984. Rapid internalization of the transferrin receptor in K562 cells is triggered by ligand binding or treatment with a phorbol ester. Proc Natl Acad Sci USA **81**:3005-3009.
37. Lee, L.S., and I.B. Weinstein. 1978. Tumor-promoting phorbol esters inhibit binding of epidermal growth factor to cellular receptors. Science **202**:313-315.
38. Magnum, B.E., I.M. Matrisian, and G.T. Bowden. 1980. Epidermal growth factor. Ability of tumor promotor to alter its degradation, receptor affinity and receptor number. J Biol Chem **255**:6373-6381.
39. Beguinot, L., J.A. Hanover, S. Ito, N.D. Richert, M.C. Willingham, and J. Pastan. 1985. Phorbol esters induce transient internalization without degradation of unoccupied epidermal growth factor receptors. Proc Natl Acad Sci USA **82**:2774-2778.

40. Kelleher, D.J., J.E. Pessin, A.E. Rusho, and G.L. Johnson. 1984. Phorbol ester induces desensitization of adenylate cyclase and phosphorylation of the β-adrenergic receptor in turkey erythrocytes. Proc Natl Acad Sci USA **81**:4316-4320.
41. Nambi, P., J.R. Peters, D.R. Sibley, and R.J. Lefkowitz. 1985. Desensitization of the turkey erythrocyte β-adrenergic receptor in a cell-free system. Evidence that multiple protein kinases can phosphorylate and desensitize the receptor. J Biol Chem **260**:2165-2171.
42. Bottaro, D.P., and G.L. King. 1987. Insulin receptor recycling in microvessel endothelial cells and its regulation by insulin and phorbol ester. Manuscript in preparation.
43. Haskell, J.F., E. Meezan, and D.J. Pillion. 1984. Identification and characterization of the insulin receptor of bovine retinal microvessels. Endocrinology **115**:698-704.
44. Haskell, J.F., E. Meezan, and D.J. Pillion. 1985. Identification of the insulin receptor of cerebral microvessels. Am J Physiol **248**:E115-E125.
45. Pardridge, W.M. 1986. Receptor-mediated peptide transport through the blood-brain barrier. Endocrine Rev **7**:314-330.
46. Frank, H.J.L., W.M. Pardridge, W.L. Morris, R.G. Rosenfeld, and T.B. Choi. 1986. Binding and internalization of insulin and insulin-like growth factors by isolated brain microvessels. Diabetes **35**:654-661.
47. Wallum, B.J., G.J. Taborsky, D. Porte, D.P. Figlewicz, L. Jacobson, J.C. Beard, W.K. Ward, and D. Dorsa. 1987. Cerebrospinal fluid insulin levels increase during intravenous insulin infusions in man. J Clin Endocrinol Metab **64**:190-194.

THE ROLE OF PHOSPHOLIPID METABOLISM IN INSULIN ACTION

Robert V. Farese and Denise R. Cooper

University of South Florida College of Medicine
and J. A. Haley Veterans Hospital
Tampa, FL

A. PHOSPHOLIPID PATHWAYS AND THEIR PERTURBATION BY HORMONES

There are two major mechanisms whereby hormones and other agonists alter phospholipid metabolism and generate intracellular signaling substances in their respective target tissues, viz., phospholipase activation and phospholipid synthesis. The most widely popularized mechanism involves the activation of a specific phospholipase C which hydrolyzes phosphatidylinositol-4,5-bisphosphate (PIP_2).[1] This hydrolysis generates inositol-1,4,5-trisphosphate (IP_3) and diacylglycerol (DAG), which, respectively, mobilize Ca^{++} from intracellular stores and activate protein kinase C[2] and other possibly related kinases. This hydrolytic mechanism is probably operative in the action of most agonists which operate via cell surface receptors and use Ca^{++} as a major intracellular signaling substance. In addition to PIP_2 hydrolysis, other types of phospholipase C may be activated, causing the hydrolysis of phosphatidylcholine (PC),[3] phosphatidylinositol (PI) or a PI-glucosamine complex (PI-glycan).[4] While it is clear that cell surface receptors are coupled to the PIP_2 phospholipase C through GTP-binding proteins (which may or may not be inhibited by pertussis toxin), little is known about the mechanisms whereby receptors activate other forms of phospholipase C.

The second general mechanism whereby hormones and agonists alter phospholipid metabolism and generate intracellular signaling substances is phospholipid synthesis. Many polypeptide hormones,[5] including insulin,[5-8] are known to rapidly increase *de novo* phosphatidic acid (PA) synthesis. This is associated with sizeable increases in the mass of PI, phosphatidylinositol-4'-PO_4 (PIP), and PIP_2, and it was therefore originally thought that newly synthesized PA is primarily metabolized through CDP-diacylglycerol to inositol-phospholipids. However, we have recently documented in several tissues that the pathway proceeds primarily and directly from PA to DAG, and thence to PC, which also increases as a result of increases in *de novo* PA synthesis.[5,7,9] By stimulating this pathway, there may be increases in DAG[7,8,10] in the absence of increases in IP_3 and Ca^{++} mobilization.[8,11]

B. PHOSPHOLIPID-DEPENDENT INTRACELLULAR SIGNALING SYSTEMS

As stated above, phospholipase C-mediated hydrolysis of PIP_2 leads to the generation of IP_3, which in turn mobilizes Ca^{++} from intracellular stores. This increase in cytosolic Ca^{++} activates a number of processes which are stimulated either directly by Ca^{++} or a Ca^{++}-calmodulin complex.

The increases in DAG resulting from either hydrolysis of PIP_2, PC, the PI-glycan, or from *de novo* PA synthesis may activate C-kinase[2] and a closely-related enzyme, protease-activated kinase II (PAK-II).[12] C-kinase requires Ca^{++} and phospholipids for activation, but DAG lowers this Ca^{++} requirement so that it is met by resting cystolic Ca^{++} levels.[2] PAK-II is also activated by DAG and phospholipids, but this enzyme does not require Ca^{++} for its activation, and the activation by DAG cannot be explained by simply changing the enzyme's requirement for Ca^{++}, which in fact may inhibit PAK-II.[12] Whether or not PAK-II is a form of C-kinase or a fully separate kinase is presently uncertain.

Current dogma suggests that DAG is present in intracellular membranes and recruits C-kinase from cytosol to membranes. This recruitment or "translocation" is therefore thought to reflect activation of C-kinase and is generally taken as evidence thereof. However, we have recently found (see below and Farese, R. V.-unpublished) that insulin-stimulated increases in DAG and phospholipids are associated with increases in the activity of cytosolic, as well as membrane-bound, C-kinase, and it is possible that the cytosolic form of C-kinase may also be activated by DAG after certain types of stimuli. It is further possible (see 13) that cytosol-to-membrane translocation is seen only with either tumor promoters, which intercalate almost exclusively into cellular membranes, or with increases in endogenously generated DAG that are accompanied by increases in cytosolic Ca^{++}. Accordingly, increases in DAG in the absence of increases in Ca^{++} may result in a C-kinase activation pattern which differs from that of simple translocation.

Phospholipase C-mediated hydrolysis of a recently described PI-glycan[4] leads to generation of a phosphoinositol-glucosamine complex along with either DAG,[14] or a 1-alkenyl or 1-alkyl analog of DAG.[15] The phosphoinositol-glucosamine complex has been postulated to act as an intracellular signaling substance for activation of cAMP phosphodiesterase (PDE), pyruvate dehydrogenase (POH) and perhaps other enzymes.[4,14] DAG generated by hydrolysis of the PI-glycan may also activate C-kinase. However, Mato and Jarett[15] have found that a 1-alkenyl, 2-acyl-glycerol analog of DAG is produced instead of DAG in some cells, and such analogs of DAG may not activate C-kinase.[16]

Hydrolysis of PC by phospholipase C has recently been observed in some systems,[3] and this hydrolysis would generate DAG and phosphocholine. Recent studies in our laboratory[17] suggest that PC hydrolysis may occur during insulin action and serve as a source of DAG.

We have recently obtained evidence in BC3H-1 myocytes,[17] and rat hepatocytes and adipose tissue (unpublished observations) that newly synthesized PA is preferentially metabolized to DAG. Thus, although DAG generation has largely been thought to result mainly from phospholipase C acting upon PIP_2, PI, and PC, it is clear that newly synthesized PA (via action of PA phosphatase) is another major source of DAG, particularly during the action of insulin and certain other polypeptide hormones. It should be recognized that the DAG derived from *de novo* PA synthesis may be anatomically and functionally distinct from that derived from hydrolysis of PIP_2 or other phospholipids.

C. EFFECTS OF INSULIN ON PHOSPHOLIPASE C ACTIVATION

Most agonists which increase ^{32}P-incorporation into PA and PI have been found to activate the phospholipase C which hydrolyzes PIP_2, (and, in some instances, PI) as evidenced by increases in IP_3, inositol-bisphosphate (IP_2) and inositol-monophosphate (IP). However, although insulin stimulates ^{32}P-incorporation into PA and PI, and although insulin increases PI, PIP, and PIP_2, which provide substrate for this phospholipase C, insulin does not increase IP_3, IP_2, or IP significantly in BC3H-1 myocytes.[8] In adipose tissue,[18] we did observe transient increases in IP_3, IP_2 and IP_1; however, after the first few minutes of incubation, neither we[10,18] nor others[11] have observed increases in the inositol-phosphates, despite observing increases in mass or precursor ($^{32}PO_4$ or ^{3}H-inositol) incorporation into inositol-phospholipids. In conjunction with early, transient increases in inositol-phosphates in adipose tissue, we observed transient increases in the rate of disappearance of prelabeled PIP_2, PIP, and PI.[18] Honeyman[19] has made similar observations concerning the hydrolysis of inositol-phospholipids during insulin action. It is clear, however, that these hydrolytic changes are transient and small, and may reflect an abortive attempt of insulin to activate a phospholipase C which hydrolyzes inositol-phospholipids.

In addition to adipose tissue, we have observed very small, and probably insignificant, increases in inositol-phosphate production in rat hepatocytes, and, on occasion, small, fleeting increases in BC3H-1 myocytes (unpublished observations). The significance of these small changes in inositol-phosphates is questionable, but they are mentioned here for the sake of being complete. In both BC3H-1 myocytes[8] and in hepatocytes (unpublished observations), insulin does not increase cytosolic Ca^{++}, as measured by Quin 2 fluorescence, and this further minimizes the importance of finding small increases in IP_3 in these tissues.

The increases in inositol-phosphates observed during insulin action would be expected to be associated with increases in DAG. However, as with inositol-phosphates, these increases must be small and are unlikely to account for the increases in DAG that are seen with insulin treatment. As shown in BC3H-1 myocytes and adipose tissue,[7,8] insulin increases DAG mass by 50-100% within 1-2 minutes, and these increases persist for 60 minutes. Therefore, we must look to other potential sources of DAG, e.g., *de novo* PA synthesis, and hydrolysis of other phospholipids such as PC and the PI-glycan.

To study phospholipase C-mediated hydrolysis of PC-PE or the PI-glycan as sources of DAG, we have used tritiated arachidonic acid or myristic acid to prelabel phospholipids over a 2-hour period.[17] Subsequent addition of insulin provokes rapid 3-fold increases in [^{3}H]DAG. These increases in [^{3}H]DAG are maximal within 0.5 minutes and diminish after 10 minutes of insulin treatment (see below). The transient nature of this DAG labeling differs from the more persistent labeling of DAG observed with [^{3}H]glycerol. Thus, it appears that insulin increases DAG through at least two mechanisms, viz., *de novo* PA synthesis and hydrolysis of pre-existing phospholipids. The source of [^{3}H]DAG after labeling phospholipids with arachidonic acid or myristic acid is not fully certain. [Note - some of this [^{3}H]DAG may also be derived from *de novo* PA synthesis, but newly synthesized PA is usually poorly labeled with arachidonate.] [^{3}H]Arachidonic acid labels PC to the greatest extent, and PI and PE to lesser extents. With myristate, PC is heavily labeled (> 90%), and there is lesser labeling in PE and PA, and slight labeling of PI. With both fatty acids, we could not detect appreciable labeling of the PI-glycan after 2 hours of labeling (note - after 24 hours, labeling of the PI-glycan by [^{3}H]myristate, but not [^{3}H]arachidonate, is detectable), and the PI-glycan appears to be an unlikely source for the [^{3}H]DAG derived from [^{3}H]arachidonic acid or [^{3}H]myristic acid in our 2-hour labeling experiments. The most likely sources for this [^{3}H]DAG appear to be PC and PE. The possibility that insulin increases phospholipase C-mediated hydrolysis of PC and PE may also be relevant to the unexplained increases in PI (and PIP-PIP_2) mass observed during insulin treatment,[6-8,11] as PI does not seem to be derived significantly from newly synthesized PA.[17] Accordingly, hydrolysis of PC or PE by phospholipase C (or phospholipase D) could generate DAG (or PA), which could then be metabolized to PI. Although experimental proof for this is lacking, PC-PE hydrolysis seems to be the only plausible source to explain the increases in PI mass.

It has recently been reported that insulin increases the generation of a phosphoinositol-glucosamine complex, apparently through activation of a specific phospholipase C, which hydrolyzes a PI-glycan.[4,14] Indeed, a substrate containing inositol and glucosamine has been identified in thin layer chromatograms of lipid extracts of BC3H-1 myocytes,[4,14] and we have verified this finding (unpublished observations). Mato and Jarett[15] have also isolated a PI-glycan which contains phosphoinositol, glucosamine, glycerol, an ether-linked alkene at the 1-position, and a palmitoyl group at the 2-position of glycerol backbone. All investigators have observed an initial decrease and a subsequent increase in the PI-glycan following insulin treatment. These findings suggest that insulin increases the hydrolysis of a PI-glycan, and this is followed by its resynthesis, presumably from PI. This hydrolysis, catalyzed by specific phospholipase C, would therefore generate the phosphoinositol-glucosamine complex along with either DAG or an analog of DAG, 1-alkenyl (or 1-alkyl), 2-acyl-glycerol.

D. EFFECTS OF INSULIN ON *DE NOVO* PHOSPHOLIPID SYNTHESIS

As stated above, insulin rapidly increases the synthesis and contents of PA, PI, PIP, and PIP_2 in BC3H-1 myocytes[7,8] and rat adipose tissue.[6,8,11] After a short lag, the contents of PC and PE are also measurably increased.[6-8] These findings suggested to us that insulin increases the *de novo* synthesis of PA, which is then converted primarily to CDP-DAG and thence to PI, PIP and PIP_2, and secondarily to DAG and thence to PC, PE, MAG and TAG. More recent studies in the BC3H-1 myocyte[17] with [^{3}H]glycerol have confirmed the fact that insulin dramatically increases the rate of *de novo* PA synthesis approximately 60-fold within 1 minute. Moreover, this newly synthesized PA is primarily converted directly to DAG, and thence to PC, PE, TAG, and MAG, rather than to CDP-DAG, PI, PIP, and PIP_2. (Similar effects of insulin on [^{3}H]glycerol incorporation have been observed in adipose tissue - unpublished observations). The poor [^{3}H]glycerol labeling of PI in these experiments is surprising since PI mass increases rapidly in response to insulin. This discrepancy between PI mass and [^{3}H]glycerol labeling suggests that the PI mass is derived from pre-existing phospholipids rather than from newly synthesized PA. As stated above, the most likely source would be PC and PE in a pool which is not labeled by [^{3}H]glycerol. Thus, the *de novo* phospholipid synthesis effect may involve simultaneous increases in PA-DAG-PC synthesis, along with increased hydrolysis of PC to DAG and subsequent conversion to PI. Obviously, this phospholipid effect would traffic large amounts of lipids through DAG.

In hepatocytes, insulin does not increase PI content appreciably (unpublished observations), but does increase [^{3}H]glycerol incorporation into PA, DAG and PC.[20] In this tissue, the *de novo* PA synthesis effect may not be attended by an increase in PC-PE hydrolysis which is sufficiently large to increase the mass or $^{32}PO_4$ incorporation into PI.

E. SUMMARY OF INSULIN EFFECTS ON PHOSPHOLIPID METABOLISM

It appears that there are several effects of insulin on phospholipid metabolism, resulting in the generation of DAG and other putative intracellular signaling substances. In some cases, there appear to be small, fleeting increases in phospholipase C-mediated hydrolysis of PIP_2, but the significance of this is questionable. Other phospholipid effects on *de novo* PA synthesis and phospholipase C-mediated hydrolysis of PC-PE and the PI-glycan seem to be more important during insulin action. Within seconds, insulin provokes a dramatic increase in the rate of *de novo* PA synthesis, which persists for the first few seconds or minutes. Thereafter, the rate of PA synthesis subsides somewhat, but is nevertheless sufficiently increased to maintain or further increase the levels of DAG and other lipids. During the initial phase of insulin treatment, there appears to be simultaneous activation of several types of phospholipase C which act upon PC-PE and the PI-glycan. Phospholipase C activation also generates DAG, which can then be used for synthesis of PA and, eventually, PI, PIP, and PIP_2. The increase in PI content may be important for replenishing the PI-glycan. It appears that increases in DAG during the first few minutes of insulin treatment are derived both from increases in *de novo* PA synthesis and hydrolysis of PC-PE and the PI-glycan; at later times of insulin treatment, the primary source of DAG seems to be *de novo* PA synthesis, rather than PC-PE hydrolysis.

F. CONSEQUENCES OF PHOSPHOLIPID EFFECTS OF INSULIN

DAG and phospholipids are known to activate both protein kinase C[2] and PAK-II kinase.[12] Presumably, the DAG which is generated in response to insulin treatment would also be effective for activation of these enzymes. The fatty acid composition of the DAG produced during insulin action is not entirely clear, but it apparently contains myristate and arachidonate. There does not appear to be a requirement for specific fatty acids in the activation of C-kinase by DAG.[16]

We have observed that insulin increases C-kinase activity in BC3H-1 myocytes,[21] rat hepatocytes[20] and rat adipocytes (unpublished observations). In BC3H-1 myocytes, this activation of C-kinase by insulin was shown to be quite complex, as follows. In the membrane fraction, a 70-80% increase was observed in C-kinase activity at 1 minute of insulin treatment, and this was found to subside between 1 and 10 minutes and increase again thereafter. In the cytosol, a steady gradual increase in C-kinase activity was observed over the first 15 minutes of insulin treatment.

The early and later insulin-induced increases in C-kinase activity in membrane fractions may be related to the fact that DAG is obligatorily synthesized in membranes and would be expected to bind and recruit C-kinase to these membranes. This binding of DAG to C-kinase reportedly increases enzyme activity by decreasing the enzyme's requirement for Ca^{++}.[2] The mechanism for the increase in cytosolic C-kinase activity after insulin treatment is presently uncertain. Under conditions of the C-kinase assay (i.e., Ca^{++} and phospholipids added in excess), it would not be expected that Ca^{++} limitation is an important factor in determining apparent enzymatic activity; thus, changes in DAG would not be expected to be important if DAG only changes the Ca^{++} requirement of the enzyme. However, in preliminary experiments we have found that insulin-induced increases in [^{3}H]glycerol-labeled DAG are associated with chromatographically purified C-kinase preparations from cytosol as well as membranes, and it is possible that this endogenously produced DAG is non-covalently bound to the enzyme, regardless of its cellular location, and alters its kinetic activities both *in vivo*, as would be expected at physiological (nanomolar) Ca^{++} concentrations, and *in vitro*, in the assay which contains excessive (0.5 mM) levels of Ca^{++}. [Note - PAK-II kinase is activated by DAG despite the fact that this enzyme does not require Ca^{++}.[12]] In addition, C-kinase activity could be altered through other mechanisms, including limited proteolysis, changes in phosphorylation of the enzyme through autophosphorylation or other kinases or phosphatases. In any event, insulin-induced increases in cytosolic C-kinase[20,21] or PAK-II kinase[12] activity may be important for phosphorylation of proteins in cellular compartments which are unaccessible to membrane-bound C-kinase. In short, insulin may alter the phosphorylation of a variety of cellular proteins through activation of both membrane-bound and cytosolic C-kinase and PAK-II kinase.

Our ability to observe stimulatory effects of insulin on C-kinase activity in BC3H-1 myocytes differs[21] with the report of Spach et al.,[22] who failed to observe effects of insulin on C-kinase activity. The reason for this discrepancy is unknown. Possible reasons include the fact that we used histone III-S as substrate for the enzyme, whereas Spach et al.[22] used a specific H1 peptide. Other differences in assay conditions or insulin concentrations used to stimulate the myocytes may also be responsible for the discrepancy. In addition, we employed higher insulin concentrations, which were required to fully activate glucose transport, and we fed our cells with 25 mM glucose for 16 hours before experiments to diminish basal DAG synthesis and C-kinase activity.

In addition to demonstrating that insulin increases C-kinase-mediated phosphorylation of histone III-S, we have found that insulin increases the activity of cytosolic C-kinase for phosphorylating another substrate, vinculin.[23] Oddly, there was no effect of insulin on the phosphorylation of this substrate by membrane fractions, despite the fact that the same membrane fractions showed increased activity for phosphorylating histone III-S. These findings indicate that there may be greater complexity in C-kinase activation than had been anticipated. Thus, C-kinase may be activated differently by DAG and/or other factors in various cellular compartments, and this may result in changes or variations in the ability to recognize and phosphorylate specific substrates. The latter possibility is supported by the finding that TPA appears to alter substrate recognition by C-kinase.[21]

In addition to C-kinase, phospholipids and DAG apparently activate PAK-II kinase.[12] As stated above, this activation occurs through a mechanism which is not related to Ca^{++}, and involves a DAG-induced change in the K_m of the enzyme. This kinase is very similar to C-kinase, both in molecular weight and chromatographic characteristics. This kinase may also contribute to insulin-induced increases in phosphorylation of S6 ribosomal protein, but there may be another, different S6 kinase which is also activated by insulin.[25] Needless to say, there presently is considerable confusion concerning the identities and interrelationship of a number of insulin-sensitive kinases.

Increases in the activity of C-kinase and related kinases may have important consequences during insulin treatment. For example, in BC3H-1 myocytes, the phorbol tumor promoter, 12-O-tetradecanoyl phorbol-13 acetate (TPA) has been reported to have insulin-like effects on glucose transport, amino acid transport, and pyruvate dehydrogenase activity.[26] These effects of TPA on glucose transport are equal to or greater than those of insulin in BC3H-1 myocytes, and furthermore, there is no additivity when insulin is added to maximally stimulating concentrations of TPA.[26] It therefore appears that stimulation of glucose transport and certain other metabolic processes by insulin and TPA may occur through activation of a common effector pathway in the BC3H-1 myocyte. Obviously, since insulin increases DAG and C-kinase activity in these cells, and since TPA mimics DAG and activates C-kinase, it is reasonable to suggest that both insulin and TPA converge on this common pathway at the level of C-kinase. In adipocytes, however, TPA provokes only mild increases in glucose transport as compared to insulin.[27,28] This suggests that activation of C-kinase cannot fully explain insulin effects on glucose transport, and presumably other processes, in this tissue. This interpretation, while reasonable, is not fully certain, since it is now clear that insulin and TPA alter C-kinase in decidedly different ways.[29-31] Further, there is a growing body of evidence to indicate that activation of C-kinase is not an all-or-none phenomenon, and that there are considerable differences in this activation when TPA and other activators are used.[13,20,21,29-31] In addition, TPA has been recognized to activate many metabolic processes (adenylate cyclase, Ca^{++} redistribution, membrane polarization, phospholipase activity, etc.), quite unpredictably in a variety of tissues. These more recent findings indicate that either observance of similarities, or failure to observe complete concordance, between effects of physiological agonists and TPA cannot be taken as definitive evidence for involvement or non-involvement (respectively) of C-kinase in the action of the physiological agonists. The complexity of this problem not only revolves around the fact that C-kinase activation seems to alter substrate recognition, depending upon the activator, but it is also now recognized that there are multiple molecular forms of C-kinase which may be activated differently by various activators.[32,33]

Effects of insulin on S6 phosphorylation,[22] Na^+-K^+ exchange,[34] glucose transport[35] and certain other processes[36] have been reported to remain intact in cells which are "desensitized" with "chronic" TPA treatment. The rationale for these experiments is that exposure of cells to TPA for several hours results in: (a) a nearly complete loss of C-kinase-mediated phosphorylation of histones; (b) loss of cellular responsiveness to TPA; and (c) decreases in immunoreactive C-kinase. Thus, it is reasonable to suggest that effects of insulin or other agonists which are evident after "TPA-desensitization" must be mediated by an enzyme other than C-kinase. However, Cochet et al.[24] have recently shown that substrate recognition is drastically modified by TPA treatment; thus, although there is almost a complete loss of C-kinase-mediated histone phosphorylation after TPA treatment, the ability of C-kinase to phosphorylate other substrates, including vinculin and several other proteins, remains fully apparent. In other words, the loss of C-kinase after TPA treatment is more apparent than real, and either TPA changes substrate recognition by C-kinase, or TPA fails to deplete all forms of C-kinase. In the BC3H-1 myocyte, we too have found that although the cytosolic C-kinase-mediated phosphorylation of histone III-S is lost after 20-minute or 18-hour TPA treatment, phospholipid- and Ca^{++}-dependent phosphorylation of vinculin remains unchanged.[23] Our findings confirm the fact that such TPA does not fully deplete C-kinase. (Along these lines, it is of interest that 2 major proteins which display immunoreactivity to C-kinase antibodies persist after chronic TPA treatment, and only a lesser 80K immunoreactive protein is lost.[36]) Thus, these "TPA desensitization" or "C-kinase depletion" experiments cannot be considered to be conclusive for evaluating the importance of C-kinase activation in actions of insulin and other hormones.

It should be recognized that increases in DAG may serve not only to activate C-kinase and related kinases, but DAG itself (since it lacks a polar head group) may cause local increases in the curvature of membrane phospholipid bilayers, and thus may both alter the biological activity of resident proteins and promote fusogenicity between adjacent membranes. This change in the physical characteristics of cellular membranes may be important for moving glucose transporters from intracellular locations to the plasma membrane where they promote glucose transport.[37,38]

The release of a phosphoinositol-glucosamine complex, which results from activation of a specific phospholipase C which hydrolyzes the PI-glycan,[4,14] has been postulated to result in activation of cAMP phosphodiesterase and pyruvate dehydrogenase. In this hydrolytic sequence, peptides which may be attached to the PI-glycan may also be released and subsequently activate certain enzymes.[39] It is of further interest to note that extracts which contain the phosphoinositol-glucosamine complex and possibly other "chemical mediators" have been found to activate certain enzymes, such as pyruvate dehydrogenase, cAMP phosphodiesterase and glycogen synthase when added to intact cells, but are ineffective for activating glucose transport in these cells.[40] The latter observation suggests that glucose transport may be activated by the DAG-C-kinase system, rather than by mediators derived from phospholipid head groups.

G. CONCLUDING REMARKS

There seems to be little doubt that insulin rapidly and dramatically alters phospholipid metabolism in many of its target tissues. There are several alterations, including increases in *de novo* PA synthesis and phospholipase C-mediated phospholipid hydrolysis. As a result of these alterations, there are increases in DAG and other intracellular signaling substances, e.g., the phosphoinositol-glucosamine complex. Furthermore, there appear to be changes in protein kinases which are activated by DAG. The changes in DAG and other lipids and phospholipids may also directly alter a variety of metabolic processes. Challenges for the future are to: (a) determine the mechanisms whereby insulin alters phospholipid metabolism; (b) further define the mechanism of activation and importance of changes in DAG-activated protein kinases; (c) determine whether there are other intracellular signaling substances which derive from insulin-induced changes in phospholipid metabolism; and (d) determine how and which metabolic processes are controlled by DAG, other lipids or phospholipids, or their derivatives during insulin action.

REFERENCES

1. M. J. Berridge, and R. F. Irvine, Inositol trisphosphate, a novel second messenger in cellular signal transduction, Nature 312:315 (1984).
2. Y. Nishizuka, Studies and perspectives of protein kinase C, Science 233:305 (1986).
3. J. M. Besterman, V. Duronio, and P. Cuatrecasas, Rapid formation of diacylglycerol from phosphatidylcholine: a pathway for generation of a second messenger, Proc. Natl. Acad. Sci. USA 83:6785 (1986).

4. A. R. Saltiel, J. A. Fox, P. Sherline, and P. Cuatrecasas, Insulin-stimulated hydrolysis of a novel glycolipid generates modulators of cAMP phosphodiesterase, Science 233:967 (1986).
5. R. V. Farese, *De novo* phospholipid synthesis as an intracellular mediator system, in: "Phospholipids and Cellular Regulation," J. Kuo, ed., CRC Press, Boca Raton, FL (1985).
6. R. V. Farese, R. E. Larson, and M. A. Sabir, Insulin acutely increases phospholipids in the phosphatidate-inositide cycle in rat adipose tissue, J. Biol. Chem. 257:4042 (1982).
7. R. V. Farese, D. E. Barnes, J. S. Davis, M. L. Standaert, and R. J. Pollet, Effects of insulin and protein synthesis inhibitors on phospholipid metabolism, diacylglycerol levels, and pyruvate dehydrogenase activity in BC3H-1 cultured myocytes, J. Biol. Chem. 259:7094 (1984).
8. R. V. Farese, J. S. Davis, D. E. Barnes, M. L. Standaert, J. S. Babischkin, R. Hock, N. K. Rosic, and R. J. Pollet, The *de novo* phospholipid effect of insulin is associated with increases in diacylglycerol, but not inositol phosphates or cytosolic Ca^{2+}, Biochem. J. 231:269 (1985).
9. R. V. Farese, M. A. Sabir, and R. E. Larson, Comparison of changes in inositide and noninositide phospholipids during acute and prolonged adrenocorticotropic hormone treatment *in vivo*, Biochem. 21:3318 (1982).
10. R. V. Farese, M. A. Sabir, and R. E. Larson, Effects of adrenocorticotropin and cycloheximide on adrenal diglyceride kinase, Biochem. 20:6047 (1981).
11. S. R. Pennington, and B. R. Martin, Insulin-stimulated phosphoinositide metabolism in isolated fat cells, J. Biol. Chem. 260:11039 (1985).
12. M. I. Gonzatti-Haces, and J. A. Traugh, Ca^{2+}-independent activation of protease-activated kinase II by phospholipids/diolein and comparison with Ca^{2+}/phospholipid-dependent protein kinase, J. Biol. Chem. 261:15266 (1986).
13. S. Pontremoli, E. Melloni, M. Michetti, F. Salamino, B. Sparatore, O. Sacco, and B. L. Horecker, Differential mechanisms of translocation of protein kinase C to plasma membrane in activated human neutrophils, Biochem. Biophys. Res. Commun. 136:228 (1986).
14. A. R. Saltiel, P. Sherline, and J. A. Fox, Insulin-stimulated diacylglycerol production results from the hydrolysis of a novel phosphatidylinositol glycan, J. Biol. Chem. 262:1116 (1987).
15. J. Mato, and L. Jarett, personal communication.
16. B. R. Ganong, C. R. Loomis, Y. A. Hannun, and R. M. Bell, Specificity and mechanism of protein kinase C activation by sn-1,2-diacylglycerols, Proc. Natl. Acad. Sci. USA 83:1184 (1986).
17. R. V. Farese, T. S. Konda, J. S. Davis, M. L. Standaert, R. J. Pollet, and D. R. Cooper, Insulin rapidly increases diacylglycerol by activating *de novo* phosphatidic acid synthesis, accepted for publication, Science (1987).
18. R. V. Farese, J. Y. Kuo, J. S. Babischkin, and J. S. Davis, Insulin provokes a transient activation of phospholipase C in the rat epididymal fat pad, J. Biol. Chem. 261:8589 (1986).
19. T. W. Honeyman, personal communication.
20. D. R. Cooper, H. Hernandez, J. Y. Kuo, and R. V. Farese, Insulin increases *de novo* synthesis of phosphatidic acid and diacylglycerol and protein kinase C activity in rat hepatocytes, submitted for publication.
21. D. R. Cooper, T. S. Konda, M. L. Standaert, J. S. Davis, R. J. Pollet, and R. V. Farese, Insulin increases membrane and cytosolic protein kinase C activity in BC3H-1 myocytes, in press, J. Biol. Chem. (1987).
22. D. H. Spach, R. A. Nemenoff, and P. J. Blackshear, Protein phosphorylation and protein kinase activities in BC3H-1 myocytes, J. Biol. Chem. 261:12750 (1986).
23. D. R. Cooper, C. M. Galaretta, L. F. Fanjul, L. Mojsilovic, M. L. Standaert, R. J. Pollet, and R. V. Farese, Insulin but not phorbol ester treatment increases phosphorylation of vinculin by protein kinase C in BC3H-1 myocytes, accepted for publication, FEBS Lett. (1987).
24. C. Cochet, C. Souvignet, M. Keramidas, and E. M. Chambaz, Altered catalytic properties of protein kinase C in phorbol ester treated cells, Biochem. Biophys. Res. Commun. 134:10031 (1986).

25. D. Tabarini, J. Heinrich, and O. M. Rosen, Activation of S6 kinase activity in 3T3-L1 cells by insulin and phorbol ester, Proc. Natl. Acad. Sci. USA 82:4369 (1985).
26. R. V. Farese, M. L. Standaert, D. E. Barnes, J. S. Davis, and R. J. Pollet, Phorbol ester provokes insulin-like effects on glucose transport, amino acid uptake, and pyruvate dehydrogenase activity in BC3H-1 cultured myocytes, Endocrinology 116:2650 (1985).
27. G. Cherqui, M. Caron, D. Wicek, O. Lascols, J. Capeau, and J. Picard, Insulin stimulation of glucose metabolism in rat adipocytes: possible implication of protein kinase C, Endocrinology 118:1759 (1986).
28. D. Kirsch, B. Obermaier, and H. U. Haring, Phorbol esters enhance basal D-glucose transport but inhibit insulin stimulation of D-glucose transport and insulin binding in isolated rat adipocytes, Biochim. Biophys. Acta 128:824 (1985).
29. J. S. Ramsdell, G. R. Pettit, and A. H. Tashjian, Jr., Three activators of protein kinase C, bryostatins, dioleins, and phorbol esters, show differing specificities of action of GH_4 pituitary cells, J. Biol. Chem. 261:17073 (1986).
30. Z. Kiss, and Y. Luo, Phorbol ester and 1,2-diolein are not fully equivalent activators of protein kinase C in respect to phosphorylation of membrane proteins *in vitro*, FEBS Lett. 198:203 (1986).
31. O. Shinohara, M. Knecht, and K. J. Catt, Differential actions of phorbol ester and diacylglycerol on inhibition of granulosa cell maturation, Biochem. Biophys. Res. Commun. 133:468 (1985).
32. L. Coussens, P. J. Parker, L. Rhee, T. L. Yang-Feng, E. Chen, M. D. Waterfield, U. Francke, and A. Ullrich, Multiple, distinct forms of bovine and human protein kinase C suggest diversity in cellular signalling pathways, Science 233:859 (1986).
33. K.-P. Huang, H. Nakabayashi, and F. L. Huang, Isozymic forms of rat brain Ca^{2+}-activated and phospholipid-dependent protein kinase, Proc. Natl. Acad. Sci. USA 83:8535 (1986).
34. F. Vara, and E. Rozengurt, Stimulation of Na^+/H^+ antiport activity by epidermal growth factor and insulin occurs without activation of protein kinase C, Biochem. Biophys. Res. Commun. 130:646 (1985).
35. K. Kitagawa, H. Nishino, and A. Iwashima, Effect of protein kinase C activation and Ca^{2+} mobilization on hexose transport in Swiss 3T3 cells, Biochim. Biophys. Acta 887:100 (1986).
36. P. J. Blackshear, R. A. Nemenoff, J. B. Hovis, D. L. Halsey, D. J. Stumpo, and J.-K. Huang, Insulin action in normal and protein kinase C-deficient rat hepatoma cells. Effects on protein phosphorylation, protein kinase activities, and ornithine decarboxylase activities and messenger ribonucleic acid levels, Mol. Endo. 1:44 (1987).
37. E. Karnieli, M. J. Zarnnowski, P. J. Hissin, I. A. Simpson, L. B. Salans, and S. W. Cushman, Insulin-stimulated translocation of glucose transport systems in the isolated rat adipose cell, J. Biol. Chem. 256:4772 (1981).
38. K. Suzuki, and T. Kono, Evidence that insulin causes translocation of glucose transport activity to the plasma membrane from an intracellular storage site, Proc. Natl. Acad. Sci. USA, 77:2542 (1980).
39. J. Larner, G. Galasko, K. Cheng, A. A. DePaoli-Roach, L. Huang, P. Daggy, and J. Kellogg, Generation by insulin of a chemical mediator that controls protein phosphorylation and dephosphorylation, Science 206:1408 (1979).
40. L. Jarett, E. H. A. Wong, S. L. Macaulay, and J. A. Smith, Insulin mediators from rat skeletal muscle have differential effects on insulin-sensitive pathways of intact adipocytes, Science 227:533 (1985).

GLUCOSE TRANSPORTERS: OVERVIEW AND IMPLICATIONS FOR THE BRAIN

Eddy Karnieli,

Faculty of Medicine, Technion
and Rambam Medical Center
Haifa Israel

W. Timothy Garvey

Department of Medicine
University of California, San Diego
La Jolla, CA 92093

I. INTRODUCTION

Binding of insulin to its receptor initiates a series of biochemical events which culminate in a variety of cellular actions. In this chapter we will review some of the biochemical mechanisms underlying insulin's ability to stimulate glucose transport in target tissues such as adipose and muscle. Furthermore, we will examine the role of the glucose transport effector system in pathophysiologic insulin-resistant states and modifications which prevent the insulin response in insulin insensitive tissues such as liver and brain.

II. GLUCOSE TRANSPORT IN INSULIN SENSITIVE TISSUES

A fundamental action of insulin is its ability to stimulate glucose metabolism in various tissues. The first step in the intracellular metabolism of glucose is its entry across the plasma membrane and this process is under stringent regulation in fat and muscle. The extreme sensitivity of fat cells to insulin, and the accessibility of viable tissue, made this the tissue of choice for examining insulin's effects on cellular glucose transport as early as the 1960's (1-5).

In adipocytes, insulin acts very rapidly to stimulate glucose transport even though there is a lag time of up to 45 sec at 37°C (6,7). Exposure of intact cells to a maximally stimulating hormone concentration results in a 10-30 fold increase in transport within 10-15 min, with a t 1/2 of 2.5-4 min at 37°C (8,9). Insulin stimulation of glucose transport could occur in the fat cell either via an increase in the affinity of the transporter for glucose or by an increase in transporter number. Kinetic analyses using several glucose analogs have uniformly shown (10-13) that insulin promotes glucose transport by increasing Vmax, while the apparent affinity or Km of the transporter for glucose is unaffected by the hormone. However, a recent report provided evidence that transporter affinity changes in rat adipocytes (14), and that insulin may stimulate glucose transport through both increasing Vmax and decreasing Km. As will be discussed below, the insulin-induced increase in Vmax is at least partially due to increased numbers of glucose transporters in the cell's plasma membrane (11).

III. THE TRANSLOCATION THEORY

Plasma membranes prepared from insulin-stimulated adipocytes sho enhanced glucose transport activity when compared with plasma membranes from basal cells (15,16). When studies to quantitate glucose transporters were carried out using the D-glucose-inhibitable cytochalasin B binding assay, Wardzala et al (11) found that insulin had also increased transporter density in plasma membranes over basal. The source of these additional glucose transporters observed in the presence of insulin was unknown.

Later, independent studies by Cushman and Wardzala (17) and by Suzuki and Kono (18) concurrently led to the discovery of an intracellular pool of adipocyte glucose transporters, which was associated with the low density microsomal membrane fraction enriched with enzymes of the golgi apparatus (18,19). In the studies by Cushman and co-workers (8,11,17), the cytochalasin B binding assay was used to quantitate the number of glucose transporters in subcellular membrane fractions which were prepared by a modification (8) of the method of McKeel and Jarett (16). In plasma membranes prepared from basal cells, the concentration of transporters was low, about 5 pmol/mg membrane protein, while the number of transporters in the low density microsomes was about 16-fold higher, 80 pmol/mg membrane protein (8,19). However, in insulin-stimulated cells, the cellular distribution of glucose transporters was dramatically altered. Insulin induced a five fold increase in plasma membrane-associated transporters and decreased transporters in low density microsomes by around 60% (8,19). Kono and colleagues (18,20,21) used a linear sucrose gradient to separate the various subcellular fractions, and measured D-glucose transport in membranes reconstituted into artificial liposomes. Similarly, these studies showed that insulin altered the cellular distribution of glucose transport activity. These two groups using different methodologies and techniques both concluded that insulin stimulates glucose transport by inducing the translocation of glucose transporters from a large intracellular pool to the plasma membrane. This translocation was rapid (t 1/2 = 2.5 min), reversible, and hormone-concentration dependent (8). The process was further shown to be energy and temperature dependent, protein synthesis independent (20), and affected by high pH and hyperosmolarity (21).

Further validation of the translocation theory in adipocytes has come from studies in which antibodies to the purified human erythrocyte glucose transporter were used to detect glucose transporters (22). In those studies, plasma membranes and low density microsomes from basal and insulin-stimulated adipocytes were incubated with antibodies raised against the purified human erythrocyte glucose transporter on Western blots. A 45-50K protein was found to cross react with the antiserum, and the relative amounts of this protein in the membrane fractions were in approximate agreement with the number of transporters determined by cytochalasin B binding. A similar mechanism for insulin-induced recruitment of transporters has been shown in other insulin-sensitive tissues such as rat diaphragm (23,24) and cardiac muscle (25). Recently, we have demonstrated the existance of a similar insulin-induced translocation process in human adipose cells (26).

Another set of studies (27) addressed the contention that transporters were recruited from a specialized region of the plasma membrane which cofractionates with low-density microsomes rather than coming from a separate intracellular pool. In these studies, intact adipocytes were first preincubated with 50 mM ethylidene glucose, (a poorly permeant glucose analog which can at concentrations above 10 mM inhibit ^{3}H-cytochalasin B binding to glucose transporters) and then covalently labeled with ^{3}H-cytochalasin B using UV irradiation. When subcellular membrane fractions were analyzed by SDS-PAGE, only the labeling of the plasma membrane associated transporters was inhibited, while labeling of the low density microsomal transporters was unaffected. These studies, therefore further support the notion that the intracellular pool of transporters is not associated with the plasma membrane (27).

Thus, the translocation theory is now largely accepted as a model for insulin's stimulatory effect on glucose transport. According to this model as shown in Fig 1, the association of insulin with its receptor (step 1) generates an as yet undefined signal (step 2), which promotes the rapid translocation of glucose transporters from an intracellular pool to the plasma membranes (step 3). Steps 4-5 represent the binding and fusion of the transporter protein with the plasma membrane which is probably a multistep and complex process, and it is possible that further activation of the transporter may be necessary even after arrival at the plasma membrane (i.e., through phosphorylation/dephosphorylation processes). When finally the transporter becomes exposed to extracellular glucose, the specific transport process can begin (step 6). Upon dissociation of insulin from its receptor (step 7), reversal of this phenomenon occurs, and the transporters rapidly (t 1/2 of 10 min) return to their intracellular depot (8).

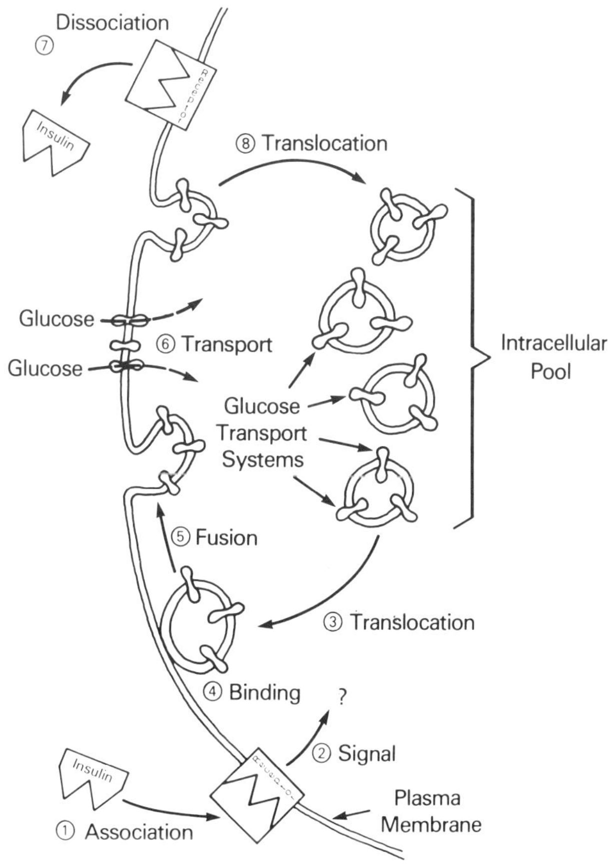

Fig. 1. Translocation theory for glucose transport/from Karnieli et al (8

IV. BIOCHEMICAL CHARACTERISTICS OF THE GLUCOSE TRANSPORTERS

The mechanism by which insulin modulates the movement of transporters in the cell is still largely unknown. A more detailed understanding of insulin's ability to promote glucose transport in adipocytes must await the biochemical characterization, isolation, and purification of glucose transporters. The recent findings that cytochalasin B forms covalent linkages with the glucose transporter when exposed to a high-intensity UV light source (27) has made this a useful probe to identify the glucose carrier and follow it through multi-step purification strategies.

Horuk et al (28) used this technique to photolabel rat adipocyte transporters which were then subjected to two dimensional electrophoresis. In the first phase, they resolved membrane proteins cross-linked with ^{3}H-cytochalasin B on SDS-PAGE. The glucose transporter containing region of the SDS gel (40-55 kDa) was then excised and the proteins eluted and concentrated by moving boundary electrophoresis (28). The extracted proteins were then subjected to isoelectric focusing in the second phase of purification of the glucose transporter. Using this technique these investigators found that two distinct D-glucose-inhibitable cytochalasin B binding proteins were present in low-density microsomes prepared from basal adipocytes. These proteins focused with isoelectric points at pH 6.4 and 5.6. When the same studies were performed in basal plasma membranes, only the pH 5.6 form was observed. Further, insulin recruited only the pH 5.6 isoform from the low density microsomes to the plasma membranes with no effect on the pH 6.4 form of the transporter. Therefore, these studies demonstrate that transporters are biochemically and functionally heterogeneous. The basis for the charge heterogeneity was at least partially due to differences in post-translational glycosylation since treatment of membranes with neuraminidase to remove terminal sialic acid residues altered the isoelectric point of the pH 5.6 isoform (to pH 6.1) but not the pH 6.4 form of the transporter (28). Similar functional and charge heterogeneity of transporters has subsequently been demonstrated in human adipocytes as well (29).

The amino acid sequence of the glucose transporter from human hepatoma cells was originally deduced from analysis of a complementary DNA clone by Mueckler et al (30). These investigators found that the glucose transporter is a single 492 amino acid polypeptide which may span the lipid bilayer 12 times based on hydrophobicity plots, and appears to contain only a single extramembranous site for N-linked glycosylation. A cDNA encoding the glucose transporter has also been established from rat brain (31). This clone also predicts a 492 amino acid protein which shares 97.6% homology with the transporter in (HepG2) hepatoma cells. Both the hepatoma cell and rat brain cDNAs hybridize with a single 2.8 kb messenger RNA (mRNA) species in rat adipocytes, HepG2 hepatoma cells, IM9 leukemia cells, and human kidney tissue (30-32). Thus the transporter is probably generated by a single and similar gene in the different tissues studied, and mRNA from insulin responsive and non-responsive tissues may be indistinguishable. However, in liver, high levels of transport were associated with little or no mRNA hybridizing with transporter cDNA, suggesting that a genetically unrelated protein may be responsible for hexose transport (31) in normal liver.

Haspel et al (32) suggested that in 3T3 cells the primary translation product resolves as a polypeptide of 38,000 daltons on SDS-PAGE, which is then processed to a 42,000 daltons precursor containing N-linked oligosaccharides. The molecular weight of the mature glycosylated polypeptide was 55,000 daltons which is in the range of 43,000-55,000 daltons observed by other investigators in a variety of tissues (22,30,33,34).

In addition to post-translational glycosylation, other cellular processes could also modify the structure of glucose transporters. A potential role for Ca^{+}- and phospholipid-dependent protein kinase (protein kinase C) in the stimulation of glucose transport has been recently addressed by Witters et al (35). They have shown in vitro that protein kinase C phosphorylated purified erythrocyte glucose transporters and that exposing the intact human erythrocytes to phorbol ester induced the phosphorylation of a membrane protein which was identified by immunoprecipitation as the glucose transporter. This work suggests that protein kinase C could phosphorylate glucose transporters in vivo, however, the specific role of this process in the various steps of the translocation model (Fig. 1) is as yet unknown.

V. GLUCOSE TRANSPORTER FUNCTION

Although the translocation hypothesis has now been largely accepted, several discrepancies still remain to be resolved. For example, insulin induces a 10-30 fold stimulation of 3-O-methyglucose uptake in intact cells, however, this is accompanied by only a 4-6 fold increase in plasma membrane glucose transporters as measured by cytochalasin B binding. Simpson et al (19) have attempted to account for this discrepancy by suggesting that the plasma membrane fraction might be contaminated with transporters from the intracellular pool. However, it remains possible that insulin may also activate previously quiescent plasma membrane transporters, or that insulin may lead to enhanced activity as well as increased number of cell surface transporters to explain its full effect on glucose transport in the intact cell.

Recently, several studies have demonstrated that glucose transport activity can be modulated independently from the number of glucose transporters. Smith et al (36) examined the effects of adenosine and isoproterenol on 3-O-methylglucose transport and the subcellular distribution of glucose transporters in maximally insulin-stimulated adipocytes. These investigators found that adenosine depletion (using adenosine deaminase) alone induced about a 30% reduction in the insulin stimulated rate of 3-O-methylglucose transport, while in combination with isoproterenol a decrease of about 70% in transport activity was observed. These agents also reduced the number of plasma membrane glucose transporters but in neither case were these changes as great as the decrement in 3-O-methylglucose transport activity (36). In other words, reduced rates of glucose transport could not totally be explained by the relatively small decrease in transporter number. These studies suggest that cAMP may act at two different sites to regulate insulin-stimulated glucose transport: one locus of action appears to be the translocation process itself (Fig. 1, step 3) and another site might be the regulation of transporter intrinsic activity (step 6) at the plasma membrane level.

Recent studies by us (37) suggest that modulation of transporter activity in the rat adipocyte may be associated with the reversal of diabetes by insulin treatment. In these studies, the maximal insulin-stimulated 3-O-methylglucose transport rate in 8-day insulin-treated diabetic rats was found to be 3-fold higher than that observed in non-diabetic control animals even though there was only a minimal (10-20%) increase in plasma membrane glucose transporters from maximally-stimulated cells. Preliminary data show that these changes in glucose transport are associated with a significant decrease in Km, suggesting changes in the functional capacity of the transporters (38). We have also observed a discrepancy between glucose transport rates and the number of plasma membrane transporters in human adipocytes (39). In cells isolated from the subcutaneous femoral fat pads of regionally obese female patients, increasing cell size was associated with a progressive decrease in the density of plasma membrane glucose transporters and surprisingly with an increase in glucose transport rates (39). Furthermore, when human omental cells were obtained from female and male subjects undergoing elective abdominal operations, we found that cells obtained from male patients exhibited higher transport rates compared with cells prepared from the females, even though there were similar numbers of transporters in plasma membrane fractions [1].

In these previous studies of glucose transporter activity, 3-O-methylglucose transport rates in the intact cell were correlated with the concentration of transporters in the plasma membrane. However, this approach provides only an indirect assessment of transporter functional activity. Further, the activity of the transporters in the intracellular pool can not be measured. In order to resolve these problems, we have recently combined both the cytochalasin B binding assay and the measurement of reconstituted transport activity (40) to study transporters in individual membrane subfractions. From these combined measurements, transporter intrinsic activity can be calculated by dividing glucose transport rates in synthetic liposomes by the number of glucose transporters in the same membrane fraction quantitated by the cytochalasin B binding assay. In our preliminary studies, we found that the intrinsic activity of both intracellular and plasma membrane transporters prepared from diabetic rat adipocytes was actually increased compared with that in control rats. Whereas, in the intact cell, the activity of plasma membrane transporters is apparently diminished in the diabetic rats (see below). Thus, accumulating evidence supports the hypothesis that the glucose transport rate in intact cells is the net expression of both transporter number and the modulation of transporter activity.

VI. GLUCOSE TRANSPORTERS AND INSULIN RESISTANT STATES

The role of glucose transporters has recently been examined in several pathophysiological states characterized by insulin resistance. Theoretically, postreceptor defects in insulin action at the level of the glucose transport system may be due to either 1) decreased number of cellular glucose transporters, 2) impaired translocation of transporters between cellular compartments, or 3) reduced functional activity of transporters. Each of these mechanisms has been demonstrated in various models of insulin resistance and are delineated in Table 1. Other potential defects in the generation of the insulin signal (step 2 in Fig. 1) or in the incorporation of transporters into the plasma membrane (step 4 and 5 in Fig. 1), or post-translational modifications (35,41) which could modulate transporter function have not yet been demonstrated and are speculative at present. In the next sections we will examine several interesting pathophysiological states characterized by insulin resistance due to abnormalities in the glucose transport system.

VIa. INSULIN RESISTANCE IN DIABETES

In Type II Noninsulin-Dependent Diabetes Mellitus (NIDDM), peripheral insulin resistance is a major metabolic abnormality contributing to hyperglycemia. In recent years, studies in NIDDM and obese patients have shown that a defect distal to receptor binding in the insulin action sequence is a major abnormality underlying insulin's reduced ability to stimulate glucose uptake (42-46). In adipocytes isolated from these patients, decreased basal and insulin-stimulated glucose transport activity found in vitro corresponded well to the in vivo expression of the postreceptor defect, and there was similar convergence of in vitro (47,48) and in vivo

[1] M. Armoni, R. Rafaeloff, A. Eitan, A. Barzilai, nd E. Karnieli, paper submitted for publication.

Table 1

Mechanisms of Reduced Insulin Effect at the Level of the Glucose Transport system*

Defects in Glucose Transporters	Adipose tissue	Insulin-Insensitive tissue
1. <u>Decreased number</u>		
a) Absolute		Neurons (?)
1) Cell surface and intracellular	NIDDM Diabetic Rat[1] Fasted rat High fat/low CHO fed rat	
2) Intracellular		Erythrocyte Liver
b) Relative	Human obesity Aged obese rat	
2. <u>Impaired Translocation</u>		
	Treatment with: - Glucose plus insulin[2] - Dexamethasone	Brain micro-vessels
3. <u>Decreased Function</u>		
	Isoproterenol Obesity? Diabetes? Female versus male[3] Aged obese rat	
4. <u>Unknown</u>		
a) Signal Generation		
b) Plasma membrane fusion processes		
c) Molecular modification		

<u>Table 1 legend</u>

* Assuming the glucose transport system in the young 150-200 gr rat model as control.
1. Streptozotocin induced diabetes.
2. In primary adipocyte culture.

(49-51) findings in NIDDM in the response to insulin treatment. Insulin's impaired stimulatory action on glucose transport has been also characterized (52) in recently-diagnosed patients with Insulin-Dependent Diabetes Mellitus (IDDM).

In diabetes, several postreceptor defects in the glucose transport system have been demonstrated (53,54). We (37,54) found that insulin resistance in the streptozotocin-treated diabetic rat model is associated with roughly a 50% depletion of the intracellular pool of glucose transporters in adipocytes. Consequently, the number of translocating transporters appearing in the plasma membrane prepared from insulin-stimulated cells is diminished. This mechanism of cellular insulin resistance is also operative in the high fat/low carbohydrate fed rat (55) and the fasted-refed rat models (56) and produces a quantitatively similar decrease in glucose transport capability. In each case, insulin resistance is associated with the cellular depletion of glucose transporters, with no appreciable impairment in the translocation process. We have also obtained recent evidence in NIDDM patients (57,58) that subcutaneous adipocytes are depleted of glucose transporters which explains in part the profound insulin resistance present in these cells. These data further support the notion that a decrease in the intracellular pool of transporters is a principal defect impairing insulin's ability to stimulate glucose transport in multiple models of insulin resistance.

We have also observed that the functional activity of transporters can be impaired in untreated diabetes and improved following therapy. In streptozotocin-treated diabetic rats, glucose transport rates are decreased to a greater extent than plasma membrane glucose transporters in maximally insulin-stimulated adipocytes compared with that in control animals (37,54). More recent studies in diabetic rats show that insulin therapy for 8 days will restore the cellular content of transporters to normal, and lead to a supranormal 3-fold enhancement of glucose transport rates in intact cells compared with that in controls (37). Thus, it appears that the functional activity of transporters is impaired in untreated diabetic rats and enhanced following insulin treatment. We concluded that there may exists co-factors which regulate plasma membrane transporter function. We have also recently found that the functional activity of transporters may be reduced in adipocytes isolated from untreated NIDDM patients (57,58). In particular, those transporters which are recruited to the plasma membrane appear to be functionally defective since insulin doubles the number of surface transporters but only minimally increases glucose transport activity. In diabetes, transporter activity could be reduced either by a modification intrinsic to the transporter per se or due to some other cellular process which modulates transporter function. As previously mentioned, preliminary data suggest that adipocyte transporters from diabetic rats may have reduced activity in vivo but show increased activity when reconstituted into synthetic liposomes compared with that in control animals (59). This implies that some other cellular process may depress transporter function in diabetic rats.

VIb. OBESITY

In the aged obese rat, marked hyperinsulinemia reflects profound peripheral insulin resistance, which is manifested in adipocytes by decreased glucose transport rates (60). Enlarged cells from 800 gr rats contain ~2.5 fold more glucose transporters per cell than do small cells from 180 gr rats, although this increase is far less than would be expected since the larger cells are roughly 10-fold greater in size. In this model, the concentration of transporters in the plasma membrane under basal conditions is similar to that found in the insulin-stimulated state in the small cells. When the larger cells are exposed to insulin, there is little, if any, stimulatory effect on glucose transport activity, nor is there any effect on the subcellular distribution of glucose transporters (60).

In human omental adipose cells prepared from obese patients undergoing n elective surgery (8), the total cellular number of transporters has been found to be similar to that in adipocytes obtained from lean patients. Thus, increasing cell size in human obesity is not accompanied by an increase in cellular transporters which could be viewed as a relative depletion. However, at least two differences exist between human obesity and the aged obese rat model. In the human adipocyte, cell enlargement is associated with a decrease in the concentration of glucose transporters per mg protein in both plasma and low density microsomal membrane fractions. Also, while insulin induces the translocation of about 30-60% of transporters from the intracellular pool to the plasma membrane in each patient examined, only a minimal effect of insulin on glucose transport activity was found in the intact cell (8). Since transport activity in cells obtained from obese humans and aged obese rats is not enhanced to the extent predicted from the increase in transporter density (per cell surface area), the functional activity of glucose transporters may be reduced. Therefore, in diabetes as well as in obesity, cofactors may inhibit the function of glucose transporters and contribute to the overall postreceptor defect in insulin action (61).

VIc. ROLE OF GLUCOSE, INSULIN, AND DEXAMETHASONE IN THE REGULATION OF GLUCOSE TRANSPORTERS

The factors which regulate the glucose transport system and the mechanisms by which these factors can induce target tissue defects are not yet clearly understood. However, investigators have suggested that postreceptor defects in insulin action could be caused by insulin deficiency (53,54,62), hyperinsulinemia (63-64) or hyperglycemia (64-67) in obese and diabetic animals.

Garvey et al (63,64) have recently shown in primary cultured rat adipocytes that D-glucose and insulin act synergistically over a short time frame (6-10h) to decrease insulin responsiveness by impairing translocation of intracellular transporters to the cell-surface, rather than by reducing the total number of cellular glucose carriers. The same mechanism has been demonstrated in cells made insulin resistant with short term dexamethasone treatment (68). Diminished translocation efficiency for glucose transporters represents a new cellular mechanism for the impaired stimulatory action of insulin on glucose transport. Interestingly, sulfonylurea treatment of rat adipocytes and muscle cells (69-71) has been shown to enhance insulin-stimulated 3-O-methylglucose flux by increasing recruitment efficiency of microsomal transporters to the plasma membrane. Thus, alterations in translocation efficiency may be one mechanism mediating both hypersensitization and desensitization of the insulin-responsive glucose transport system.

VII. GLUCOSE TRANSPORT IN INSULIN INSENSITIVE TISSUES

The purpose of this section is to overview recent studies on glucose transport in insulin insensitive tissues, with particular emphasis on the brain. We will examine how modifications of the glucose transport system, which produce insulin resistance in target tissues, can also completely eliminate insulin responsiveness in tissues such as brain and liver.

VIIa. GLUCOSE TRANSPORT IN THE BRAIN

Glucose is the most important substrate for energy metabolism in the brain and, under normal conditions, is responsible for over 90% of oxidative metabolism (72,73). The first step in the intracellular metabolism of glucose is its entry into the cell (74). However, the parenchyma of the mammalian central nervous system is isolated from the systemic circulation by a unique capillary endothelium, possessing tight cell junctions, which consitutes the blood-brain barrier (75-77). It has become well established that glucose crosses the blood-brain barrier by passive facilitated diffusion with characteristic saturability, stereo-specificity, and competitive inhibition by other hexoses (78-80). Therefore, glucose must first pass the blood-brain barrier to enter the brain's extracellular space and then cross neuronal and glial cell plasma membranes before being metabolized, with the potential for regulation of transport at each step. These considerations have complicated the investigation of glucose uptake by the brain and have necessitated a multifaceted approach. For example, brain glucose transport has been studied in vivo with intravascular administration of label (pulse or constant infusion) accompanied by either blood sampling (indicator dilution method), tissue sampling (Oldendorf brain uptake index method), or external monitoring using radiography or position emission tomography. In vitro studies have also been carried out both at the level of the brain parenchyma using brain slices, cultured cells, and synaptosome preparations, and at the level of the blood-brain barrier in isolated brain microvessels. Many of these studies have been previously reviewed (74-76).

Most studies show that insulin has no direct effect on brain glucose transport, either at the level of neurons or the blood-brain barrier (74,81-90). Although specific insulin receptors (91) and insulin (92) are widely distributed in the central nervous system, the slow rate at which insulin penetrates the brain (8 4,93-96) would preclude any immediate regulation of glucose transport in the brain parenchyma. Insulin can, however, stimulate intracellular metabolism of glucose (81,97-102) which indirectly increases the net uptake of glucose from blood to brain without acting on the transport mechanisms per se. Perhaps this latter consideration, or the possibility that transport is insulin-sensitive only in certain domains or cell types (103) in the brain, explain insulin's ability to stimulate glucose uptake in a few studies (99,100,104-106).

Direct studies of glucose transport in brain parenchyma must be performed independent of the blood-brain barrier which has necessitated the use of various in vitro preparations, including brain slices, cultured cells, and synaptosomes. Studies using cortical brain slices show that facilitated glucose transport is extremely rapid but two factors complicate quantitative assessment. First, labeled substances must diffuse through the extracellular space to reach cell membranes and the rate of diffusion can be rate-limiting with respect to the rate of membrane transport (107). Therefore, measurement of maximal transport rates and affinity constants may reflect diffusion kinetics rather than the saturation kinetics of membrane transport. Secondly, rates of membrane transport exceed the rates of phosphorylation and at physiologic hexose concentrations the intracellular concentrations of free hexoses can be higher than in other tissues (7 4,78,107). This will result in back-diffusion of unphosphorylated hexose and consequently cis-trans rates of transport will be underestimated. In many insulin target tissues such as muscle and fat, transport and not hexokinase activity is rate-limiting for overall glucose metabolism, however, the reverse situation in nervous tissue would appear advantageous given the brain's dependence on a steady supply of glucose for energy metabolism.

Studies using cultured cells are of interest since cell membranes are in direct contact with the medium and techniques exists for isolating neurons separate from glial cells in the absence of blood-brain barrier endothelium. In highly enriched neuronal cell cultures, available evidence suggests that glucose transport occurs by saturable facilitated diffusion, that basal uptake rates are relatively high with no stimulation by insulin, and that hexose phosphorylation and not transport is rate-limiting for glucose metabolism (86,95,108). In contrast, there has been one study using primary cultured glia from rat brain in which basal glucose transport rates were relatively low and insulin led to a 90% increment (103). Although extrapolating data from cells which develop in vitro to the in vivo situation should be done with caution, this latter finding may explain why some investigators find a small stimulatory effect on overall brain glucose transport (99,100,104-106). Studies using transformed cells (i.e., gliomas, neuroblastomas) may not be representative of normal neurons since transformation itself is associated with alterations in hexose transport (109). Finally, synaptosomes (sealed presynaptic nerve terminals) have been used for in vitro studies. This preparation displays rapid but saturable glucose uptake and, again, transport does not appear to be rate limiting for glucose metabolism (110,111). Primary cultured neurons and glial cells as well as synaptosome preparations all possess high affinity glucose transport with low Km values (0.2-1.0 mM) for 2-deoxyglucose (86,103,108,110,111) relative to peripheral tissues such as muscle or fat (~5.0 mM).

Most in vivo studies of glucose uptake by the brain predominantly reflect transport across the blood-brain barrier (78-82). The results indicate that glucose transport across this functional barrier occurs by saturable facilitated diffusion which in most studies is not acutely regulated by insulin; however, kinetic parameters such as the Km of substrate uptake (2-28 mM) are variable depending upon techniques used, species studied, and whether steady-state conditions were present (78). In recent years, the isolated brain microvessel preparation has been developed to study blood-brain barrier nutrient transport in vitro. Glucose uptake in cortical microvessels occurs rapidly via saturable facilitated diffusion (88,89), which in one study (102) exhibited an extremely low value for substrate Km (0.1 mM). Again, hexokinase rather than transport appears to be rate limiting for glucose metabolism in these studies since free glucose accumulated intracellularly in the presence of a physiological media glucose concentration (89), and insulin was unable to promote glucose transport (88-90) despite stimulatory effects on intracellular glucose metabolism (102). Although these features are characteristic of brain glucose transport at other loci, uptake studies in brain microvessels should be reviewed critically since the cells can be leaky following mechanical disruption of the cortex and fail to exclude vital dyes, and since the labeled substrate can quickly come into equilibrium with the intracellular water space making it difficult to measure initial rates of uptake (80).

In summary, the study of brain glucose transport has required the use of multiple methodological approaches, each with its own pitfalls and limitations, and, therefore, results are sometimes inconsistant. However, on balance, several general conclusions seem warranted: 1) A functional blood-brain barrier located in microvessel endothelium is interposed between the brain parenchyma and the circulatory system, 2) glucose transport occurs via carrier-mediated facilitated diffusion, which has inherent saturability and specificity, both at the level of the blood-brain barrier and brain cells, 3) the transport systems may exhibit higher substrate affinities (with lower Km values) than in peripheral tissues, 4) glucose transport does not appear to be rate-limiting for glucose metabolism, and 5) insulin does not stimulate glucose transport (with the possible exception of glial cells) but may enhance intracellular glucose metabolism. Finally, these generic statments may not apply to all cellular components or specialized domains within the central nervous system.

VIIb. GLUCOSE TRANSPORT PROTEINS IN THE BRAIN AND LIVER

The mechanisms responsible for insulin's inability to stimulate brain glucose transport are not known. One possibility is that the insulin receptor, which has unique structural (112) and ligand binding properties

(113) relative to peripheral tissues, does not propagate the insulin signal and is uncoupled from the glucose transport system. On the other hand, certain properties intrinsic to the glucose transport effector system may underlie insulin insensitivity. Within the context of the translocation model, the same mechanisms which produce resistance in insulin target tissue, namely, alterations in glucose transporter number, function, cellular distribution, or capacity for translocation (Table 1), could also explain the lack of responsiveness in insulin insensitive tissues. One example is the liver. Studies performed in vivo (114), in perfused liver (115), and in isolated hepatocytes (116) indicate that hepatic glucose transport is not stimulated by insulin even though liver cells are known to possess specific low-affinity carriers for facilitated diffusion (116). Recently, Ciaraldi et al (117) have measured the concentration and cellular distribution of glucose transport proteins in isolated hepatocytes by performing the cytochalasin B binding assay in subcellular membrane fractions. In liver, most of the transporters were located in the plasma membrane (42 $\pm$ 5 pmol/mg protein) and only a small amount were present intracellularly (4 $\pm$ 3 pmol/mg in low-density microsomes), the reverse of the situation in basal adipocytes. Presumably, there is no insulin response in hepatocytes since there are no intracellular glucose transporters available for recruitment to the cell surface.

The subcellular distribution and biochemical characteristics of glucose transporters have been studied in rat and pig brain microvessels (90,118), another tissue lacking a glucose transport response to insulin (88-90). In these studies, isolated cortical microvessels were preincubated with and without insulin, homogenized, and subjected to a differential centrifugation protocol to isolate membrane subfractions (90). In basal cells, there were ample numbers of glucose transporters in the plasma membrane as measured by the cytochalasin B binding assay (35 $\pm$ 6 pmol/mg). However, in contradistinction to the liver, there was a large pool of intracellular transporters residing in both low-density microsomal (41 $\pm$ 10 pmol/mg) and high-density microsomal (55 $\pm$ 6 pmol/mg) membrane subfractions (90). As expected, there was no translocation of intracellular carriers to the cell surface when the cells were incubated with insulin. Therefore, the lack of insulin responsiveness was due to a translocation block (i.e., the large number of glucose transporters could not be recruited to the plasma membrane) and not due to depletion of the intracellular pool as in hepatocytes.

It is conceivable that structural modifications of the transporter determine whether or not translocation can occur. The glucose transporter in rat and pig cerebral microvessel preparations has an apparent molecular weight on SDS-PAGE gels of 53-55 kDa, whether identified by cytochalasin B photolabeling or immunologic detection (90,118), which is in the molecular weight range of transporters in peripheral tissues (40-55 kDa). Other recent evidence suggests that the primary structure of the transporter may be identical in brain and the periphery. As described previously, complementary DNA (cDNA) clones encoding the glucose transporter have been established from human (HepG2) hepatoma cells (30) and rat brain (31), and both cDNA predict 492 amino acid proteins which share 97.6% homoglogy and both hybridize to a single 2.8 kb mRNA species in rat adipocytes and rat brain. Thus, there appears to be a single, very similar or identical mRNA transcript for the glucose transporter in insulin sensitive and insensitive tissues; however, different post-translational modifications of the transporter could still occur. In rat (28) and human (29) adipocytes, isoelectric focusing of cytochalasin B photolabeled transporters revealed both a translocating pH isoform focusing at pH 5.6 and a non-translocating isoform focusing at pH 6.4 in intracellular membrane fractions, while only he pH 5.6 isoform of the transporter was observed in plasma membranes.

The basis for the charge heterogeneity was partially due to the glycosylation state since treatment with glycosidases altered the isoelectric point of only the pH 5.6 transporter isoform (to pH 6.0 or pH 6.1). In rat brain microvessels, only a pH 6.0 isoform of the glucose transporter is observed on isoelectric focusing gels both in microsomal and plasma membranes (90). Similarly, hepatocytes possess only a pH 6.05 transporter isoform (117). It remains possible that differences in the extent of post-translational glycosylation not only contribute to the charge heterogeneity of transporters in adipocytes, but also produce unique pH isoforms in insulin-insensitive tissues. Whether the structural modifications which alter charge also affect the function of the transporter in microvessels (i.e. decrease the Km for glucose, eliminate capacity for translocation) remains to be determined.

Although insulin does not appear to affect glucose transport rates across the blood-brain barrier, other regulatory factors may exist. For example, using different methodologies, it has been shown that brain uptake of glucose is depressed in chronic hyperglycemia (87,119,120), and that glucose transport and glucose metabolism are specifically diminished in brain microvessels from diabetic rats (121). Interestingly, lowering blood glucose in the diabetic rat either by insulin therapy (which raises blood insulin levels) or by fasting (which lowers blood insulin) restores glucose transport to normal, suggesting that chronic alterations in glycemia regulate microvessel transport rather than insulin per se. When numbers of glucose transporters were assessed in rat brain microvessels, it was found that diabetes decreases glucose carriers in all subcellular membrane fractions including the plasma membrane (121). Therefore, chronic hyperglycemia may regulate microvessel transport activity in conjunction with the cellular content of glucose transport proteins.

Glucose transporters have been less well studied in the brain parenchyma. Based on the previous studies in insulin insensitive tissues, one could hypothesize that: 1) as in the liver, there are large numbers of plasma membrane glucose transporters with a markedly depleted intracellular pool, or 2) there are intermediate numbers of both plasma membrane and intracellular glucose transporters which lack the capacity for translocation as in brain microvessels. However, two studies indicate that neuronal cells may be unique. Dick et al (118) measured glucose transporters in a total membrane fraction (particulate fraction) from rat and pig cerebral cortex and found that their concentrations were extremely low (4-7 pmol/mg) compared to similar measurements in microvessels (~62 pmol/mg). Also, Heidenreich et al (108) have recently obtained preliminary evidence in primary cultured chick neurons that the concentration of glucose transporters was low (<5 pmol/mg) in a plasma membrane enriched fraction as well as in a lower density membrane subfraction. Thus, neurons may have low numbers of plasma membrane carriers, similar to basal adipocytes, and also have a small intracellular pool as observed in hepatocytes. However, adequate neuronal uptake of glucose could be guaranted by a relatively large cell surface area, and if the low Km for substrate uptake (86,103,108,110,111) led to more rapid glucose transport by existing plasma membrane carriers. It is unknown whether structural alterations could enhance substrate affinity or alter the cellular distribution and content of glucose transporters in neurons.

ACKNOWLEDGEMENT

We wish to thank our colleagues Michal Armoni, Thomas P. Huecksteadt, and Ronit Rafaeloff for their contribution in some of the studies described in this manuscript. We are grateful to Mr. Cleon Tate for his excellent secretarial assistance.

REFERENCE

1. Winegred, A.I. and Renold, A.E. (1958). Studies on rat adipose tissue *in vitro*. J. Biol. Chem. 233:267-272.

2. Crofford, O.B. and Renold, A.E. (1965). Glucose uptake by incubated rat epididymal adipose tissue. Rate limiting steps and site of insulin action. J. Biol. Chem. 240:14-21.

3. Crofford, O.B. and Renold, A.E. (1965). Glucose uptake by incubated rat epididymal adipose tissue. Characteristics of the glucose transport system and action of insulin. J. Biol. Chem. 240:3237-3244.

4. Levine R. and Goldstein, M. (1955). On the mechanism of action of insulin. Recent Prog. Horm. Res. 11:343-380.

5. Park, C.R., Reinwein, D., Henderson, M.J., Cardenas, E. and Morgan, H.E. (1959). The action of insulin on the transport of glucose through the cell membrane. Am. J. Med. 26:674-684.

6. Haring, H.V., Kemmler, W., Renner, R. and Hepp, K.D. (1978). Initial lag-phase in the action of insulin on glucose transport and cAMP levels in fat cells. FEBS Lett. 95:177-180.

7. Ciaraldi, T.P. and Olefsky, J.M. (1979). Coupling of insulin receptors to glucose transport: A temperature dependent time lag in activation of glucose transport. Arch. Biochem. Biophys. 193:221-231.

8. Karnieli, E., Zarnowski, M.J., Hissin, P.J., Simpson, I.A., Salans, L.B. and Cushman, S.W. (1981). Insulin-stimulated translocation of glucose transport systems in the isolated rat adipose cell: time-course, reversal, insulin concentration dependency and relationship to glucose transport activity. J. Biol. Chem. 256:4772-4777.

9. Ciaraldi, T.P., and Olefsky, J.M. (1980). Relationship between deactivation of insulin stimulated glucose transport and insulin dissociation in isolated rat adipocytes. J. Biol. Chem. 255:327-330.

10. Vinten, J., Gliemann, J. and Osterlind, K. (1976). Exchange of 3-O-methylglucose in isolated fat cells: Concentration dependence and effect of insulin. J. Biol.. Chem. 251:794-800.

11. Wardzala, L.J., Cushman, S.W., and Salans, L.B. (1978). Mechanism of insulin action on glucose transport in the isolated rat adipose cell. J. Biol. Chem. 253:8002-8005.

12. Olefsky, J.M. (1978). Mechanisms of the ability of insulin to activate the glucose transport system in rat adipocytes. Biochem. J. 172:137-145.

13. Whitesell, R.R., and Gliemann, J. (1979). Kientic parameters of transport of 3-O-methylglucose and glucose in adipocytes. J. Biol. Chem. 245:5276-5286.

14. Whitesell, R.R., and Abumrad, N.A. (1985). Increased affinity predominates in insulin stimulation of glucose transport in the adipocyte. J. Biol. Chem. 260:2984-2899.

15. Martin, D.B., and Carter, J.R. (1970). Insulin stimulated glucose uptake by subcellular particles from adipose tissue. Science 67:873-874.

16. McKeel, D.W., and Jarret, L. (1970). Preparation and characterization of plasma membrane fractions from isolated fat cell. J. Cell Biol. 44:417-432.

17. Cushman, S.W., and Wardzala, L.J. (1980). Potential mechanism of insulin action on glucose transport in the isolated rat adipose cell: apparent translocation of intracellular transport systems to the plasma membrane. J. Biol. Chem. 255:4758-4662.

18. Suzuki, K., and Kono, T. (1980). Evidence that insulin causes translocation of glucose transport activity to the plasma membrane from an intracellular storage site. Proc. Natl. Acad. Sci. USA. 77:2542-2545.

19. Simpson, I.A., Yver, D.R., Hissin, P.J., Wardzala, L.J., Karnieli, E., Salans, L.B., and Cushman, S.W. (1983b). Insulin-stimulated translocation of glucose transporters in the isolated rat adipose cell: characterization of subcellular fractions. Biochim. Biophys. Acta. 763:393-407.

20. Kono, T., Suzuki, K., Dansey, L.E., Robinson, F.W., and Blevins, T.L. (1981). Energy-dependent and protein synthesis-independent recycling of the insulin-sensitive glucose transport mechanism in fat cells. J. Biol. Chem. 256:6400-6407.

21. Toyoda, N., Robinson, F.W., Smith, M.M., Flanagan, J.E., and Kono, T. (1986). Apparent translocation of glucose transport activity in rat epididimal adipocytes by insulin-like effects of high pH or hyperosmolarity. J. Biol. Chem. 261:2117-2122.

22. Wheeler, T.J., Simpson, I.A., Sogin, D.C., Hinkle, P.C., and Cushman, S.W. (1982). Detection of the rat adipocyte glucose transporter with an antibody against the human red cell glucose transporter. Biochem. Biophys. Res. Commun. 105:89-95.

23. Wardzala, L.J., and Jeanrenaud, B. (1981). Potential mechanism of insulin action on glucose transport in isolated rat diaphragm. Apparent translocation of intracellular transport untis to the plasma membrane. J. Biol. Chem. 256:7090-7093.

24. Wardzala, L.J., and Jeanrenaud, B. (1983). Identification of D-glucose inhibitable cytochalasin-B binding site as the glucose transporter in rat diaphragm plasma and microsomal membranes. Biochim. Biophys. Acta 730:49.

25. Watanabe, T., Smith, M.M., Robinson, F.W., and Kono, T. (1984). Insulin action on glucose transport in cardiac muscle. J. Biol. Chem. 259:13117-13122.

26. Karnieli, E., Brazilai, A., Rafaeloff, R. and Armoni, M. (1986). Distribution of glucose transporters in membrane fractions isolated from human adipose cells: relation to cell size. J. Clin. Invest. 78:1051-1055.

27. Oka, Y., and Czech, M.P. (1984). Photoaffinity labeling of insulin-sensitive hexose transporters in intact rat adipocytes: direct evidence that laten transporters become exposed to the extracellular pace in response to insulin. J. Biol. Chem. 259:8125-8133.

28. Horuk, R., Matthaei, S., Olefsky, J.M., Baly, D.L., Cushman, S.W., and Simpson, I.A. (1986). Biochemical and functional heterogeneity of rat adipocyte glucose transporters. J. Biol. Chem. 261:1823-1828.

29. Matthaei, S., Garvey, W.T., Horuk, R., Hueckstaedt, T.P., and Olefsky, J.M. (1987). The human adipocyte glucose transport system: biochemical and functional heterogeneity of hexose carriers. J. Clin. Invest. In press.

30. Mueckler, M., Caruso, C., Baldwin, S.A., Panico, M., Blench, I., Morris, H.R., Allard, W.J., Lienhard, G.E., and Lodish, H.F. (1985). Sequence and structure of a human glucose transporter. Science 229:941-945.

31. Birnbaum, M.J., Haspel, H.C., and Rosen, O.M. (1986). Cloning and characterization of a cDNA endoding the rat brain glucose transporter protein. Proc. Natl. Acad. Sci. USA. 83:5784-5788.

32. Haspel, H.C., Birnbaum, M.J., Wilk, e.W., and Rosen, O.M. (1985). Biosynthesis precursors and in vitro translation products of the glucose transporter of human hepatocarcinoma cells, human fibroblasts, and murine preadipocytes. J. Biol. Chem. 260:7219-7225.

33. Gorga, F.R., Baldwin, S.A., and Leinhard, G.E. (1979). The monosaccharide transporter from human erythrocytes is heterogeneously glycosylated. Biochem. Biophys. Res. Commun. 91:955-961.

34. Shanahan, M.F., Olson, S.A., Weber, M.J., Lienhard, G.E., and Gorga, J.C. (1982). Photolabeling of glucose-sensitive cytochalasin B binding proteins in erythrocyte, fibroblast and adipocyte membranes. Biochem. Biophys. Res. Commun. 107:38-43.

35. Witters, L.A., Vater, C.A., and Lienhard, G.E. (1985). Phosphorylation of the glucose transporter in vitro, and in vivo by protein kinase C. Nature 315:777-778.

36. Smith, U., Karoda, M. and Simpson, I.A. (1984) Counter-regulation of insulin-stimulated glucose transport by cathechalamines in the isolated rat adipose cell. J. Biol. Chem. 259:8758-8763.

37. Karnieli, E., Armoni, M., Cohen, P., Kanter, Y., and Rafaeloff, R. (1987). Reversal of insulin resistance in diabetic rat adipocytes by insulin therapy: restoration of the pool of glucose transporters and enhancement of glucose transport activity. Diabetes. In press.

38. Rafaeloff, R., Armoni, A., and Karnieli, E. (1986) Insulin therapy manipulates the affinity of glucose transporters in adipocytes isolated from diabetic rats. Diabetes 35(Suppl. 1):79A (Abstr).

39. Karnieli, E., R. Moscona, B. Hirshovitz, Y. Illouz, R. Rafaeloff, and M. Armoni. (1986). Discrepancy between glucose transport and transporters in subcutaneous human adipocytes. Diabetes 35(Suppl. 2):52A (Abstr).

40. Kono, T. (1983). Recycling of insulin-sensitive glucose transporter in rat adipocytes. Methods in Enzymology 98:431-444.

41. Haspel, H.C., Wilk, E.W., Birnbaum, M.J., Cushman, S.W., and Rosen, O.M. (1986). Glucose deprivation and hexose transporter polypeptides of murine fibroblasts. J. Biol. Chem. 261:6778-6789

42. Reaven, G.M., Bernstein, R., Davis, B., and Olefsky, J.M. (1976). Non-ketotic diabetes mellitus: Insulin deficiency or insulin resistance? Am. J. Med. 60:80-88.

43. Kolterman, O.G., Gray, R.S., Griffin, J., Burstein, P., Insel, J., Scarlett, J.A., and Olefsky, J.M. (1981). Receptor and post-receptor defects contribute to the insulin resistance in non-insulin dependent diabetes mellitus. J. Clin. Invest. 68:957-969.

44. Rizza, R.A., Mandarino, L.J., and Gerich, J.E. (1981). Mechanisms of insulin resistance in man: Assessment using the insulin dose response curve in conjunction with insulin receptor binding. Am. J. Med. 70:169-176.

45. Ciaraldi, T.P., Kolterman, O.G., Scarlett, J.A., Kao, M., and Olefsky, J.M. (1982). Role of the glucose transport system in the post-receptor defect of non-insulin dependent diabetes mellitus. Diabetes 31:1016-1022.

46. Kashiwagi, A., Verso, M.A., Andrews, J., Vasquez, B., Reaven, G., and Foley, J.E. (1983). In vitro insulin resistance of human adipocytes isolated from subjects with noninsulin-dependent diabetes mellitus. J. clin. Invest. 72:1246-1254.

47. Scarlett, J.A., Kolterman, O.G., Ciaraldi, T.P., Kao, M., and Olefsky, J.M. (1983). insulin treatment reverses the post-receptor defect in adipocyte 3-O-methyl glucose transport in Type II diabetes mellitus. J. Clin. Endocrinol. Metab. 56:1195-1201.

48. Foley, J.E., Kashiwagi, A., Verso, M.A., Reaven, G., and Andrews, J. (1983). Improvement in in vitro insulin action after one month of insulin therapy in obvese non insulin-dependent diabetes. J. Clin. Invest. 72:1901-1909.

49. Garvey, W.T., Olefsky, J.M., Griffin, J., Hamman, R.F., and Kolterman, O.G. (1985). The effect of insulin treatment on insulin secretion and insulin actionin Type II diabetes mellitus. Diabetes 34:222-234.

50. Scarlett, J.A., Gray, R.S., Griffin, J., Olefsky, J.M., and Kolterman, O.G. (1982). Insulin treatment reverses the insulin resistance of Type II diabetes mellitus. Diabetes Care 5:353-363.

51. Andrews, W.J., Vasquez, B., Nagulesparan, M., Klimes, I., Foley, J.E., and Unger, R. (1984). Insulin therapy in obese NIDDM induces improvements in insulin action and secretion that are maintained for two weeks after insulin withdrawal. Diabetes 33:634-642.

52. Hjollund E., Pederson, O., Richelsen, B., Beck-Nielsen, H., and Schwartz, S.N. (1985). Glucose transport and metabolism in adipocytes from newly diagnosed untreated insulin-dependent diabetics: severly impaired basal and post insulin binding activities. J. Clin. Invest. 76:2091-2096.

53. Kobayashi, M., Olefsky, J.M. (1979). Effects of streptozotocin-induced diabetes on insulin binding, glucose transport, and intracellular glucose metabolism in isolated rat adipocytes. Diabetes 28:87-95.

54. Karnieli, E., Hissin, P.J., Simpson, I.A., Salans, L.B., and Cushman, .W. (1981). A possible mechanism of insulin resistance in the rat

adipose cell in streptozotozin-induced diabetes mellitus. Depletion of intracellular glucose transport systems. J. Clin. Invest. 68:811-814.

55. Hissin, P.J., Karnieli, E., Simpson, I.A., Salans, L.B., and Cushman, S.W. (1982). A possible mechanism of insulin resistance in the rat adipose cell with high fat/low carbohydrate feeding. Depletion of intracellular glucose transport systems. Diabetes 31:589-592.

56. Kahn, B.B., and Cushman, S.W. (1984). Effects of fasting and refeeding on the distribution of glucose transporters in isolated rat adipocytes. Diabetes 33(Suppl. 1):71A (abstr).

57. Garvey, W.T., Huecksteadt, T.P., and Olefsky, J.M. (1987). Role of glucose transport proteins in the insulin resistance of Type II diabetes mellitus. Clin. Res. 35:105A.

58. Armoni, M., Rafaeloff, R., Kanter, Y., Moscona, R., and Karnieli, E. (1987). The distribution of glucose transporters in NIDDM. Endocrinology 120:(abstr).

59. Karnieli, E., Lima, F.B., and Huecksteadt, T. (1987). The impact of diabetes on the intrinsic activity of glucose transporters. Diabetes 36:(Suppl 1) (abstr).

60. Hissin, P.J., Foley, J.e., Wardzala, L.J., Karnieli, E., Simpson, I.A., Salans, L.B., and Cushman, S.W. (1982). Mechanism of insulin-resistant glucose transport activity in the enlarged adipose cell of the aged obese rat. Relative depletion of intracellular glucsoe transport systems. J. Clin. Invest. 70:780-790.

61. Dean, B., Peluso, I., and Harrison, L.C. (1984). A post-binding inhibitor of insulin action: increased concentrations in the plasma of non-insulin dependent diabetic subjects. Diabetes 33:450-454.

62. Reaven, G.M., Sageman, W.S., Swenson, R.S. (1977). Developoment of insulin resistance in normal dogs following alloxan-induced insulin deficiency. Diabetologia 13:459-462.

63. Garvey, W.T., Olefsky, J.M., and Marshall, S. (1986). Insulin induces progressive insulin resistance in cultured rat adipocytes: Sequential effects at receptor and multiple postreceptor sites. Diabetes 35:258-267.

64. Garvey, W.T., Olefsky, J.M., Matthaei, S., and Marshall, S. (1987). Glucose and insulin co-regulate the transport system in primary cultured adipocytes: A new mechanism of insulin resistance. J. Biol. Chem. 262:189-197.

65. Van-Putten, J.P.M., and Krans, H.M.J. (1985). Glucose as a regulator of insulin-stimulated hexose transport in 3T3 adipocytes. J. Biol. Chem. 260:7996-8001.

66. Yamada, K., Tilloston, L.G., and Isselbacher, K.J. (1985). Regulation of hexose carriers in chick embrio fibroblasts: effects of glucose starvation and role of protein synthesis. J. Biol. Chem. 258:9786-9792.

67. Sasson, S., and Cerase, E. (1986). Substrate regulation of the glucose transport system in rat skeletal muscle: characterization and kinetic analysis in isolated soleus muscle and skeletal muscle cells in culture. J. Biol. Chem. 261:16827-16833.

68. Carter-Su, C., and Okamoto, K. (1985). Effect of glucocorticoids on hexose transport in rat adipocytes: evidence for decreased transporters in the plasma membrane. J. Biol. Chem. 260:11091-11098.

69. Zuber, M.X., Wang, S.M., Thammavaram, K.V., Reed, D.K., and Reed, B.C. (1985). Elevation of the number of cell-surface insulin receptors and the rate of 2-deoxyglucose uptake by exposure of 3T3-L1 adipocytes to tolbutamide. J. Biol. Chem. 260:14045-14052.

70. Jacobs, d.B., and Jung, C.Y. (1985). Sulfonylurea potentiates insulin-induced recruitment of glucose transport carrier in rat adipocytes. J. Biol. Chem. 260:2593-2596.

71. Wang, P.H., Beguinot, F., and Smith, R.J. (1986). Sulfonylurea effects in cultured skeletal muscle cells: Augmentation of insulin and insulin-like growth factor I and II action. Diabetes 35(Suppl. 1):53A (Abstr).

72. Scheinberg, F.P. (1965). Observation on cerebral carbohydrate metabolism in man. Ann. Int. Med. 62:367-371.

73. Owen, O.E., Morgan, A.P., Kemp, H.G., Sullinva, J.M., Herrera, M.G., and Cahill, G.F. (1967). Brain metabolism during fasting. J. Clin. Invest. 46:1589-1595.

74. Elbrink, J., and Bihler, I. (1975). Membrane transport: its relationship to cellular metabolic rates. Science 188:1177-1184.

75. Broman, T. (1941). The possibilities of the passage of substances from the blood to the central nervous system. (Is there a blood-brain barrier and a blood-cerebrospinal fluid barrier?). Acta Psychiatr. Neurol. 16:1-25.

76. Brightman, M.W., and Reese, T.S. (1969). Functions between intemately apposed cell membranes in the vertebrate brain. J. Cell. Biol. 40:648-677.

77. Crone, C. (1965). Facilitated transfer of glucose from blood into brain tissue. J. Physiol. London 181:103-113.

78. Lund-Andersen, H. (1979). Transport of glucose from blood to brain. Physiol. Rev. 59:305-352.

79. Gjedde, A. (1983). Modulation of substrate transport to the brain. Acta Neurol. Scand. 67:3-25.

80. Pardridge, W.M. (1983). Brain metabolism: a perspective from the blood-brain barrier. Physiol Rev. 63:1481-1535.

81. Rafaelsen, O.J. (1961). Action of insulin on glucsoe uptake of rat brain slices and isolated rat cerebellium. J. Neurochem. 7:45-51.

82. Buschiazzo, P.M., Terrell, E.B., and Regen, D.M. (1970). Sugar transport across the blood-brain barrier. Am. J. Physiol. 219:1505-1513.

83. Betz, A.L., Gillse, D.D., Yudilevich, D.L., and Drewes, L.R. (1973). Kinetics of unidirectional glucose transport into the isolated dog brain. Am. J. Physiol. 225:586-592

84. Goodner, C.J. and Berrie, M.A. (1977). The failure of rat hypothalamic tissue to take up labelled insulin in vivo or to respond to insulin in vitro. Endocrinol. 101:605-612.

85. Hom, F.G., Goodner, C.J. and Berrie, M.A. (1984). A (^{3}H)2-deoxyglucose method for comparing rates of glucose metabolism and insulin responses among rat tissues in vivo. Diabetes 33:141-152.

86. Gorus, F.K., Hooghe-Peters, E.L., and Pipeleers, D.G. (1984). Glucose metabolism in murine fetal cortical brain cells: lack of insulin effects. J. Cell. Physiol. 121:45-50.

87. Brooks, D.J., Gibbs, J.S.R., Sharp, P., Herold, S., Turton, D.R., Luthra, S.K., Kohner, E.M., Bloom, S.R., and Jones, T. (1986). Regional cerebral glucose transport in insulin-dependent diabetic patients sutided using [^{11}C]3-O-methyl-D-glucose and positron emission tomography. J. Cereb. Blood Flow Metab. 6:240-244.

88. Goldstein, G.W., Csejtey, J. and Diamond, I. (1977). Carrier mediated glucose transport in capillaries isolated from rat brain. J. Neurochem. 28:725-728.

89. Betz, A.L., Csejtey, J. and Goldstein, G.W. (1979). Hexose transport and phosphorylation by capillaries isolated from rat brain. Am. J. Physiol. 236:C96-C102.

90. Matthaei, S., Olefsky, J.M., Garvey, W.T., and Horuk, R. (1987). Biochemical characterization and subcellular distribution of the glucose transporter from rat brain microvessels. Biochem. J., In press.

91. Havrankova, J., Roth, J., and Brownstein, M. (1978). Insulin receptors are widely distributed in the central nervous system of the rat. Nature (Lond) 272:827-829.

92. Havrankova, J., Schmechel, D., Roth, J. and Brownstein, M. (1978). Identification of insulin in the brain. Proc. Natl. Acad. Sci USA 75:5737-5741.

93. Haugaard, N., Vaughan, M., Haugaard, E.S., and Stadie, W.C. (1954). Studies of radioactive injected labeled insulin. J. Biol. Chem. 208:549-563.

94. Margoles, R.V. and Altszuler, N. (1967). Insulin in the cerebrospinal fluid. Nature (Lond) 215:1375-1376.

95. Sloviter, H.A. and Yamada, H. (1971). Absence of direct action of insulin on metabolism of the isolated perfused rat brain. J. Neurochem. 18:1269-1274.

96. Woods, S.C. and Porte, D. (1977). Relationship between plasma and cerebrospinal fluid insulin levels of dogs. Am. J. Physiol. 233:E331-E334.

97. Nelson, S.R., Schultz, D.W., Passonneau, J.V., and Lowry, O.H. (1968). control of glycogen levels in the brain. J. Neurochem. 15:1271-1279.

98. Mellerup, E.T., and Rafaelsen, O.J. (1969). Brain glycogen after ntracisternal insulin injection. J. Neurochem. 16:777-781.

99. Prasannan, K.B. (1972). Effect of insulin on glucose metabolism in cerebral cortex slices under aerolic and anaerobic conditions. J. Neurochem. 19:1825-1828.

100. Daniel, P.M., Love, E.R. and Pratt, O.E. (1975). Insulin and the way the brain handles glucose. J. Neurochem. 25:471-476.

101. Daniel, P.M., Love, E.R. and Pratt, O.E. (1977). The influence of insulin upon the metabolism of glucose by the brain. Proc. R. Soc. London Ser. B. 196:85-104.

102. Pillion, D.J., Haskell, J.F., and Meegan, E. (1982). Cerebral cortical microvessels: an insulin-sensitive tissue. Biochem. Biophys. Res. Commun. 104:686-692.

103. Clarke, D.W., Boyd, F.T., Kappy, M.S., and Raizada, M.K. (1984). Insulin binds to specific receptors and stimulates 2-deoxy-D-glucose uptake in cultured glial cells from rat brain. J. Biol. Chem. 259:11672-11675.

104. Phillips, M.E. and Coxon, R.V. (1976). Effect of insulin and phenobarbitol on the uptake of 2-deoxyglucose by brain slices and hemidiaphragms. J. Neurochem. 27:643-645.

105. Gottstein, V. (1975). The effect of insulin on cerebral glucose uptake in normal and diabetic human subjects. In Brain Work. D.H. Ingvar and N.A. Lassen, Editors. Munksgaard, Copenhagen.

106. Hertz, M.M., Paulson, O.B., Barry, d.I., Christiansen, J.S., and Svendsen, P.A. (1981). Insulin increases glucose transfer across the blood-brain barrier in man. J. Clin. Invest. 67:597-604.

107. Lund-Andersen, H. and Kjeldsen, C.S. (1977). Uptake of glucose analogues by rat brain cortex slices: membrane transport versus metabolism of 2-deoxy-D-glucose. J. Neurochem. 29:205-211.

108. Heidenreich, K.A., Gilmore, P.R., and Garvey, W.T. (1987). Insulin receptors and glucose transport in primary neuronal cultures. Diabetes 36(Suppl. 1):abstract.

109. White, M.K., Bramwell, M.E. and Harris, H. (1981). Hexose transport in hybrids between malignant and normal cells. Nature 294:232-235.

110. Diamond, I. and Fishman, R.A. (1973). High affinity transport and phosphorylation of 2-deoxy-D-glucose in synaptosomes. J. Neurochem. 20:1533-1542.

111. Heaton, G.M. and Bachelard, H.S. (1973). The kinetic properties of hexose transport into synaptosomes from guinea pig cerebral cortex. J. Neurochem. 21:1099-1108.

112. Heidenreich, K.A., Zahniser, N.R., Berhanu, P., Brandenburg, D., and Olefsky, J.M. (1984). Structural differences between insulin receptors in the brain and peripheral target tisues. J. Biol. Chem. 258:8527-8530.

113. Gammeltoft, S., Staun-Olsen, P., Ottensen, B., and Fahrenbrug, J. (1984). Insulin receptors in rat brain cortex. Kinetic evidence for a receptor subtype in central nervous system. Peptides 5:937-944

114. Bergman, R.N. (1977). Integrated control of hepatic glucose metabolism. Fed. Proc. Fed. Am. Soc. Exp. Biol. 36:265-270.

115. Williams, T.F., Exton, J.H., Park, C.R., and Regen, D.M. (1968). Stereospecific transport of glucose in the perfused rat liver. Am. J. Physiol. 215:1200-1209.

116. Baur, H., and Heldt, H.W. (1977). Transport of hexoses across the liver-cell membrane. Eur. J. Biochem. 74:397-403.

117. Ciaraldi, T.P., Horuk, R., and Matthaei, S. (1986). Biochemical and functional characterization of the rat liver glucose-transport system. Biochem. J. 240:115-123.

118. Dick, A.P.K., Harik, S.I., Klip, A., and Walker, D.M. (1984). Indentification and characterization of the glucose transporter of the blood-brain barrier by cytochalasin B binding and immunological reactivity. Proc. Natl. acad. Sci. USA 81:7233-7237.

119. Gjedde, A. and Crone, C. (1981). Blood-brain glucose transfer: repression in chronic hyperglycemia. Science 214:456-457.

120. McCall, A.L., Millington, W.R., and Wurtman, R.J. (1982). Metabolic fuel and amino acid transport into the brain in experimental diabetes mellitus. Proc. Natl. Acad. Sci. USA 79:5406-5410.

121. McCall, A.L., Gould, J.B. and Ruderman, N.b. (1984). Diabetes-induced alterations of glucose metaoblism in at cerebral microvessels. Am. J. Physiol. 247:E462-E467.

122. Matthaei, S., Horuk, R., and Olefsky, J.M. (1986). Blood-brain glucose transfer in diabetes mellitus: decreased number of glucose transporters at blood-brain barrier. Diabetes 35:1181-1184

ALTERATION OF INSULIN RECEPTOR BINDING AND PROTEIN KINASE ACTIVITY IN RAT LIVER AND PLACENTA BY ß-NAPHTHOFLAVONE

Shoou-Lih Wang, Mohan K. Raizada and Kathleen T. Shiverick

Department of Pharmacology & Experimental Therapeutics and Department of Physiology
University of Florida
Gainesville, FL 32610

INTRODUCTION

Insulin has been shown to be a significant fetal growth factor during late gestation.[1,2] The development of insulin receptors in a number of fetal tissues is characterized by an increase in binding activity with gestational age.[3-6] Human placenta is a rich source of insulin receptor which has been extensively characterized for its physico-chemical and protein kinase properties.[7] Exposure to polyaromatic compounds during pregnancy has been associated with low birth weight in rodents,[8,9] monkeys[10] and humans.[11] This laboratory has found that late feto-placental growth was markedly impaired after the administration of ß-naphthoflavone (ßNF) and other polyaromatic compounds during mid-gestation.[9] Recent evidence suggests an interaction of polyaromatic compounds with growth factor receptors. In human pregnancy, exposure to halogenated aromatic compounds and cigarette smoke has been associated with a decrease in EGF receptor protein kinase activity in the placenta.[12] TCDD (2,3,7,8-tetrachlorodibenzo-p-dioxin) administered to newborn mice decreased EGF binding to liver plasma membranes, increased membrane protein kinase activities and elicited symptoms characteristic of excess EGF.[13,14] At present, little is known about the interaction of polyaromatic compounds with other growth factor receptors in development.

The objectives of this study were to characterize the insulin receptor in the rat placenta and to investigate whether the adverse effects of ßNF on feto-placental growth may be associated with alterations in placental insulin receptors.

MATERIALS AND METHODS

Chemicals

BSA fraction V, was purchased from U.S. Biochemical Co. (Cleveland, OH). Porcine insulin, chicken insulin, glucagon, PMSF, adenosine 5'-triphosphate, cytidine 5'-triphosphate, poly-(Glu_4,Tyr), N-acetyl-D-glucosamine, SDS-PAGE protein standard kit and ßNF were from Sigma Chemical Co. (St. Louis, MO). Human growth hormone was kindly supplied by NIH (Bethesda, MD). Relaxin was a gift from Dr. Michael Fields, Department of Dairy Science, University of Florida. Desoctapeptide insulin was from Eli Lilly Laboratory (Indianapolis, IN). Insulin-like growth factor-I (IGF-I) was purchased from Amgen Biological (Thousand oaks, CA). ßNF was recrystallized from ethanol. Chemicals for SDS-PAGE were purchased from Bio-Rad (Hempstead, NY). Agarose-bound wheat germ agglutinin was obtained from Vector Laboratories, Inc. (Burlingame, CA). [^{125}I]-Human insulin labelled at tyrosine B-26 (specific activity 2000 Ci/mmole) and [γ-^{32}P]-ATP (specific activity 3,000 Ci/mmole) were purchased from Amersham Co. (Arlington Heights, IL).

Animals

Pregnant rats were purchased from Holtzman Co. (Madison, WI) and housed in wire cages on a 12-hr light cycle. Day 0 of gestation was designated as the day on which sperm was detected in the vaginal smear. ßNF was administered 15 mg/kg i.p. in corn oil to pregnant rats on gestation days 10 or 17.

[^{125}I]-Insulin Binding

Microsomal membranes of placental tissue, fetal and maternal liver were prepared by differential centrifugation as described by Pilistine et al.[15] Protein concentration of microsomal membrane was measured by the method of Lowry et al.[16] with BSA as a standard.

Microsomal membranes (250 µg protein) were incubated in triplicate with [^{125}I]-insulin (40,000 cpm, 0.05 nM), and 0.1 M sodium phosphate buffer, pH 7.5 containing 1.0% BSA (w/v) (buffer A) in a final reaction volume of 200 µl for 30 min at 25°C for the measurement of total binding. Nonspecific binding was determined in the presence of 2.5 µM unlabelled porcine insulin. The reaction was terminated by addition of 0.5 ml of ice-cold buffer A. Membrane-bound [^{125}I]-insulin was separated immediately by centrifugation at 10,000xg for 3 min in an Eppendorf microcentrifuge followed by aspiration of the supernatant; the pellet was washed with another 0.5 ml of ice-cold buffer A, recentrifuged for 1 min and the supernatant was aspirated. The resultant pellets were counted in a Beckman Gamma 5500 counter. Specific binding was obtained by subtracting the radioactivity of nonspecific binding from total binding and expressed as a ratio of the specific binding vs unbound [^{125}I]-insulin (bound/free or B/F).

[^{125}I]-Insulin degradation was tested frequently during the course of experiments by a trichloroacetate precipitation method.[17] The extent of degradation was used to correct the total radioactivity added in the reaction mixture. Scatchard analysis was performed as described in the standard assay except that 0 to 10 µM unlabelled insulin was added to the incubation mixture.[18]

Cross-linking of [^{125}I]-Insulin to Insulin Receptors

The method of Czech et al.[19] was used for covalent binding of [^{125}I]-insulin to membrane receptor using 0.5-5.0 mM disuccinimidyl suberate (DSS) as the cross-linking agent. Briefly, the insulin binding reaction was performed as follows: 2.0 mg placental membrane protein on gestation day 11, 19 or liver membrane protein was incubated with [^{125}I]-insulin (750,000 cpm, 0.2 nM), and buffer A in a total volume of 1.0 ml for 30 min at 25°C. Nonspecific binding was conducted similarly except 2.5 µM unlabelled porcine insulin was added to the reaction mixture. The reaction was terminated by adding 3.0 ml of cold buffer A. [^{125}I]-Insulin bound protein was separated immediately by centrifugation at 35,000xg for 20 min, the pellet was washed with 3.0 ml cold buffer A and recentrifuged. The resultant pellet was resuspended in 1.0 ml buffer A and then incubated with 2.5 mM DSS dissolved in 1.0 µl of DMSO at 4°C for 15 min. The reaction mixture was quenched by adding 2.5 ml of 0.5 mM Tris-HCl, containing 1 mM EDTA, pH 7.4, centrifuged at 35,000xg for 20 min and washed with 2.5 ml of 5 mM Tris-HCl and 1 mM EDTA, pH 7.4 and recentrifuged for two times. The pellet was saved for SDS-PAGE. A parallel test of dissociation of bound [^{125}I]-insulin from its receptor was performed before and after cross-linking experiments to assure the linkage between [^{125}I]-insulin and insulin receptor. The washed pellet was resuspended to proper volume of buffer A containing 2.5 µM of unlabelled insulin. Aliquots of resuspended sample were removed at different time periods, centrifuged, supernatant aspirated and the resultant pellets were counted.

Wheat Germ Agglutinin Chromatography

Insulin receptors were purified from placenta and liver membranes by wheat germ agglutinin (WGA) chromatography.[6,20]. Microsomal membranes were solubilized in 50 mM HEPES, 10 mM $MgSO_4$, 1 mM PMSF and 1% Triton X-100, pH 7.6. The solubilized proteins (20-30 mg) were recycled three times over a column containing 3.5 ml agarose bound wheat germ agglutinin at 4°C. The column was washed with 40 ml washing buffer (50 mM HEPES, 150 mM NaCl and 0.1% Triton X-100, pH 7.6) and the receptors were eluted from the column with 10 ml of the same buffer containing 0.3 M N-acetyl-D-glucosamine and collected 2.0 ml per fraction. The eluates were monitored for protein concentration and ones with highest absorbance at 280 nm were combined and protein concentration was determined using the Bio-Rad microassay (Manual of Bio-Rad Protein Kit).

Insulin Receptor Phosphorylation

Insulin receptor phosphorylation was performed by a modification of the method of Lowe et al.[6] Lectin-purified receptor preparations (100 µl containing 12 µg protein) were preincubated in the absence or presence of 1.0 µM porcine insulin in a final volume of 150 µl 50 mM HEPES buffer, pH 7.6 with 2 mM PMSF. After 30 min at 22°C, phosphorylation was initiated by the addition of 50 µl reaction mixture to give final concentrations of 5 µM [^{32}P]ATP (specific activity 20 µCi/nmole), 1 mM cytidine-5-triphosphate, 3 mM $MnCl_2$, 20 mM $MgCl_2$ and 1 mM sodium vanadate. After 10 min at 22°C, the reaction was terminated by the addition of an equal volume of stopping solution (0.17 M Tris-HCl, 10% SDS and 100 mM dithiothreitol, pH 6.8) and heating at 100°C for 10 min. Aliquots (120 µl) were analyzed by 7.5% SDS-PAGE followed by autoradiography. The intensity of [^{32}P]-labelled protein bands shown on X-ray film was quantitated by Soft-Laser densitometer, model SF-TRFF (Biomed Instrument, Inc., Fullerton, CA).

RESULTS

Characterization of [^{125}I]-Insulin Binding to Placenta, Maternal and Fetal Liver

The specific binding of [^{125}I]-insulin to membranes prepared from placenta, maternal and fetal liver increased linearly with protein concentrations of 0.2 to 1 mg over a 30 min time period at 25°C. Data in Fig. 1 show that values of % B/F in placenta were lower than maternal or fetal liver. Specific binding of insulin to membrane preparations from placenta and maternal liver decreased progressively from mid to late gestation, with binding on day 18 only 50% of that observed on day

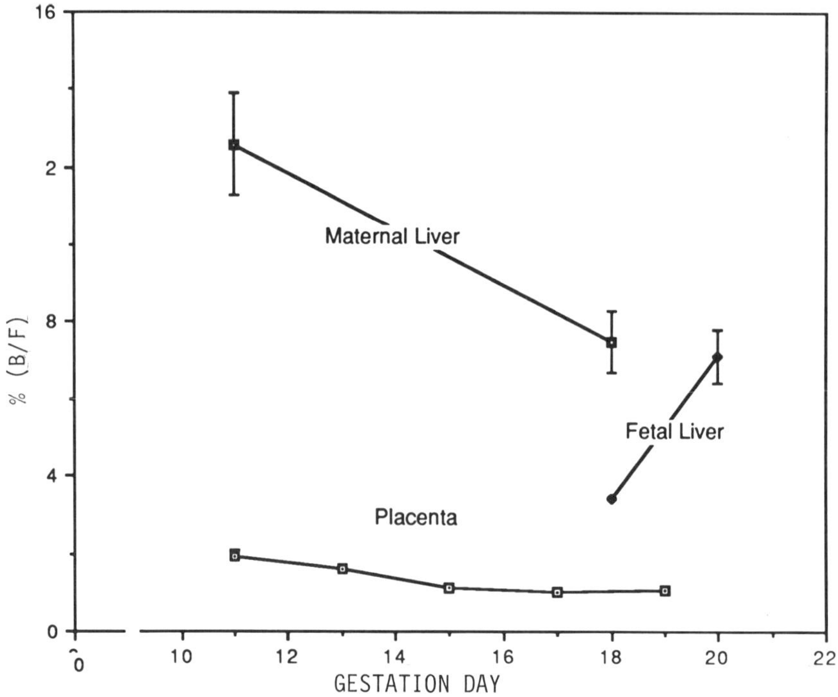

Fig. 1. Specific binding of insulin to membrane preparations from rat placenta, maternal and fetal liver during gestation.

11. In contrast, binding to fetal liver increased 2-fold from gestation day 18 to 20. In placental membranes, unlabelled porcine and chicken insulin showed typical displacement curves (IC_{50}, 65 nM) for competition with [^{125}I]-insulin, while IGF-1 was much less potent with an IC_{50} of 2.12 mM (Fig. 2). In data not shown, growth hormone, glucagon, relaxin and desoctapeptide insulin had no inhibitory effect on tracer binding. Scatchard analysis of specific binding to membranes from maternal liver and placenta demonstrated curvilinear plots (Fig. 3). Estimates of high affinity binding from the linear first portion of the Scatchard plots indicate that dissociation constants (K_d) were similar for placental and liver membranes, while the number of binding sites was substantially greater for liver. In data not shown, Scatchard analysis of binding to placenta membranes on gestation days 11 and 18 showed that K_d values were similar, while the number of binding sites was 50% greater on day 11 placenta.

In separate experiments, receptors in placenta and maternal liver membranes were covalently cross-linked with DSS. Radiolabeled proteins were solubilized and detected by SDS-PAGE and autoradiography (Fig. 4). A single radioactive band with M_r 130,000 was observed in membranes from liver (Lane E) as well as placentas on gestation days 11 (Lane A) and 18 (Lane C). The greater intensity of the radioactive band from placenta on day 11 compared with day 18 is consistent with a higher number of binding sites at midgestation.

Effects of ß-Naphthoflavone on Feto-placental Growth

In initial experiments ßNF was administered to pregnant rats on days 9-14. During this treatment period, there was no evidence of an adverse effect of ßNF on maternal weight gain, fetal resorption rate, fetal body weight or placental weight.

Study of animals on day 20 of gestation, however, showed 25-35% reductions in fetal and placental weights in ßNF-treated litters (Table 1). Thus late feto-placental growth was impaired significantly after ßNF administration during mid-gestation.

Table 1. Effects of ß-Naphthoflavone on Feto-Placental Growth

	Placenta Wt. g	Fetal Wt. g
Control (4)	0.67±.03	3.94±.02
ßNF (7)	0.44±.02*	3.00±.09*

Pregnant rats received ßNF (15 mg/kg) on gestation days 9-14 or corn oil vehicle. Animals were studied on day 20. Data are expressed as the mean ± SE of (N) number of dams. Placenta and fetal weights are expressed as the average weight per litter.

* $p < 0.05$.

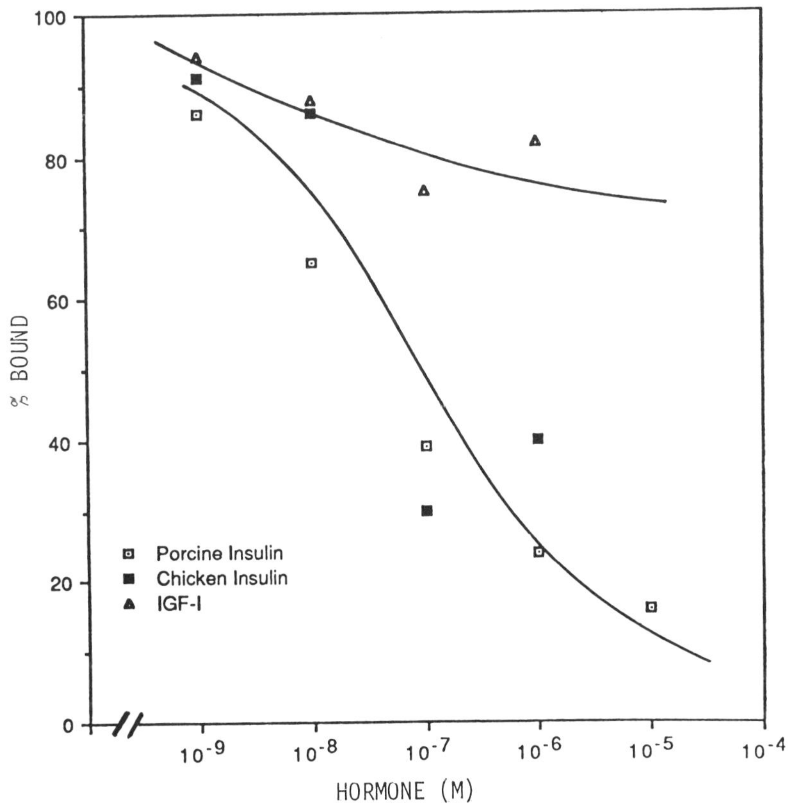

Fig. 2. Specificity of [^{125}I] insulin binding to membrane preparations from rat placenta.

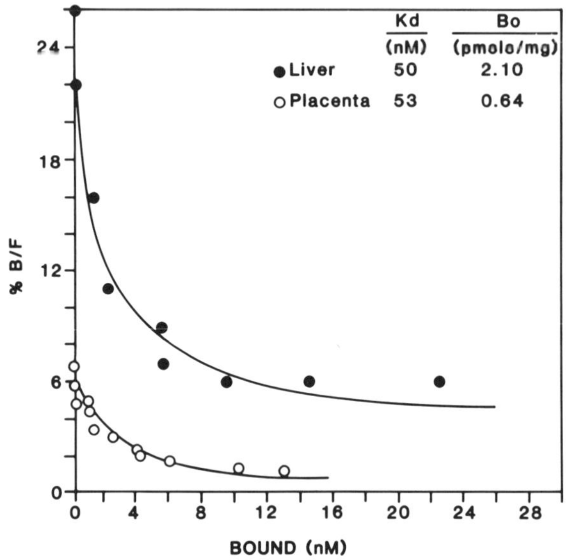

Fig. 3. Scatchard plots of [^{125}I]-insulin binding to membranes of rat placenta and maternal liver.

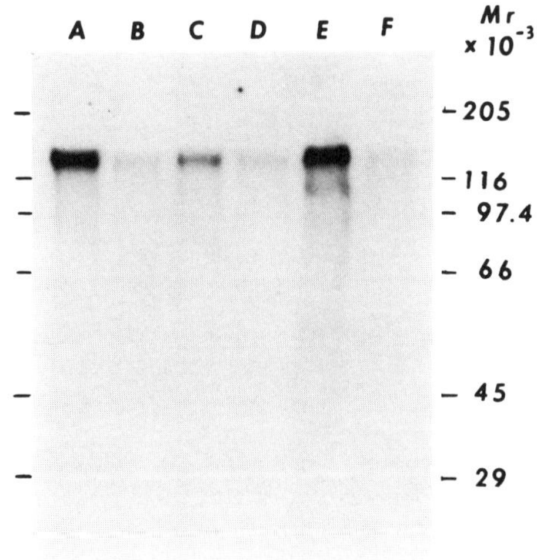

Fig. 4. Autoradiogram of SDS-PA gel which characterizes the insulin receptor subunit covalently cross-linked with [^{125}I]-insulin.

Effects of ßNF on Insulin Binding

Data in Fig. 5 compare the effects of a single dose of ßNF on insulin binding to membranes prepared from maternal liver (A) and placenta (B). Tissues were studied 24 hr after the administration of ßNF at mid (day 11) and late (day 18) gestation. Insulin binding to maternal liver preparations was decreased 45% on day 18 following ßNF treatment, while binding on day 11 was not different from control. In placental preparations, however, insulin binding was decreased 40% in membranes prepared from both day 11 and 18 placentas. For comparison with these tissues, fetal liver showed no effect of ßNF treatment on insulin binding on day 18 of gestation.

Insulin Receptor Autophosphorylation

Membrane receptors from placenta and maternal liver were solubilized and partially purified by WGA affinity chromatography for study of intrinsic protein kinase activity. Insulin stimulated the phosphorylation of a M_r 95K protein in receptor preparations from maternal liver and no significant gestational difference was observed between days 11 and 18 (Fig. 6). Densitometric scans of autoradiograms to quantitate autophosphorylation indicated that ßNF treatment did not markedly alter the extent of phosphorylation of the 95K ß-subunit of the liver receptor. However, insulin stimulated the phosphorylation of an additional 90K protein band in liver membrane proteins from ßNF-treated animals.

A comparison of autophosphorylation in placental membrane proteins from days 11 and 18 shows a major gestational difference in protein kinase activity (Fig. 7). Insulin actively stimulated the phosphorylation of a 95K protein band in day 11 placental preparations, while no autophosphorylation was observed in day 18 membrane proteins. Data in Fig. 7 also show the effects of ßNF treatment on autophosphorylation of the placental insulin receptor. Following ßNF treatment, the intensity of the 95K protein band was decreased 40% from control in preparations from day 11 placenta, while no change was observed in the profile of phosphorylated proteins. For day 19 membrane proteins, however, the absence of protein kinase activity made it impossible to detect changes associated with ßNF treatment.

DISCUSSION

While the insulin receptor of rat liver has been well characterized, little is known about the nature of the insulin receptor in rat placenta. The present study characterized the ontogeny of the insulin receptor in rat hemochorial placenta in comparison with maternal liver during gestation. The binding of [^{125}I]-insulin to placental membranes was not due to its binding to IGF-I receptors since IGF-I competed for [^{125}I]-insulin binding with a potency of less than 0.001%. These data complement previous observations on rat placental IGF receptors which showed that insulin bound to the type I receptor with very low potency, and was not recognized by the type II receptor.[15] Although specific binding of insulin to rat placenta is low, evidence for insulin gene expression in the rat yolk sac during the second half of gestation suggests a role for insulin in placental function.[21] The receptor α- and ß-subunits were similar in rat liver and placenta and K_d values were similar for both tissues. The observation that specific binding of [^{125}I]-insulin to placenta and maternal liver membranes decreased from gestation day 11 to 18 suggests that pregnancy-related factors, probably hormonal, play a role in

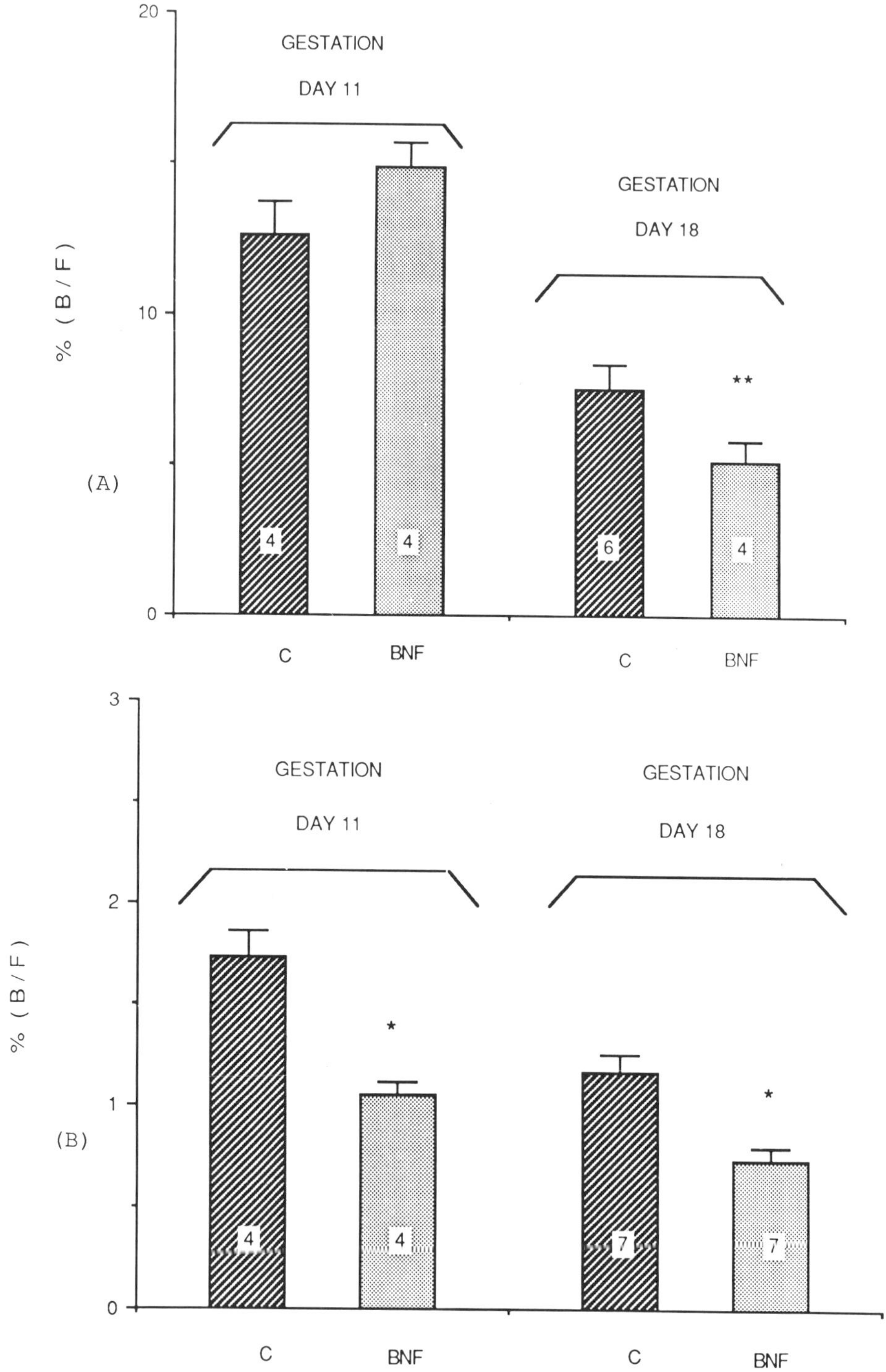

Fig. 5. Effects of ßNF on insulin binding to membrane preparations from rat maternal liver (A) placenta(B).

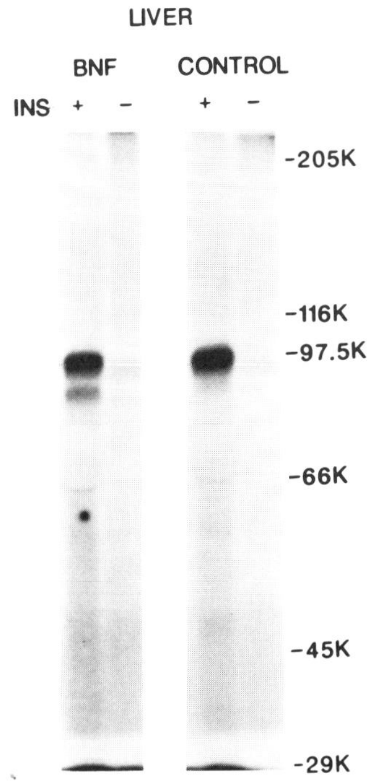

Fig. 6. Autoradiograms of SDS-PA gels for insulin stimulated phosphorylation of proteins in solubilized, lectin-purified preparations of maternal liver membrane (3.6 μg protein).

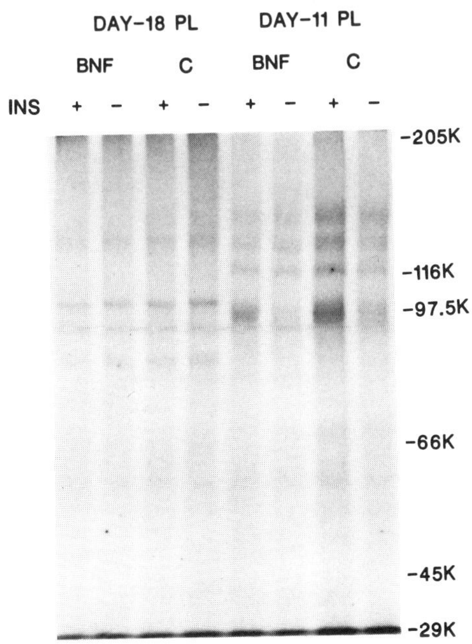

Fig. 7. Autoradiograms of SDS-PA gel for insulin stimulated phosphorylations of proteins in solubilized, lectin-purified preparations of placental membranes (3.6 μg protein).

regulation of the insulin receptor. A comparison of mid- and late-gestation placenta showed that protein kinase activity was far more extensive for receptor preparations from day 11 placenta, data which suggest that α- and ß-subunits are coupled and more functional during midgestation.

The acute administration of ßNF was associated with significantly decreased binding of [^{125}I]-insulin to membranes prepared from placenta on gestation days 11 and 18, as well as from maternal liver on day 18. The absence of an effect of ßNF on liver membrane binding on day 11 is unexplained, but further suggests the existence of gestation-dependent regulatory factors. Alterations in hepatic binding of insulin and EGF have been reported following acute exposure to the hepatocarcinogens 2-acetylaminofluorene[22,23] and diethylnitrosamine[24] which reflected an apparent decrease in the number of receptors. Although alterations in liver insulin receptors have been associated with chronic exposure to the tumor promoters TCDD[25] and phenobarbital,[26] it is difficult to distinguish receptor changes that are due to long-term alterations in growth state from direct chemical mediated events, including toxicity. In several cell lines, benzo(a)pyrene and other inducers of cytochrome P_1-450 have been reported to show acute inhibition of EGF receptor binding which was mediated by the aryl hydrocarbon (Ah) receptor.[27,28,29] While the dose of ßNF administered in the present study clearly induced Ah hydroxylase activity in maternal liver and placenta,[30] the absence of an alteration in insulin binding to liver membranes on day 11 gestation makes uncertain the relationship between Ah hydroxylase induction and decreased binding.

The presence of intrinsic tyrosine kinase activity in receptors for insulin, EGF and several other polypeptide growth factors has been proposed to represent a general mechanism in transmembrane signaling of hormones and growth factors.[31] In the present study, although ßNF administration did not alter autophosphorylation of the hepatic receptor ß-subunit, insulin-stimulated the phosphorylation of an additional 90K protein band in lectin-purified liver membrane preparations from ßNF-treated animals. Studies are in progress to determine whether this hepatic 90K protein is a ßNF-induced membrane protein or degraded insulin receptor. In this regard, previous studies with the hepatocarcinogen diethylnitrosamine have shown an acute, dose-dependent decrease in ligand binding and autophosphorylation of both EGF and insulin receptors in liver membranes.[24] In our studies of placental insulin receptor, ßNF administration was associated with significantly decreased ligand binding and decreased autophosphorylation in midgestation. At the same timé, the absence of autophosphorylation in purified membrane preparations from day 18 placenta raises questions as to the functional significance of a decrease in ligand binding during late gestation following ßNF treatment. Study of EGF receptors in term human placenta, however, have reported that exposure to cigarette smoke and halogenated aromatic compounds was associated with biochemical alterations in protein kinase activity, with little or no change in ligand binding.[12] A dissociation between insulin binding and receptor kinase has been reported in skeletal muscle,[32] streptozotocin induced diabetes[33] and obese insulin resistant mice.[34]

Although the mechanisms which underlie these xenobiotic-related changes are not understood, short-term alterations in receptor number may involve receptor internalization, degradation or synthesis.[35] In addition, recent evidence for resistance to insulin action through altered receptor kinase activity, termed desensitization, provides a potential mechanism for post-binding receptor defects.[33,34,36] In vitro studies with purified receptors further suggest the modulation of protein kinase activity through interaction with protein kinase C,[37] src kinase[38] and calmodulin.[39] In this regard, an acute effect of TCDD has been reported to be stimulation of protein kinase activities, particularly kinase C in hepatic membranes.[14] Thus complex interactions among multiple signalling systems may result in synergistic or antagonistic actions. Experiments are in progress to characterize the biochemical mechanisms which underline ßNF-related changes in insulin receptor binding and protein kinase activity.

ACKNOWLEDGEMENTS

The authors are indebted to Theresa Medrano for expert technical assistance and Mrs. Judy Adams for manuscript preparation. Mohan K. Raizada is an Established Investigator of the American Heart Association.

REFERENCES

1. J. B.Susa, K. L. McCormick, J. L. Widness, D. B. Singer, W. H. Oh, K. Adamsons, and R. Schwartz, Chronic hyperinsulinemia in the fetal rhesus monkey: effects on fetal growth and composition, Diabetes, 28:1058 (1979).

2. J. M. Fletcher, J. Falconer, and J. M. Bassett, The relationship of body and placental weight to plasma levels of insulin and other hormones during development in fetal rabbits, Diabetologia 23:124 (1982).

3. A. V. Thorsson and R. L. Hintz, Insulin receptor in the newborn, increase in receptor affinity and number, New England J. Medicine 297:908 (1977).

4. A. Sandra and R. J. Przybylski, Ontogeny of insulin binding during chick skeletal myogenesis in vitro, Developmental Biology 68:546 (1979).

5. N. D. Neufeld, M. Scoll, and J. A. Kaplan, Ontogeny of the mammalian insulin receptor. Studies of human and rat fetal liver plasma membranes, Developmental Biology 78:151 (1980).

6. W. L. Lowe, F. T. Boyd, D. W. Clarke, M. K. Raizada, C. Hart, and D. Leroith, Development of brain insulin receptors: Structural and functional studies of insulin receptors from whole brain and primary cell cultures, Endocrinology 119:25 (1986).

7. T. W.Siegel, S. Ganguly, S. Jacobs, O. M. Rosen, and C. S. Rubin, Purification and properties of the human placental insulin receptor, J. Biol. Chem. 256:9266 (1981).

8. S. Shum, S., N. M. Jensen, and D. W. Nebert, The murine Ah locus: In utero toxicity and teratogenesis associated with genetic differences in benzo(a)pyrene metabolism, Teratology 20:365 (1979).

9. K. T. Shiverick, E. Ortiz, C. Fuhrman-Lane, and P. Crowley, Effects of ß-naphthoflavone and 3-methylcholanthrene administered to pregnant rats on steroid

metabolism in the isolated basal zone of the placenta, J. Pharmacol. Exp. Therap. 210:761 (1984).

10. J. R. Allen and D. A. Barsotti, The effects of transplacental and mammary movements of PCBs on infant rhesus monkeys, Toxicology 6:331 (1976).

11. T. K. Wong, R. B. Everson, and S. T. Hsu, Potent induction of human placental monooxygenase activity by previous dietary exposure to polychlorinated biphenyls and their thermal degradation products, Lancet 1:721 (1985).

12. G. I. Sunahara, T. Tiernan, R. M. Philpot, T. Wong, R. B. Everson, K. G. Nelson, and G. W. Lucier, Placental markers of exposure to toxic halogenated aromatics and cigarette smoke, Environmental Health Perspectives, in press (1987).

13. B. V. Madhukar, D. W. Brester, and F. Matsumura, Effects of in vivo administered 2,3,7,8-tetrachlorodibenzo-p-dioxin on receptor binding of epidermal growth factor in the hepatic plasma membrane of rat, guinea pig, mouse and hamster, Proc. Nat. Acad. Sci. 81:7407 (1984).

14. D. W. Bombick, B. V. Madhukar, D. W. Brewster, and F. Matsumura, TCDD(2,3,7,8-tetrachlorodibenzo-p-dioxin) causes increases in protein kinases particularly protein kinase in the hepatic plasma membrane of the rat and the guinea pig, Biochem. Biophys. Res. Commun. 127:295 (1985).

15. S. J. Pilistine, A. C. Moses, and H. N. Munro, Insulin-like growth factor receptors in rat placenta membranes, Endocrinol. 115:1060 (1984)

16. O. H. Lowry, N. J. Rosebrough, A. L. Farr, and R. J. Randall, Protein measurement with the Folin phenol reagent, J. Biol. Chem. 193:265 (1951).

17. N. Freinkel, and C. J. Goodner, Carbohydrate metabolism in pregnancy. In: The metabolism of insulin by human placental tissue, J. Clin. Invest. 39:116 (1960).

18. G. Scatchard, Attraction of proteins for small molecules and ions, Ann. N.Y. Acad. Sci. 51:660 (1949).

19. M. P. Czech, J. Massague, and P. F. Pilch, The insulin receptor: structural features, Trends Biochem. Sci. 6:222 (1981).

20. J. A. Hedo, L. C. Harrison, and J. Roth, Binding of insulin receptors to lectins: Evidence for common carbohydrate determinants on several membrane receptors, Biochem. 20:3385 (1981).

21. L. Muglia and J. Locker, Extrapancreatic insulin gene expression in the fetal rat, Proc. Natl. Acad. Sci. USA 81:3635 (1984).

22. Z. Josefsberg, B. I. Carr, D. Hwang, G. Barseghian, C. Tomkinson, and A. Lev-Ran, Effect of 2-acetylaminofluorene on the binding of epidermal growth factor to microsomal and golgi fractions of rat liver cells, Cancer Res. 44:2754 (1984).

23. A. Lev-Ran, Z. Josefsberg, B. I. Carr, G. Barseghian, and D. Hwang, Effects of the hepato- carcinogen 2-acetylaminofluorene on insulin binding to microsomal and golgi fractions of rat liver cells, J. Natl. Cancer Inst. 73:505 (1984).

24. B. I. Carr, A. Roitman, D. L. Hwang, G. Barseghian, and A. Lev-Ran, Effects of diethylnitrosamine on hepatic receptor binding and autophosphorylation of epidermal growth factor and insulin in rats, J. Natl. Cancer Inst. 77:219 (1986).

25. F. Matsumura, D. W. Brewster, B. V. Madhukar, and D. W. Bombick, Alteration of rat hepatic plasma membrane functions by 2,3,7,8-tetrachlorodibenzo-p-dioxin, Arch. Environ. Contam. Toxicol. 13:509 (1984).

26. D. L. Hwang, A. Roitman, A. Lev-Ran, and B. I. Carr, Chronic treatment with phenobarbital decreases the expression of rat liver EGF and insulin receptors, Biochem. Biophys. Res. Comm. 135:501, (1986).

27. V. Ivanovic and I. B. Weinstein, Benzo(a)pyrene and other inducers of cytochrome P_1-450 inhibit binding of epidermal growth factor to cell surface receptors, Carcinogenesis 3:505 (1982).

28. S. O. Karenlampi, H. J. Eisen, Q. Hankinson, and D. W. Nebert, Effects of cytochrome P_1-450 inducers on the cell-surface receptors for epidermal growth factor, insulin and phorbol 12,13-dibutyrate, J. Biol. Chem. 258:10378 (1973).

29. L. G. Hudson, W. A. Toscano, and W. F. Greenlee, Regulation of epidermal growth factor binding in a human keratinocyte cell line by 2,3,7,8-tetrachlorodibenzo-p-dioxin, Tox. Appl. Pharm. 77:251 (1985).

30. A. S. Salhab, M. O. James, S-L. Wang, and K. T. Shiverick, Positional metabolism of benzo(a)pyrene in rat placenta and maternal liver: comparison of induction effects, Drug. Metab. Disp. 14:471 (1986).

31. E. Van Obberghen and S. Gammelltoft, Insulin receptors: structure and function, Experientia 42:727 (1986).

32. D. E. James, A. Zorzano, M. Boni-Schnetzler, R. A. Nemenoff, A. Powers, P. F. Pilch, and N.B. Ruderman, Intrinsic differences of insulin receptor kinase activity in red and white muscle, J. Biol. Chem. 261:14939 (1986).

33. T. Kadowaki, M. Kasuga, Y. Akanum, D. Ezaki, and F. Takuku, Decreased autophosphorylation of the insulin receptor-kinase in streptozotocin-diabetic rats, J. Biol. Chem. 259:14208 (1984).

34. Y. LeMarchand-Brustel, T. Gremeau, R. Ballotti, and E. Van Obberghen, Insulin receptor tyrosine kinase is defective in skeletal muscle of insulin-resistant obese mice, Nature 315:676 (1985).

35. M. P. Czech, New perspectives on the mechanism of insulin action, Recent Prog. Hormone Res. 40:347 (1984).

36. F. Grigorescu, J. S. Flier, and C. R. Kahn, Defect in insulin receptor phosphorylation in erythrocytes and fibroblasts associated with severe insulin resistance, J. Biol. Chem. 259:15003 (1984).

37. G. E. Bollag, R. A. Roth, J. Beaudoin, D. Mochly-Rosen, and D. E. Koshland, Protein kinase C directly phosphorylates the insulin receptor *in vitro* and reduced its protein-tyrosine kinase activity, Proc. Natl. Acad. Sci. USA 83:5822 (1986).

38. K-T. Yu, D. K. Werth, I. H. Pastan, and M. P. Czech, src Kinase catalyzes the phosphorylation and activation of the insulin receptor kinase, J. Biol. Chem. 260:5838 (1985).

39. C. B. Graves, R. D. Gale, F. P. Laurino, and J. M. McDonald, The insulin receptor and calmodulin: calmodulin enhances insulin-mediated receptor kinase activity and insulin stimulates phosphorylation of calmodulin, J. Biol. Chem. 261:10429(1986).

EVOLUTION OF INSULIN AND INSULIN RECEPTORS

Derek LeRoith, William L. Lowe, Jr. and
Charles T. Roberts, Jr.

Section of Molecular and Cellular Physiology
Diabetes Branch, NIDDK, National Institutes of Health
Bethesda, Maryland 20892

Introduction

Insulin traditionally has been considered to be a unique product of the vertebrate pancreas. More recent studies, however, have suggested that there may be extrapancreatic sources of insulin and that insulin may act on tissues other than its classic target tissues. Of specific interest to us has been the suggestion that nervous tissue may be an extrapancreatic source of insulin synthesis and, furthermore, that nervous tissue may be a specific target for insulin. To pursue these questions, we and others have chosen a phylogenetic approach in our studies. In this review we will first discuss the evolutionary origins of insulin-related molecules including their presence in non-vertebrate species. These findings strongly suggest that insulin or a related molecule can be produced by tissues other than a pancreas. In the second part, we will describe studies on the phylogenetic conservation of the brain insulin receptor. Finally, we discuss the phylogenetic and developmental conservation of the structurally unique brain insulin receptor.

Evolutionary Origins of Insulin

1. Vertebrates

The insulins of vertebrate species show an extensive degree of evolutionary conservation, at both the level of nucleic acid sequence as well as primary structure of the protein. Although the sequence differences between hagfish insulin[1] (a primitive vertebrate) and the mammalian insulins (e.g. rat or human) may appear significant, closer analysis reveals a gradual progression from the phylogenetically more primitive molecules to the insulins of more advanced species. This is reflected in the high degree of immunological cross-reactivity exhibited by these "mainstream" vertebrate insulins and probably results from the necessity of each of these molecules to interact successsfully with the even more evolutionarily conserved insulin receptor molecule (as discussed below).

An interesting exception to this overall conservation of vertebrate insulin structure is the group of insulins found in hystricomorph rodents[2,3]. The amino acid sequences of a number of these variant insulins have now been determined, including those for guinea pig[4], chinchilla[5], casiragua[6], porcupine[7], coypu[2], and cais[8]. In addition, the structure of the cDNA coding for guinea pig insulin has recently been elucidated[9,10]. A recent analysis of the amino acid differences between the various hystricomorph insulins and several "mainstream" mammalian insulins such as pig, rat, and bovine insulin[11] reveals that, while the hystricomorph sequences vary significatly from other vertebrate insulins, there is even more variation among the hystricomorph insulins themselves (Fig. 1). In this same study, it was found that both coypu and casiragua insulin in spite of extensive amino acid sequence divergence, still could attain the three-dimensional structure of bovine insulin (as determined by circular dichroism measurements).

	Pig	Bovine	Rat I	Guinea pig	Chinchilla	Casiragua	Coypu	Porcupine	Cuis
Pig									
Bovine	2								
Rat 1	4	6							
Guinea pig	18	19	18						
Chinchilla	6	8	7	17					
Casiragua	21	23	21	21	21				
Coypu	22	24	23	20	22	7			
Porcupine	7	6	7	15	9	22	23		
Cuis	17	19	17	16	14	20	21	17	

Fig 1. Amino acid differences between various insulin sequences (11).

Given the fact that hystricomorph insulins are not thought to form higher-order aggregates such as the dimers and hexamers which occur with other vertebrate insulins, it may be that the sequence diversity evident in the hystricomorph insulins is a direct result of the lack of constraints on certain residues involved in such intramolecular interactions. This situation would have certain ramifications for the amino acid sequences of the putative non-vertebrate insulins described below. Specifically, if the more primitive insulins were not required to participate in aggregate formation, their amino acid (and pertinent nucleic acid) sequences potentially could be significantly different from any vertebrate counterpart, although still exhibiting bio-activity and immunological cross-reactivity.

2. Multicellular Non-vertebrates

In the following discussion we focus on the presence in non-vertebrates, including unicellular eukaryotic and prokaryotic organisms, of materials related to insulin by virtue of their insulin-related bioactivity and/or immunological cross-reactivity. It should be borne in mind that, as just described above, the presence of such activities does not necessarily predict any degree of sequence similarity between these compounds and vertebrate insulins.

Using immunological approaches, insulin-related peptides have been detected in a number of insect species approaches, including the honey bee (*Apis mellifera*), fruitfly *Drosophila melanogaster*, and the blowfly *Calliphora vomitora*,[12,13,14,15,16]. Biological activities of mammalian insulin in insects include increased sugar uptake, lipid mobilization, and growth stimulation[17]. Additionally, mammalian insulin can serve as a growth factor for certain *Drosophila* cell lines and can supplant the serum requirement of *Drosophila* embryonic cell cultures. In the case of the blowfly, insulin-related material isolated from brain using classical acid-ethanol insulin extraction procedures mimicked authentic mammalian insulin in a number of immunological and biological assays, and the HPLC-purified material was found to have an insulin-like amino-acid composition. Furthermore, the blowfly insulin-related material was localized to the median neurosecretory cells of the brain by immunocytochemistry. The elevated glucose levels seen upon removal of these cells was reversed by treatment with mammalian insulin and by administration of purified blowfly insulin-related material, suggesting that the presence of an insulin-related molecule in this insect is accompanied by a physiological role similar to insulin's role in higher organisms.

Another hormone from insects shows interesting similarities to vertebrate insulins. Prothoracicotrophic hormone (PTTH) is released from insect brain and regulates metamorphosis by promoting the release of ecdysone from the prothoracic glands. Amino-acid sequence analysis of one of the forms of PTTH (4K PTTH-II) from the silkworm *Bombyx mori*[18] revealed that the amino-terminus shows significant homology to the A chains of both human insulin and insulin-like growth factor I (Fig 2). This finding suggests the possible presence in insects of an insulin gene family, similar to that which includes the insulin, insulin-like growth factor, and relaxin genes of vertebrates.

Plisetskaya et al.[19] demonstrated the presence of insulin-related material in the alimentary tract of the freshwater snails *Anodonta cygnea* and *Unis pictorum* using anti-mammalian insulin antibodies. In the case of *Anodonta,* treatment with mammalian insulin following a glucose load elevated muscle glycogen synthase activity and muscle glycogen levels; these effects were reversed by anti-insulin sera. These studies thus suggest the presence of an insulin-related molecule in molluscs and demonstrate a probable physiological role similar to the action of insulin in vertebrates.

3. Unicellular Organisms

An extremely early evolutionary origin for the insulin gene is supported by a number of studies in unicellular eukaryotes and in prokaryotes such as *Escherichia coli* [20,21]. Material which demonstrated immunological cross-reactivity with mammalian insulin antisera was isolated from the protozoan Tetrahymena as well as the fungi Neurospora and Aspergilis fumigatus using acid-ethanol extraction and gel purification protocols developed originally for vertebrate insulins (Fig 3). Sufficient amounts of these materials were obtained to allow the assay of insulin-like bioactivity in a heterologous system, namely the stimulation of incorporation of ^{3}H-glucose into lipid using rat fat-pad cells (Fig.4). Additionally, this bioactivity was inhibited by treatment with antibodies specific for mammalian insulin.

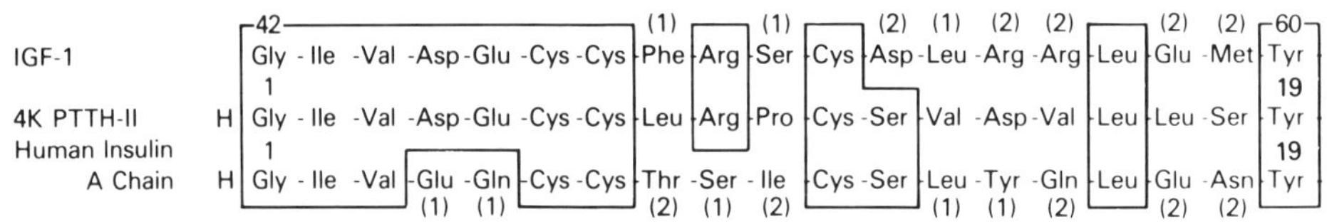

Fig 2. Amino acid sequence of Bombyx mori 4K PTTH-II: Comparison with human insulin (A chain) and insulin-like growth factor I(IGF-I). Identical amino acids are indicated by boxed sections and the numbers in parentheses note the minimum number of nucleotide base changes required for the amino acid substitution from that in 4K PTTH-II. (Adapted from [18]).

In summary, then, there is a substantial body of evidence that insulin (or at least insulin-related molecules) arose very early in evolution, as reflected by their presence today in primitive bacteria and unicellular eukaryotes. While the functions of insulin-like molecules in these primitive organisms are unknown at the present time, it is clear that the role of insulin-related peptides in the more advanced multicellular invertebrates such as insects and molluscs may be similar in many aspects to the role of insulin in vertebrates. Finally, most vertebrate insulins examined to date show a high degree of sequence conservation, possibly reflecting a common requirement for the ability to form higher-order molecular aggregates in these species. A major exception to this similarity of vertebrate

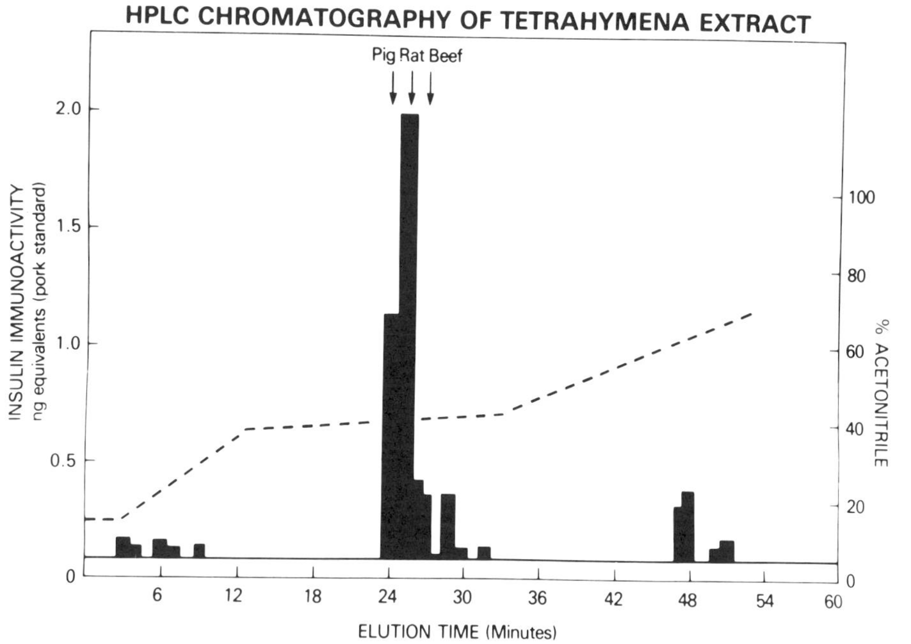

Fig 3. Insulin-related material found in Tetrahymena pyriformis. T. pyriformis grown in defined synthetic medium was extracted and purified by Sep-Pak C_{18} columns, Sephadex G-50, and ion-exchange chromatography. The immunoactive insulin-related material was then applied to an HPLC system using a μBondapak column and eluted using an elution gradient of 37-40% acetonitrile in 0.1% TFA. Fractions were lyophilized and tested for insulin immunoactivity.

insulins is found in the hystricomorphs, whose insulins are significantly divergent from both "mainstream" vertebrate insulin as well as from each other. This significant variation is possibly due to the putative 'monomeric' nature of these insulins as opposed to other mammalian insulins, and leads to the suggestion that the insulin-related proteins found in lower organisms could differ greatly in their primary structure while retaining the ability to exhibit both immunological and biological activity in a vertebrate system.

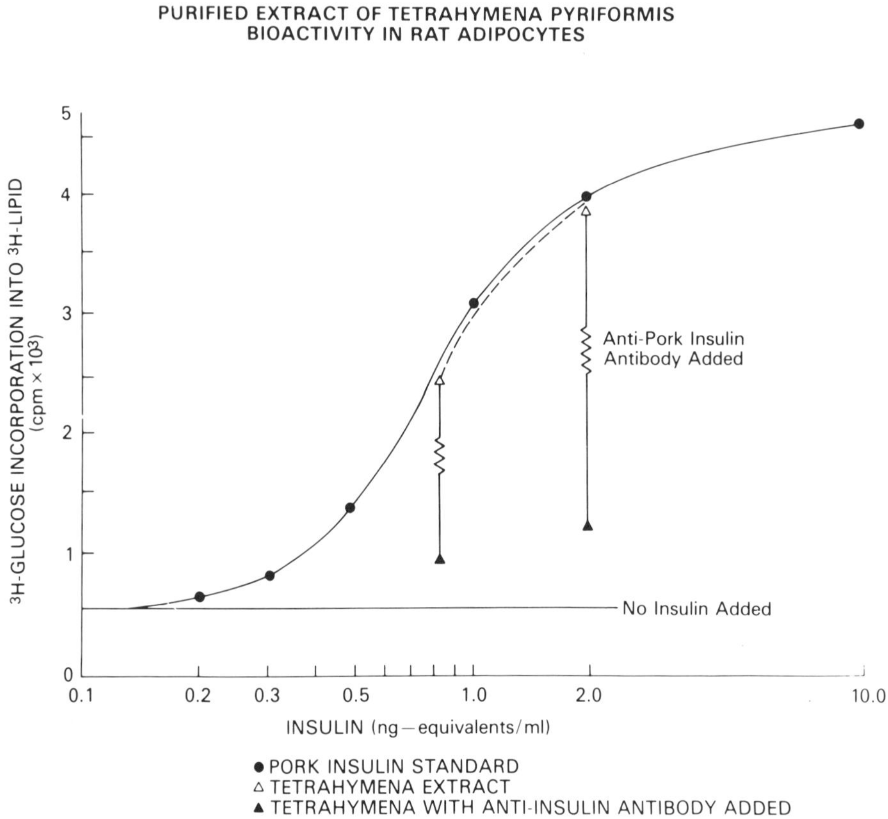

Fig 4. Insulin-related material purified from T.pyriformis was tested in a classic bioassay that measures glucose incorporation into lipids in fat cells isolated from rat epididymal fat pads.(o) Porcine insulin standard curve. (Δ) anti-porcine insulin antiserum neutralizes the biological activity of the insulin-related material from Tetrahymena. (Reproduced from references 20 and 21).

Phylogenetic conservation of the insulin receptor

In this section we will first describe the conservation of the insulin receptor throughout evolution including in Drosophila, the most primitive species known to contain receptors resembling the classic insulin receptor. Secondly, we will discuss the evidence for strong phylogenetic conservation of the unique brain insulin receptor.

Mammalian and non-mammalian receptor preparations were incubated with porcine (^{125}I)iodo insulin in the absence and presence of increasing concentrations of various insulin analogues. In most species tested the rank order of potency was chicken insulin > porcine > fish > proinsulin, suggesting functional conservation of the insulin receptor in all vertebrate species.

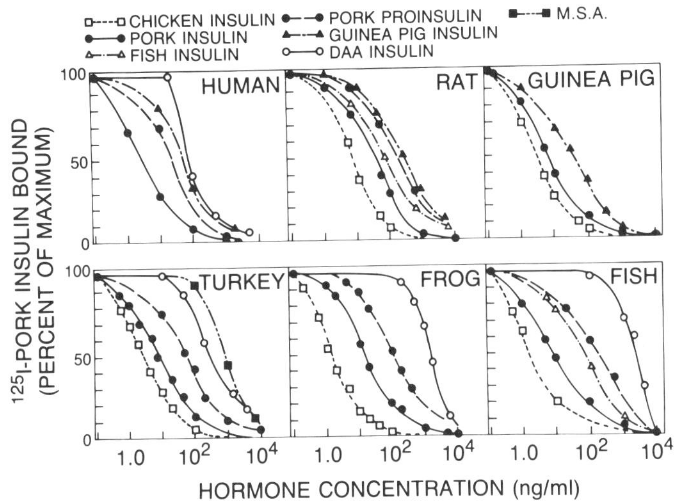

Fig 5. Competition for porcine (^{125}I)iodo-insulin binding by insulin analogues in mammalian and non-mammalian tissues.

1. <u>Vertebrate Receptors</u> The insulin receptor is a heterotetramer composed of two α and β subunits which are covalently linked by disulfide bonds. The approximate Mr's of the α and β subunits are 135 kDa and 95 kDa respectively[22,23]. Previous affinity crosslinking and photoaffinity labeling studies of the insulin receptor suggested that the α subunit contains the insulin binding site[24,25]. The β subunit, on the other hand, contains insulin-dependent tyrosine kinase activity[26] and serves as a substrate for this insulin-stimulable tyrosine kinase activity[26]. Furthermore, this auto-phosphorylation activates the kinase activity of the β subunit[27,28].

Initial studies characterizing the insulin receptor from several vertebrate species demonstrated a similarity in the binding characteristics of the receptors from these species[29,30]. Insulin binding to human lymphocytes and to liver or erythrocyte membranes from cows, frogs, fish, and turkeys was found to be pH, time and temperature dependent (Fig 5)[29,31,32]. Insulin receptors can also be characterized by the specificity of binding of different insulins and insulin analogues as measured by their ability to displace the binding of ^{125}I-porcine insulin to the insulin receptor. When the specificity of binding of various insulins to red blood cell membrane preparations from multiple species (including humans, rats, guinea pigs, turkeys, frogs, trout, and hagfish) was determined, a similar pattern was seen in all preparations. The affinities of the insulins were as follows: chicken> porcine> fish> pork proinsulin > guinea pig insulin (Fig.5)[29]. Similar results were seen with membrane preparations of liver from chickens, calves and guinea pigs[32]. In some cases, the insulin receptors bound heterologous insulins with higher affinity than homologous insulins[29,32]. In particular, in guinea pigs which contain an insulin that differs markedly from other mammalian insulins in both its biological potency and molecular structure[33,34], the insulin receptors bound typical mammalian insulins with an affinity 10-50 fold higher than they bound guinea pig insulin[29,32]. These data suggested that the insulin receptor was more highly conserved during evolution than insulin itself. Furthermore, the similar functional characteristics of these receptors from different species suggested basic similarities between them, as opposed to specializations which would allow for specific high-affinity interactions with their own endogenous insulin.

Recent structural and functional studies employing affinity crosslinking of ^{125}I-insulin to the insulin receptor as well as insulin stimulated autophosphorylation of the β subunit of the insulin receptor have further characterized the similarities between insulin receptors from multiple species. Affinity crosslinking of ^{125}I-insulin to liver membrane preparations from rats, guinea pigs, cows (R.J. Waldbillig, unpublished observations), chickens, lizards, and frogs (C.Hart, unpublished observations) followed by SDS polyacrylamide gel electrophoresis (PAGE) under reducing conditions has demonstrated the presence of an α subunit of Mr ~ 135 kDa in each case[35,36,37,38]. In each of these species, insulin stimulated the phosphorylation of a phosphoprotein with Mr ~ 95 kDa which has been identified as the β subunit of the insulin receptor[35,36,37,38]. The structural similarities between the insulin receptors from some of these species has been further confirmed by the ability of anti-insulin receptor antibodies obtained from the sera of patients with autoimmune disease and severe insulin resistance to immunoprecipitate the insulin receptors from rats, guinea pigs, and lizards[35,36,38]. These studies demonstrate the apparent conservation of the subunit structure of the insulin receptor.

2. Insulin Receptor of *Drosophila melanogaster*

More recently, Ora Rosen and coworkers have characterized the putative insulin receptor from *Drosophila melanogaster*[39,40,41]. Initial studies using lectin purified preparations demonstrated specific insulin binding with ~ 3-fold greater binding in preparations from the head as compared to the body[39]. Interestingly, the specificity of binding of the receptor differed somewhat from vertebrate receptors in that the receptor bound insulin-like growth factor-II (IGF-II) with greater affinity than either bovine pro-insulin or IGF-I [39]. Affinity crosslinking of insulin to lectin-purified preparations from adult fruit flies demonstrated a single band of Mr ~ 130 kDa consistent with previous studies in vertebrates[39]. Similar studies performed with embryos, however, demonstrated a second band with Mr ~ 100 kDa[40]. The identity of this band has not been determined. Subsequent studies demonstrated insulin-stimulable tyrosine kinase activity as measured by phosphorylation of histone H2b by lectin-purified preparations from embryos[40]. Initial attempts to demonstrate the presence of the β-subunits were, however, unsuccessful[40]. Subsequently, a genomic bank from _Drosophila melanogaster_

EFFECT OF NEURAMINIDASE ON THE STRUCTURE OF THE INSULIN RECEPTOR FROM GUINEA PIG LIVER AND BRAIN

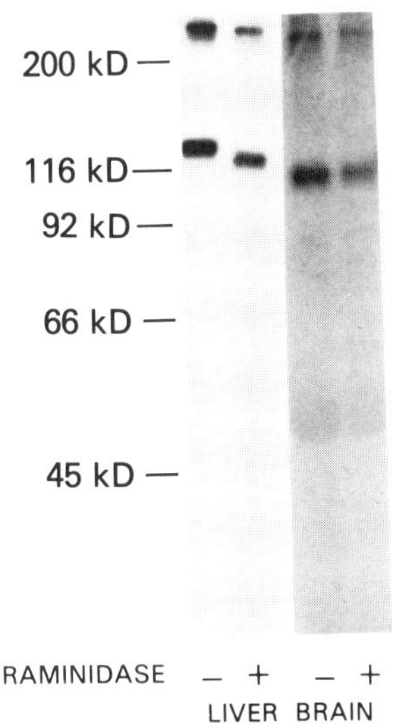

Fig 6. Electrophoretic mobility of the insulin receptor α subunit from guinea pig brain and liver.

[^{125}I]insulin was crosslinked to crude membranes using disuccinimidyl suberate and treated with neuraminidase, an exoglycosidase which cleaves terminal sialic acid residues. The receptors then were immunoprecipitated using an anti-insulin receptor antiserum and applied to SDS-PAGE under reducing conditions. The migration of the liver insulin receptor α subunit (136 kDa) was altered following neuraminidase treatment whereas that for brain (121 kDa) was unaffected.

was screened with a probe derived from the human insulin receptor cDNA. A 1.7-kb fragment from this bank which hybridized to a probe specific for the β subunit coding region was identified, isolated, and sequenced[41]. The sequence contained a 900-base pair segment which coded for a 300-amino acid peptide homologous to the kinase domain of the human insulin receptor. Overall homology at the amino acid level between the Drosophila clone and the comparable portion of the human cDNA was 53%[41]. Over a 68-amino acid stretch there was 90% homology between the two receptors[41]. Using an antibody directed against a peptide in the human insulin receptor which was conserved in the

EFFECT OF ENDOGLYCOSIDASE H ON THE STRUCTURE OF THE INSULIN RECEPTOR FROM GUINEA PIG LIVER AND BRAIN

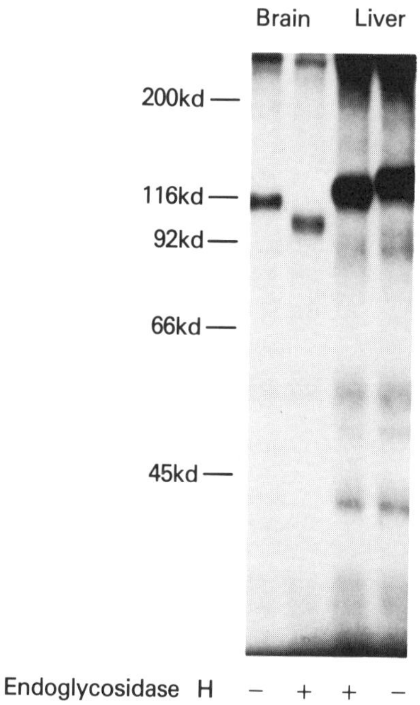

Fig 7. Effect of Endoglycosidase H on the electrophoretic mobility of the insulin receptor α subunit.

Drosophila insulin receptor, Rosen and coworkers were able to immunoprecipitate a phosphoprotein of M_r 95 kDa from Drosophila embryo lectin-purified preparations incubated with [γ-^{32}P]ATP and insulin[41]. These studies suggested the presence of a β subunit in Drosophila similar to that found in vertebrate species.

(^{125}I)insulin-crosslinked receptors from liver and brain were treated with endo H and applied to SDS-PAGE. The altered mobility of the brain and liver α subunit suggests the presence of high mannose N-linked carbohydrate branches.

3. Phylogenetic Conservation of Brain Insulin Receptors

With the demonstration of specific insulin binding in the brain a structural and functional analysis of insulin receptors in the brain was undertaken. Interestingly, studies of α subunit structure employing either photoaffinity labeling or affinity crosslinking of insulin to the α-subunit followed by SDS polyacrylamide gel electrophoresis under reducing conditions demonstrated that the rat brain insulin receptor α subunit migrated with an apparent molecular weight ~10 kDa lower than the molecular weight of the α subunit (135kDa) from peripheral, non-neural tissue derived from rat liver and fat as well as from human IM-9 lymphocytes[25,43,44]. Despite this structural difference, binding studies in which brain membrane preparations were incubated with different insulins and insulin analogues demonstrated specificities similar to those found using insulin receptors from peripheral tissues[25]. Furthermore, these receptors appeared to be functional as determined by insulin-stimulable autophosphorylation and phosphorylation of exogenous substrates[45,46], suggesting that the α and β subunits were coupled in these receptors.

Although the significance of this difference in Mr of the α subunit of the insulin receptor from brain and peripheral tissues is still unclear, the difference appears to be evolutionarily well conserved. Recent studies employing affinity crosslinking of ^{125}I-insulin to membrane preparations from liver and brain followed by SDS-PAGE have confirmed the initial observation of the M_r difference in rat brain and peripheral α-subunits[35]. Furthermore, similar findings have been demonstrated in multiple species including cows, rabbits, guinea pigs, chickens, lizards, and frogs[36,37,38]. Similar observations have also been made in humans using membrane preparations from human brain and RBC[47]. In each species (with the exception of the rabbit where further studies were not pursued) the brain insulin receptors possessed insulin-stimulable tyrosine kinase activity as measured by autophosphorylation and the phosphorylation of tyrosine-containing exogenous substrates[36,37,38,47]. Furthermore, in the studies where it was directly evaluated, the β subunit of the brain insulin receptor (90 kDa) had an Mr ~5 kDa less than the Mr of the β subunit from non-neuronal insulin receptors (95kDa). In addition to being evolutionarily well conserved, the difference in molecular weight of the α and β subunits from brain insulin receptors appears to be conserved during development[35]. In rats, the molecular weight difference between the brain and liver α and β subunits was apparent from 19 days of gestation through adulthood[35].

The smaller molecular weight of the α subunit of brain insulin receptors appears to be due to differences in glycosylation of the α subunits of brain and peripheral insulin receptors (Fig 6 and 7). Initial studies with neuraminidase (Fig 6), an exoglycosidase which cleaves terminal sialic acid residues, suggested that at least part of the structural difference was due to glycosylation differences. The migration on SDS-PAGE of the α subunit from peripheral insulin receptors was altered with neuraminidase, whereas the migration of the brain insulin receptor α subunit was unaffected by neuraminidase digestion [43,44]. This suggested either the absence of, or an alteration of, the terminal sialcylation of the brain insulin receptor α subunits. When guinea pig brain and liver insulin receptors as well as rat brain and adipocyte receptors were crosslinked or photoaffinity labeled with insulin and digested with endoglycosidase F, the bands on SDS-PAGE corresponding to the α subunits from brain and peripheral tissues comigrated (Fig 8.)[36,48]. Since this enzyme hydrolyzes the chitobiose core structure of both high mannose and complex N-linked oligosaccharides, these data suggested that the deglycosylated α subunits from brain and peripheral insulin receptors were peptides of similar molecular weight and presumably, similar in structure[36,48]. This is supported by further studies of Heidenreich and Brandenburg[48] in which the deglycosylated α subunits from brain and adipocytes were digested with Staphylococcus V8 protease. This digestion yielded identical peptides for both receptors.

As noted previously, the functional significance of this structural difference in brain and peripheral insulin receptors is, at present, unclear. Previous studies with primary cultures of neuronal and glial cells from rat brain have demonstrated some interesting functional differences between the two cell types. Insulin stimulates glucose uptake and causes down-regulation of insulin receptors in glial cells but not in neuronal cells[49,50]. In neuronal cells as opposed to glial cells, however, insulin affects monoamine metabolism[51]. Interestingly, the structure of the α subunit of the insulin receptor as determined by affinity cross-linking differs in these two cell types. Glial cells have an α subunit structure more characteristic of peripheral cells, whereas the α subunit structure of neuronal cells is similar to that of the brain[35]. This would suggest that the two structural subtypes of receptors may have some unique functions.

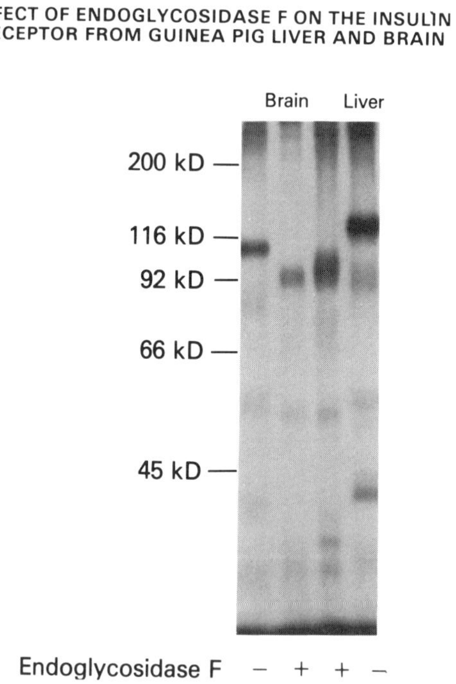

Fig 8. Effect of Endoglycosidase F on the electrophoretic mobility of the insulin receptor α subunit from guinea pig liver and brain. The altered mobility suggests the presence of high mannose and complex N-linked carbohydrate branches.

Conclusion

The studies outlined in this review suggest that insulin and insulin-related molecules are phylogenetically very old and evolutionarily well conserved. Furthermore, the presence of insulin-related materials in organisms that do not contain a pancreas adds strong support to the possibility of extrapancreatic insulin production in vertebrates.

Brain insulin receptors are structurally different from insulin receptors in peripheral non-neural tissues. Though the role of insulin in the nervous system is as yet still undetermined, the strong phylogenetic conservation of this structurally different brain insulin receptor suggests that insulin may play a role in nervous tissue function.

References

1. P.M. Hobart, L.P. Shen, R. Crawford, R.L. Pictet and W.J. Rutter, Science 210:1360-1363 (1980)
2. L.F. Smith, Diabetes 21, Suppl. 2, 457-460(1972)
3. A.E. Zimmerman and C.C. Yip, J. Biol. Chem. 249:4021-4025 (1974)
4. L.F. Smith, Am. J. Med. 40:662-666 (1966)
5. S.P. Wood, T.L. Blundell, A. Wollmer, N.R. Lazarus and R.W.J. Neville, Eur. J. Biochem. 55:532-542 (1975)
6. R. Horuk, P. Goodwin, K. O'Connor, R.W.J. Neville, and N.R. Lazarus, Nature 279:439-440 (1979)
7. R. Horuk, T.L. Blundell, N.R. Lazarus, R.W.J. Neville, D. Stone, and A. Wollmer Nature (London)286:822-824 (1980)
8. M. Bajaj, Ph.D. Thesis, Birkbeck College, University of London (1984)
9. S.J. Chan, V. Episkopou, S. Zeitlin, S.K. Karathanasis, A. Mackrell, D.F. Steiner and A. Efstratiadis, Proc. Natl. Acad. Sci. (USA) 81:5046-5050 (1984)
10. V.M. Watt, J. Biol. Chem. 260:10926-10929 (1985)
11. M. Bajaj, T.L. Blundell, R. Horuk, J.E. Pitts, S.P. Wood., L. K. Gowan, C. Schwabe, A. Wollmer, J. Gliemann and S. Gammeltoft Biochem. J. 238:345-351 (1986).
12. D. LeRoith, M.A. Lesniak, and J. Roth, Diabetes 30:70-76 (1980)
13. K.J. Kramer, C.N. Childs, R.D. Spiers and R.M. Jacobs, Insect Biochem. 12:91-98 (1982)
14. H.Duve, Gen. Comp. Endocrinol 36:102-110 (1978)
15. H. Duve and A. Thorpe, Cell Tissue Res 200:187-191 (1979)
16. H. Duve, A. Thorpe, and N.R. Lazarus. Biochem. J. 184:221-227 (1979)
17. K.J. Kramer In "Comprehensive Insect Physiology, Biochemistry and Pharmacology" (G.A. Kerkat and L.I. Gilbert, eds.) Vol 7, Ch. 10, Pergamon, Oxford (1985)
18. H.H. Nagasawa, A. Kataoka, S. Isogai, A. Tamura, H. Suzuki, A. Ishizake, A. Mizoguchi, Y. Fujiwara, and A. Suzuki, Science 226:1344-1345 (1984)
19. E. Plisetskaya, V.K. Kazakov, L. Solititskaya and L.G. Leibson Gen. Comp. Endocrinol. 35:133-145 (1978)
20. D. LeRoith, J. Shiloach, J. Roth nd M.A. Lesniak, Pro. Natl. Acad. Sci. USA 77:6184-6188 (1980)
21. D. LeRoith, J. Shiloach, J. Roth and M.A. Lesniak, J. Biol. Chem 256:6533-6536 (1981)
22. E. Van Obberghen, M. Kasuga, A. LeCam, J.A. Hedo, A. Itin and L. C. Harrison. Proc. Natl. Acad. Sci. USA 78:1052-1056 (1981)

23. M. Kasuga, J.A. Hedo, K. M. Yamada and C.R. Kahn, J. Biol. Chem. 257:10392-10399 (1982)
24. P.F. Pilch and M.P. Czech, J. Biol. Chem. 255:1722-1731 (1980)
25. C.C. Yip, M.L. Moule, and C.W.T. Yeung. Biochem. Biophys. Res. Commun. 96:1671-1678 (1980)
26.M. Kasuga, F.A. Karlsson, and C.R. Kahn, Science 215:185-187 (1982)
27. K-T. Yu and M.P. Czech J. Biol. Chem. 259:5277-5286 (1984)
28. R. Herrera and O.M. Rosen J. Biol. Chem. 261:11980-11985 (1986)
29. M. Muggeo, B.H. Ginsberg, J. Roth, D.M. Neville,Jr., P. De Meyts, and C.R. Kahn, Endocrinol. 104:1393-1398 (1979)
30. M. Muggeo, E.Van Obberghen, C.R. Kahn, J. Roth, B.H. Ginsberg, P. De Meyts, S.O. Emdin and S. Falkmer, Diabetes 28:175-181 (1979)
31. J.R. Gavin, III, P. Gorden, J.Roth, J. Archer and D.N.Buell J. Biol. Chem. 248:2202-2207 (1973)
32. W. Kemmler, R. Renner, A. Zynamon and K.D. Hepp, Biochem. et Biophys. Acta 543:349-356 (1978)
33. A.E. Zimmerman, M.L. Moule, C.C. Yip, J. Biol Chem. 249:4026-4031 (1974)
34. S.J. Chan, V. Episkopou, S. Zeitlin, S.K. Karathanasis, A. MacKrell, D.F. Steiner, and A. Efstratiadis. Proc. Natl. Acad. Sci USA 81:5046-5050 (1984)
35. W.L. Lowe, Jr. F.T. Boyd, D. W. Clarke, M.K. Raizada, C. Hart and D. LeRoith, Endocrinology 119:25-35 (1986)
36. W. Lowe, Jr, and D. LeRoith, Endocrinology 118:1669-1677 (1986)
37. J. Simon and D. LeRoith, Eur. J. Biochem. 158:125-132 (1986)
38. J. Shemer, J.C. Penhos, and D. LeRoith, Diabetologia 29:321-329 (1986)
39. L. Petruzzelli, R. Herrera, R. Garcia and O.M. Rosen, Cancer Cells 3:115-120 (1985)
40. L. Petruzzelli, R. Herrera, R. Garcia-Arenas and O. M. Rosen, J. Biol. Chem. 260:16072-16075 (1985)
41. L. Petruzzelli, R. Herrera, R. Arenas-Garcia, R. Fernandez, M.J. Birnbaum and O.M. Rosen, Proc. Natl. Acad. Sci. USA 83:4710-4714 (1986)
42. J. Havrankova, J. Roth and M. Brownstein, Nature 272:827-829 (1978)
43. K.A. Heidenreich, N.R. Zahniser, P. Berhanu, D. Brandenburg, and J.M.Olefsky, J. Biol. Chem 258:8527-8530 (1983)
44. S.A. Hendricks, C-D. Agardh, S.I. Taylor and J. Roth, J. Neurochem. 43:198-203 (1984)
45. R. W. Rees-Jones, S.A. Hendricks, M. Quarum and J. Roth, J. Biol. Chem. 259:3470-3474 (1984)
46. S. Gammeltoft, A. Kowalski, M. Fehlmann and E. Van Obberghen FEBS Lett. 172:87-90 (1984a)
47. G. Grunberger, W.L. Lowe, Jr., A. McElduff and R.P. Glick, J. Clin. Invest. 77:997-1005 (1985)
48. K.A. Heidenreich and D. Brandenburg, Endocrinology 118:1835-1842 (1986)
49.F.T. Boyd. Jr. and M.K. Raizada, Am J. Physiol 245:C283-C287 (1983)
50. M. Kappy, S. Sellinger, and M. Raizada, J. Neurochem. 42:198-203 (1984)
51. F.T. Boyd, D.W. Clarke, T.F. Muther, and M.K. Raizada, J. Biol Chem. 260:15880-15885 (1985)

EVIDENCE FOR CENTRAL NERVOUS SYSTEM INSULIN SYNTHESIS

Derrel W. Clarke,[1] Jennifer J. Poulakos,[1] Laura M. Mudd,[2]
Mohan K. Raizada,[2] David L. Cooper[3]

Departments of Pediatrics,[1] Physiology,[2] and Pathology[3]
of the University of Florida College of Medicine,
Gainesville, FL 32610

Since Havrankonva and co-workers described the widespread distribution of both insulin[1] and insulin receptors[2] in the rat central nervous system (CNS), two basic questions have remained unanswered. The first is the source of this insulin within the CNS, whether locally produced or of pancreatic origin. Second is the function of insulin within the CNS. Does insulin have similar effects centrally to those outside the CNS or does insulin have unique functions in the CNS?

This chapter will review the evidence that insulin is produced within the CNS, specifically by neurons within the CNS. Conclusive evidence for insulin synthesis within the CNS, a sequenced messenger RNA or cDNA for insulin from the whole brain, has not been identified.[3] Nevertheless, an increasingly convincing body of indirect evidence indicates endogenous CNS insulin production.

The synthesis of insulin by both neurons and pancreatic islet beta cells would be consistent with the accepted evidence for production of a variety of other peptides by both the CNS and the pancreas/gastrointestinal system (Table I).[4,5] These peptides often co-exist with neuroactive amines both within and outside of the CNS.[4] These cells have common origins as "neuroendocrine-programmed cells originating from the ectoblast"[5] and form the APUD (Amine Precursor Uptake and Decarboxylation) system[5] of endocrine and neuronal cells. Although the evidence for other pancreatic islet cells belonging to this system seems clear, especially the somatostatin- and vasoactive intestinal peptide-producing delta cells, the role of insulin-producing cells in this system remains unproven.

TABLE 1. Gut-Pancreatic-CNS Neuronal Peptides

ACTH	Glucagon
Bombesin	Neurotensin
Cholecystokinin	Pancreatic polypeptide
Endorphin	Substance P
Enkephalin	Somatostatin
Enteroglucagon	Thyrotropin releasing hormone
Gastrin	Vasoactive intestinal peptide

Effect of Diabetes on CNS Insulin Content

One of the earliest lines of evidence for CNS insulin production was the finding by Havrankova et al., later confirmed by other investigators, that relatively high concentrations of insulin are maintained in the CNS compared to plasma levels (Tables 2 and 3)[6-12,14] and that CNS insulin concentrations are not affected by alterations in plasma insulin concentrations (Table 3).[6-9] Despite the marked hypoinsulinemia produced by streptozotocin-induced or prolonged fast, CNS insulin concentrations remain similar to controls.[6-8] The marked hyperinsulinism found in the obese ob/ob mouse likewise does not lead to a corresponding increase in brain insulin levels.[6,9,14] Recently obese, hyperinsulinemic fa/fa rats have been found to actually have markedly lower brain insulin concentrations than their normoinsulinemic, non-affected Fa/Fa littermates.[14] Heterozygote fa/Fa rats have intermediate brain insulin levels.

Several possible alternative explanations could be offered. The first possibility is that CNS insulin concentrations are tightly regulated despite wide fluctuations of plasma insulin concentrations by a compensatory alteration of transport of insulin into the cerebrospinal fluid (CSF) or brain. The finding that the CSF insulin content appears to parallel plasma insulin levels in normal and diabetic animals and appears to reflect a slow integration of plasma insulin levels[15,16] would contradict this theory. Frank et al. found that isolated capillaries comprising the blood-brain barrier actively bind, internalize, and release insulin, but that the released insulin is completely degraded and therefore bioinactive.[17] Thus, neither tight regulation of CSF or brain active transport of intact insulin from plasma would seem plausible explanations for the maintenance of constant insulin concentrations. Alterations in brain insulin degradation by the altered diabetic metabolic state is a remote, unproven explanation.

Table 2. Relative Insulin Concentrations in CNS and Plasma in Euinsulinemic Mammals

	CNS (ng/gm wet wt)	Plasma ng/ml	CNS/Plasma	Ref
Rat	22.8	0.9	25.3	1
	6.0	1.4	4.3	6
	2.0	1.1	1.8	7
	4.6	1.4	3.3	8
	22.0	2.0	11.0	9
	1.33	0.85	1.6	10
	5.93	0.85	7.0	10
Guinea Pig	1.0	<0.02	>50.0	11
	1.35	<0.15	>9.0	10
	2.99	<0.15	>19.9	10
	.8	<0.01	>80.0	12
Human	3.2	0.4	8.0	9
	6.7	1.6	4.0	12

Table 3. The Effect on CNS Insulin Concentrations by Alterations of Plasma Insulin Concentrations

	Hypoinsulinemic Model					Hyperinsulinemic Model		
	Streptozotocin			Prolonged fast		ob/ob mice		fa/fa rats
CNS [Insulin]*								
model	17.8	2.9	17.5	7.1	23.0	6.5	7.0	.13
control	6.0	4.6	6.0	4.6	22.0	6.5	7.0	.33
Plasma [Insulin]**								
model	.8	.3	1.2	.3	2.0	50	50.0	3.6
control	1.4	1.4	1.6	1.4	2.5	1.0	1.5	.23
CNS model / CNS control	3.0	.6	2.9	1.5	1.0	1.0	1.0	0.4
Plasma model / Plasma Control	.6	.2	.7	.2	.8	50.0	33.3	15.7
CNS model / Plasma model	22.2	9.7	14.6	23.7	11.5	.13	.14	.39
CNS control / Plasma control	4.3	3.3	5.0	3.3	8.8	6.5	46.7	15.7
Reference	6	8	9	8	9	6	9	14

*Insulin concentration expressed as ng/gm wet brain weight
**Insulin concentration expressed as ng/ml

Immunohistochemical Localization of Insulin Within the CNS

Although immunohistochemical staining of the brain with anti-insulin antibodies cannot distinguish cells which actively internalize pancreatic insulin from cells which synthesize insulin, important speculative evidence about sites of insulin synthesis may be obtained. Havrankova et al. first localized insulin in neuronal perikarya in the olfactory bulb and frontal cortex of the immature rat brain.[1] This staining with insulin antibodies seems specific since it was blocked with pretreatment of the anti-insulin serum with insulin prior to tissue application.[1]

Dorn and co-workers have expanded these findings by demonstrating immunofluorescent staining of many neurons especially in the hypothalamus, thalamus, hippocampus, and amygdyla of the mouse brain.[18] They later reported the widespread co-localization of immunostaining of the human brain with specific antibodies for insulin and C-peptide.[13] This co-staining occurs within the soma and dendrites of the cerebral cortex, hippocampus, amygdyla, brain stem (especially the nucleii for cranial nerves IX, X, and XII), cerebellum, and hypothalmus.[13] This co-localization of both insulin and part of its synthetic precursor, C-peptide, supports the theory of endogenous CNS insulin synthesis, since co-localization of separate uptake mechanisms for each of these peptides by specific neurons is unlikely and the very existance of a transport system for a non-functional peptide such as C-peptide is improbable.

In brain cultures from newborn rat brains, Raizada demonstrated that the insulin immunostaining is restricted to approximately 5% of the cultured neuronal soma and dendrites without staining of the glial component of the culture.[19] Serum deprivation of the culture has no effect on the number or intensity of staining, while cycloheximide, a protein synthesis inhibitor, profoundly inhibits the staining. His studies therefore imply that neuronal staining for immunoreactive insulin is not due to insulin taken up from the culture media, but is probably due to neuronal insulin synthesis by a cycloheximide-sensitive mechanism. As mentioned previously, however, storage of pancreatic insulin or C-peptide from plasma by a cycloheximide sensitive mechanism cannot be entirely ruled out in any of these studies.

Unique Guinea Pig CNS Insulin

The guinea pig has proven to be an especially useful model in investigating CNS insulin production. Guinea pig pancreatic insulin shares only 65% homology with human, rat, or porcine insulins. Because of this poor homology radioimmunoassays using specific antibodies have been developed to detect guinea pig or rat/pork insulins with negligible cross-reactivity.[12] The CNS and other extrapancreatic tissues of the guinea pig contain relatively large amounts of an insulin detectable by the rat/pork radioimmunoassay which is undetectable by the same radioimmunoassay of the pancreas or plasma (Table 2).[10-12] Because of the specificity of these radioimmunoassays, it is clear that the amount of this extrapancreatic rat/pork insulin can in no way be accounted for by cross-reactivity with the relatively small amount of guinea pig pancreatic insulin. This extrapancreatic insulin also has the same elution time on Sephadex 50 column as insulin,[11] implying structural homology.

The poor structural homology of the guinea pig pancreatic insulin with the rat/pork insulin is also reflected in its poor ability to bind to the insulin receptor and stimulate insulin-mediated cellular events such as lipogenesis and glucose uptake.[10,11] The guinea pig extrapancreatic insulin,[10,11] on the other hand, has greater potency in stimulating lipogenesis, comparable to rat/pork insulin. This effect is abolished by the addition of anti-porcine insulin antibodies, but not by anti-guinea pig insulin antibodies.[11] This is in contrast to the loss of bioactivity of the guinea pig pancreatic insulin by anti-guinea pig insulin antibodies, but not by anti-porcine insulin antibodies.[11]

The guinea pig, therefore, appears to synthesize two distinct insulin molecules as identified by specific radioimmunoassays and bioassays. Since the extrapancreatic insulin is found in several tissues such as liver and brain,[11] it is not clear whether the CNS actually produces this insulin or if it is transported via nerves from these organs to the CNS. Difficult to reconcile with the concept of two insulins being produced in the guinea pig is the inability of Chan et al.[20] to demonstrate the presence of a second guinea pig insulin gene using Southern blotting with a rat insulin cDNA probe. These findings, therefore, remain unexplained.

Insulin Release in CNS Cultures

Primary cultures of CNS tissue have been developed to investigate the divergent physiologic functions of the major cellular components of the CNS, the neurons and glia. These primary CNS cultures have provided evidence of insulin synthesis by neurons within the CNS. These data, though, must be viewed with caution. Although these neurons and glia obtained from fetal or newborn animals appear to retain all of the morphologic, biochemical, and functional characteristics of their _in vivo_ counterparts, the effects of the culture conditions on gene expression and cellular maturation have not been absolutely defined. Therefore, the possible effect of the culture conditions on insulin gene expression must be always kept in mind. Nevertheless, these cultures provide valuable models to isolate cell types of the CNS and study the effects of single variables on insulin synthesis and release.

As mentioned earlier, the first culture studies implicating neuronal insulin synthesis were those of Raizada, who found immunohistochemical staining for insulin by cultured neurons, but not glia.[19] In the same study, these cultures were found to incorporate [^{3}H] valine into immunoprecipitable insulin, implying _in situ_ neuronal insulin synthesis. Birch et al. found that the media of cultured fetal mouse brain cells grown in serum free media for 2-3 weeks contained typically 100 pg of immunoreactive insulin per 6 ml of culture media.[21] Two peaks of radioimmunoassayable insulin were isolated on both high performance liquid chromatography (HPLC) and gel exclusion chromatography. These peaks had retention times similar to proinsulin and insulin. Exposing the proinsulin-like material to mild proteolysis with trypsin shifted the retention time to that of the insulin peak, as would be expected. In radioimmunoassays this proinsulin-like material competed for insulin antibody binding with a potency similar to porcine proinsulin, while the protein co-eluting with insulin was similar in potency to porcine insulin. Reduction of disulfide bonds and alkylation with iodoacetamide of porcine insulin and this insulin-like peptide led to a loss of immunoreactivity of both peptides. Thus, these mouse brain cultures appear to release peptides into the culture media which are very similar to proinsulin and insulin.

Our studies have focused on insulin release as a neurotransmitter from neuronal cultures. Depolarization of neurons with an isotonic solution containing calcium and high potassium concentrations (60mM) results in a greater than threefold stimulation of insulin release from the cells into the bathing solution.[22] Since depolarization of the neurons involves not only the alteration of cell membrane potential by the high extracellular potassium, but also the secondary influx of calcium into the neurons, it was not unexpected that the omission of either ion from the depolarization solution completely blocks the stimulated insulin release.

To eliminate any possible artifacts due to alterations of the ionic milieu, the neurons were pharmacologically depolarized in the presence of calcium ion with veratridine, a sodium ionophore. Veratridine likewise causes a 379% stimulation of insulin release into the bathing solution.[22]

Since neuronal cultures in our hands contain approximately 20% astrocytes, glial cultures were treated under similar conditions to investigate glial insulin release. Glial cultures are not stimulated to release insulin under similar depolarizing conditions,[22] implying that the released insulin is of neuronal origin.

To confirm that the released insulin is endogenously by neurons, protein synthesis was blocked by cycloheximide and pulse-labelling experiments were performed.[22] Cycloheximide completely blocks stimulated insulin release, implying that release is protein synthesis dependent. This confirmed Raizada's earlier findings that cycloheximide markedly inhibited the intensity and number of cells staining with fluorescent labelled anti-insulin antibodies.[19] Preincubation of the neurons with [^{3}H] leucine results in incorporation of the [^{3}H] leucine into immunoprecipitable insulin. A time course of depolarization-stimulated release of this [^{3}H] leucine labelled insulin results in a biphasic release after subtracting out basal [^{3}H] insulin release.[22] This biphasic response is thought to reflect the release of rapidly releasable stores in the first phase (10 minute peak for these neuronal cultures) and stimulated synthesis or processing of proinsulin in the second phase (a 30 minute peak).

To begin to verify that this immunoreactive insulin is truly insulin, the released insulin was analyzed by reversed-phase HPLC and subsequent radioimmunoassay of each fraction was performed. Two peaks of immunoassayable insulin were obtained which co-migrated with the two rat insulin standard peaks corresponding to rat I and rat II insulins. These studies would again confirm neuronal synthesis of the insulin since the horse serum in which these cells were grown has only one insulin peak by HPLC.

In summary, these studies have provided strong evidence for neuronal synthesis and release of insulin upon depolarization. This neuronal insulin appears to have similar structural characteristics as pancreatic insulin. It raises the speculation that insulin may act as a neurotransmitter in the CNS.

Insulin mRNA in the CNS

All of these previously mentioned studies have provided evidence for CNS insulin synthesis, although they all have intrinsic flaws making them nonconclusive. With new techniques in molecular biology, the identification of the messenger RNA for insulin within the CNS would eliminate lingering doubts. Unfortunately, the isolation and characterization of this insulin mRNA has not yet been performed. In fact, Giddings et al., after a thorough investigation of several areas of the rat brain, were unable to find the insulin mRNA.[3] Nevertheless, our group and others have reported the existance of mRNA in the CNS hybridizing with insulin probes.[23-26]

Dr. Young at the National Institutes of Health has recently used an oligonucleotide probe of the insulin gene to localize the insulin mRNA in the rat CNS.[26] He found by _in situ_ hybridization that neurons of the periventricular nucleus of the hypothalamus contain mRNA hybridizing with the radiolabelled insulin probe. These neurons would be in a strategic place in the brain to perhaps sense metabolic or hormonal changes in the cerebrospinal fluid and release insulin as neuromodulator/neurotransmitter. Although the conditions used in the _in situ_ hybridization appear to be stringent enough to not allow cross-hybridization of the probe with other mRNAs for insulin-like molecules, sequencing of this mRNA to confirm that it indeed is the insulin mRNA has not been performed. Other sites either hybridizing or not with the insulin mRNA are not mentioned, but this study appears to be an important beginning in understanding CNS insulin synthesis and its possible physiologic role in the CNS.

We have found that primary neuronal, but not glial, cultures contain a major 2.4 kB mRNA which hybridizes with a genomic insulin DNA probe (Figure 1a). This 2.4 kb mRNA presumably represents a preproinsulin mRNA species which has yet to be processed to the 550 base proinsulin species. The 550 base proinsulin species accounts for about 5% of all the RNA hybridizing with the insulin probe in the neuronal cultures as determined by scanning microdensitometry of the autoradiograph (Figure 1b). The pancreas similarly contains this 2.4 kB mRNA species, but by far the major insulin mRNA is the 550 base species. The reason for these tissue differences in processing of the insulin mRNA have yet to be elucidated. Although the stringency of the hybridization is sufficient to not allow cross-hybridization with insulin-like molecules we, like Young, have not sequenced this mRNA to prove that it is indeed encoding for insulin. Because of the variables introduced by cultures, as discussed previously,

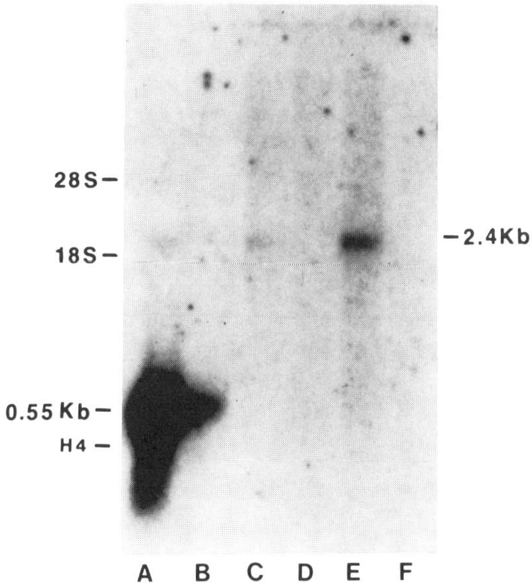

Fig. 1a. Northern blot analysis of insulin-specific RNA transcripts. All lanes represent 10 ug of RNA from A)poly (A+)pancreatic RNA, B)total pancreatic RNA, C)poly (A+) submandibular gland RNA, D)poly (A+) glial RNA, E)poly (A+) neuronal RNA, and F)total neuronal RNA which were separated by size on an agarose/formaldehyde denaturing gel and hybridized with ^{32}P-labelled human insulin cDNA probe.

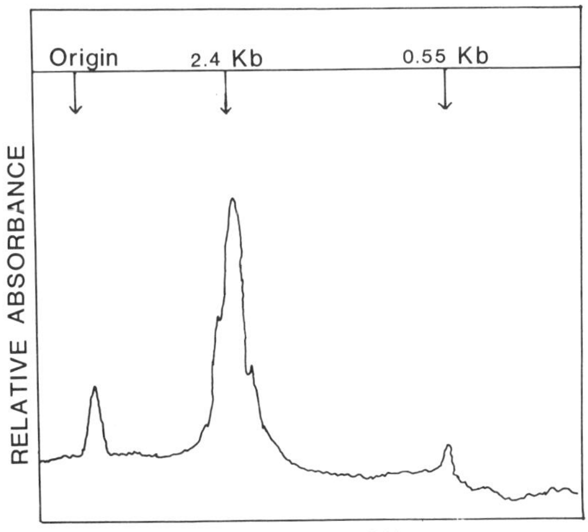

Fig. 1b. Quantitative microdensitometric analysis of Lane E from 1a.

confirmation of these findings in whole brain will still need to be done. Our preliminary studies, however, using *in situ* hybridization techniques to localize the sites of insulin mRNA, have confirmed the existance of neurons within the CNS which contain mRNA hybridizing with the rat insulin DNA probe. Using radiolabelled insulin DNA probe to hybridize to RNA in tissue slides under stringent conditions, we have found that neuroectodermal cells of the newborn rat cerebral cortex hybridize with the insulin probe (Figure 2). These pluripotential cells of the developing brain could be important sites of synthesis of insulin as a growth factor[27] or neurotransmitter.[22] Further mapping of the CNS for insulin synthesis sites are now being conducted.

Conclusions

The information collected over the last 10 years now provides impressive evidence for CNS insulin synthesis. Molecular biology techniques to isolate and sequence the insulin mRNA in the whole brain are still needed to provide definitive proof of CNS insulin synthesis. Preliminary data from these techniques appear to collaborate the indirect evidence for neuronal insulin synthesis and release.

Once CNS synthesis is proven, then the role of insulin in the CNS will take on new significance. Insulin has already been found to be important in neuronal and glial growth and development,[27-28] modulation of neuronal firing rate and catecholamine metabolism,[29-32] and as a possible neurotransmitter.[22] Proof that the CNS is more than the passive recipient of pancreatic insulin, but actually synthesizes insulin, could mean that insulin is released as a neurotransmitter in response to various metabolic and hormonal stimuli. Insulin in the CNS has already been found to have profound effects in inducing satiety,[33] modulating glucose-sensitive neuronal responses to glucose[8] and modulating peripheral carbohydrate metabolism by modulating hepatic glucose output[34] and modulating pancreatic insulin production.[35] Understanding CNS insulin synthesis and the regulation of its synthesis and release may therefore be crucial in understanding disorders of satiety such as anorexia nervosa and obesity and disorders of abnormal glucose regulation such as adult-onset diabetes mellitus.

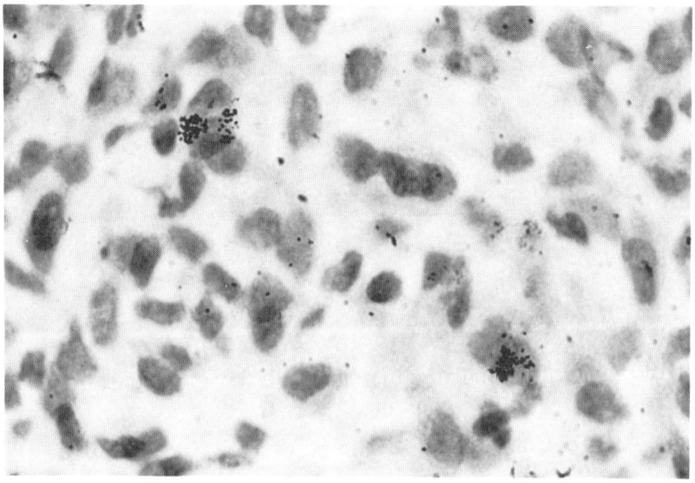

Fig. 2. In Situ hybridization of neonatal rat brain with insulin DNA probe. Neonatal rat brain tissue sections were fixed with paraformaldehyde and hybridized with ^{35}S-labelled rat insulin genomic DNA probe (1.5 kb). Autoradiographic localization of insulin mRNA to subcortical neuroectodermal cells is shown.

REFERENCES

1. J. Havrankova, D. Schmechel, J. Roth, and M. Brownstein, Identification of insulin in rat brain, Proc. Nat. Sci. USA 75:5737 (1978).
2. J. Havrankova, J. Roth, and M. Brownstein, Insulin receptors are widely distributed in the central nervous system of the rat, Nature 272:827 (1978).
3. S. J. Giddings, J. Chirgwin, and M. A. Permutt, Evaluation of rat insulin messenger RNA in pancreatic and extrapancreatic tissues, Diabetologia 28:343 (1985).
4. T. Hokfelt, O. Johansson, A. Ljungdahl, J. M. Lundberg, and M. Schultzberg, Peptidergic neurons, Nature 284:515 (1980).
5. A. G. E. Pearse, The cytochemistry and ultrastructure of polypeptide hormone-producing cells of the APUD series and the embryologic, physiologic and pathologic implications of the concept, J. Histochem. Cytochem. 17:303 (1969).
6. J. Havrankova, J. Roth, and M. Brownstein, Concentrations of insulin and of insulin receptors in the brain are independent of peripheral insulin levels: Studies of obese and streptozotocin-treated rodents, J. Clin. Invest. 64:636 (1979).
7. J. Eng and R.S. Yalow, Insulin recoverable from tissues, Diabetes 29:105 (1980).
8. Y. Oomura and H. Kita, Insulin acting as a modulator of feeding through the hypothalamus, Diabetologia 20(suppl.):290 (1981).
9. J. L. Rosenzweig, J. Havronkova, M. A. Lesniak, M. J. Brownstein, and J. Roth, Insulin is ubiquitous in extrapancreatic tissues of rats and humans, Proc. Natl. Acad. Sci. USA 77:572 (1980).
10. R. W. Stevenson, Further evidence for non-pancreatic insulin immunoreactivity in guinea pig brain, Horm. Metab. Res. 15:526 (1983).
11. J. L. Rosenzweig, M. A. Lesniak, B. A. Samuels, C. C. Yip, A. E. Zimmeraman, J. Roth, Insulin in the extrapancreatic tissues of guinea pig differs markedly from the insulin in their pancreas and plasma, Trans. Assoc. Am. Phys. 93:263 (1980).
12. J. L. Rosenzweig, D. LeRoith, M. A. Lesniak, C. C. Yip, D. N. Orth, H. R. Nankin, P. Murone, M. Berelowitz, L. A. Frohman, A. S. Liotta, D. T. Krieger, and J. Roth, Two distinct insulin-related molecules in the guinea pig: immunological and biochemical characterization of insulin-like immunoreactivity from extrapancreatic tissues of the guinea pig, Diabetologia 28:237 (1985).
13. A. Dorn, A. Rinne, H. G. Bernstein, H. J. Hahn, and M. Ziegler, Insulin and C-peptide in human brain neurons, J. Hirnforsch. 24:495 (1983).
14. D. G. Baskin, L. J. Stein, H. Ikeda, S. C. Woods, D. P. Figlewicz, D. Porte, Jr., M. R. C. Greenwood, and D. M. Dorsa, Genetically obese Zucker rats have abnormally low brain insulin content, Life Sci. 36:627 (1985).
15. S. C. Woods and D. Porte, Jr., Relationship between plasma and cerebrospinal fluid insulin levels of the dog, Am. J. Physiol. 233:E331 (1977).
16. L. J. Stein, D. M. Dorsa, D. G. Baskin, D. P. Figlewicz, H. Ikeda, S. P. Frankman, M. R. C. Greenwood, D. P. Porte, Jr., and S. C. Woods, Immunoreactive insulin levels are elevated in the cerebrospinal fluid of genetically obese Zucker rats, Endocrinology 113:2299 (1983).
17. H. J. L. Frank, W. M. Pardridge, W. L. Morris, R. G. Rosenfeld, and T. B. Choi, Binding and internalization of insulin and insulin-like growth factors by isolated brain microvessels, Diabetes 35:654 (1986).
18. A. Dorn, H.-G. Bernstein, H.-J. Hahn, M. Ziegler, and H. Rummelfanger, Insulin immunohistochemistry of rodent CNS: apparent species differences but good correlation with radioimmunological data, Histochemistry 71:60 (1981).
19. M. K. Raizada, Localization of insulin-like immunoreactivity in neurons from primary cultures of rat brain, Exp. Cell Res. 143:351 (1983).

20. S. J. Chan, V. Episkopov, S. Zeitlin, S. D. Karathanasis, A. Mackrell, D. F. Steiner, and A. Efstratiadis, Guinea pig preproinsulin gene: an evolutionary compromise?, Proc. Natl. Acad. Sci. 81:5046 (1984).
21. N. P. Birch, D. L. Christie, and A. G. C. Renwick, Proinsulin-like material in mouse foetal brain cell cultures, FEBS Let. 168:299 (1984).
22. D. W. Clarke, L. Mudd, F. T. Boyd, Jr., M. Fields, and M. K. Raizada, Insulin is released from rat brain neuronal cells in culture, J. Neurochem. 47:831 (1986).
23. G. C. Budd, B. Pansky, B. Cordell, Insulin or insulin-like peptides in the pituitary gland, J. Cell Biol. 97:404A (1983).
24. C. H. Lee, B. C. Lin, E. Costa, D. M. Chuang, Detection of mRNA species in the brain and other tissues of rat which hybridize with proinsulin gene, Fed. Proc. 43:2219 (1984).
25. D. L. Cooper and D. W. Clarke, Transcription of the insulin gene in the brain and submandibular gland of the rat, Pediatr. Res. 19:311A (1985).
26. W. S. Young, Periventricular hypothalamic cells in the rat brain contain insulin mRNA, Neuropeptides 8:93 (1986).
27. D. W. Clarke, F. T. Boyd, Jr., M. S. Kappy, and M. K. Raizada, Insulin stimulates macromolecular synthesis in cultured glial cells from rat brain, Am. J. Physiol. 249:C484 (1985).
28. D. G. Puro and E. Agardh, Insulin-mediated regulation of neuronal maturation, Science 225:1170 (1984).
29. R. A. Palovicik, M. I. Phillips, M. S. Kappy, and M. K. Raizada, Insulin inhibits pyramidal neurons in hippocampal slices, Brain Res. 309:187-191 (1984).
30. A. Sauter, M. Goldstein, J. Engel, and K. Ueta, Effect of insulin on central catecholamines, Brain Res. 260:330 (1983).
31. M. Barbaccia, D. Chuang, and D. Costa, Is insulin a neuromodulator?, Adv. Biochem. Psychopharmacol. 33:511 (1982).
32. F. T. Boyd, Jr., D. W. Clarke, T. F. Muther, and M. K. Raizada, Insulin receptors and insulin modulation of norepinephrine uptake in neuronal cultures from rat brain, J. Biol. Chem. 260:15880 (1985).
33. S. C. Woods, E. C. Lotter, L. D. McKay, and D. Porte, Jr., Chronic intracerebroventricular infusion of insulin reduces food intake and body weight of baboons, Nature 282:503-505 (1979).
34. A. J. Szabo and O. Szabo, Influence of the insulin sensitive central nervous system glucoregulator receptor on hepatic glucose metabolism, J. Physiol. 253:121 (1975).
35. S. C. Woods, D. Porte, Jr., Effect of intracisternal insulin on plasma glucose and insulin in the dog, Diabetes 24:905 (1975).

LOCALIZATION OF INSULIN TO NEURONAL CELLS

Sherin Devaskar, Ruben Schechter and Arnold Kahn

Department of Pediatrics, St. Louis University
Cardinal Glennon Children's Hospital and The Pediatric
Research Institute, St. Louis, MO

Insulin has been identified in the brain of various animal species[1], including the human[2]. Although various biologic effects for insulin have been described in the central nervous system[3,4,5], the exact origin of the peptide remains unclear. A local (i.e. central nervous system) origin for the peptide has been suggested by some groups of investigators[5,6], while others contend that insulin enters the brain from the blood vascular system [7]. For example, Frank et al, using ^{125}I-insulin, demonstrated the hormone's ability to cross the neonatal rabbit blood-brain barrier[7]. In subsequent studies, the mechanism by which insulin traverses the vascular endothelium was not clear as there was an absence of externalization (as a part of transcytosis) of the hormone at the brain capillary antiluminal membrane[8]. Baskin et al observed the uptake of insulin by the adult rat hypothalamus to be from cerebro-spinal fluid[9]. The cerebrospinal fluid insulin levels in turn have been found to correlate closely with plasma insulin concentrations[10,11]. On the other hand, insulin mRNA has been demonstrated in the brain[5,12], providing the essential biochemical basis for the local synthesis of hormone.

In previous studies, using an acid-ethanol brain extract from fetal rabbits (28d; term ~31d) and quantitating the insulin content by a radioimmunoassay[13], we estimated that there exists ~4 ng of insulin per gm of brain (wet weight). Exogenous administration of insulin raised the fetal plasma insulin concentrations considerably above control (table 1), but, failed to increase brain insulin content. Only intracranial administration of hormone succeeded in raising the brain insulin content.

Recently, employing a more sensitive enzyme-linked immunosorbant assay (ELISA), we have measured insulin content in younger fetal rabbit brains (gestational ages 22, 25 and 27d). A monoclonal anti-insulin antibody (Biogenex) at a 1:10,000 dilution was employed for this purpose after its specificity was confirmed by yielding a positive peroxidase-antiperoxidase staining of fetal pancreatic islet cells and by the absence of cross-reactivity with insulin-like growth factor I (Amgen). Figure 1 demonstrates the standard curve obtained with authentic insulin and brain extract; there being much less insulin on a weight to weight (w/w) basis in the latter when compared to the former. There were no significant differences at the various gestational ages studied[15].

In an attempt to determine the location of insulin in the brain (27d), we employed the peroxidase-antiperoxidase technique of Sternberger[14] to Bouin's cryostat and paraffin-fixed brain and fetal pancreatic slices. In the pancreas, a positive insulin-immunoreaction was observed at a 1:10,000

Table 1

Groups (n)	Plasma insulin µU/ml	Fetal Brain Insulin content ng/g
Systemic insulin:		
Control (5)	13.72±1.60	4.44±2.39
1 U (4)	103.13±34.63*	4.68±0.78
2 U (4)	288.3±51.0***	4.58±0.64
p (ANOVA)	<0.01	NS
Intracranial insulin:		
Control (5)	22.25±1.27	3.74±1.17
0.01 U (4)	36.5±13.5	16.06±2.76**
0.1 U (5)	36.33±8.10	133.07±35.76**
p (ANOVA)	NS	<0.01

t-test: p * <0.05, ** <0.01, *** <0.001, when compared to the respective control. NS = not significant.

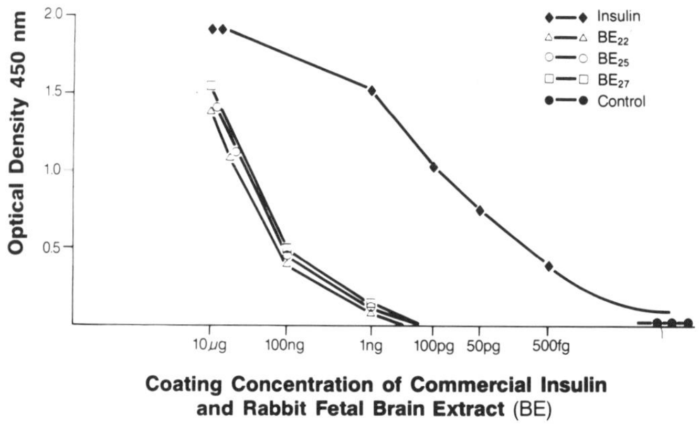

Figure 1

The dose response curves for authentic insulin and brain extract insulin as determined by the ELISA.

dilution of the anti-insulin antibody. On the other hand, at antibody dilutions as high as 1:20, no immunoreactivity was detected in the brain slices. This absence of reaction may be secondary to the fact that insulin is present in very small amounts in the brain or is altered by tissue fixation thereby masking its recognition by the antibody. We therefore, used isolated brain cells in culture as an alternative target for staining. Neuron-enriched (~80%) cultures[5] and glial cell cultures[3] were isolated as described previously. Neurons were identified by a positive immunoreaction to neuron-specific enolase[16], and glial cells by the presence of fibrillary acidic protein[3]. At a 1:100 anti-insulin antibody dilution, we demonstrated

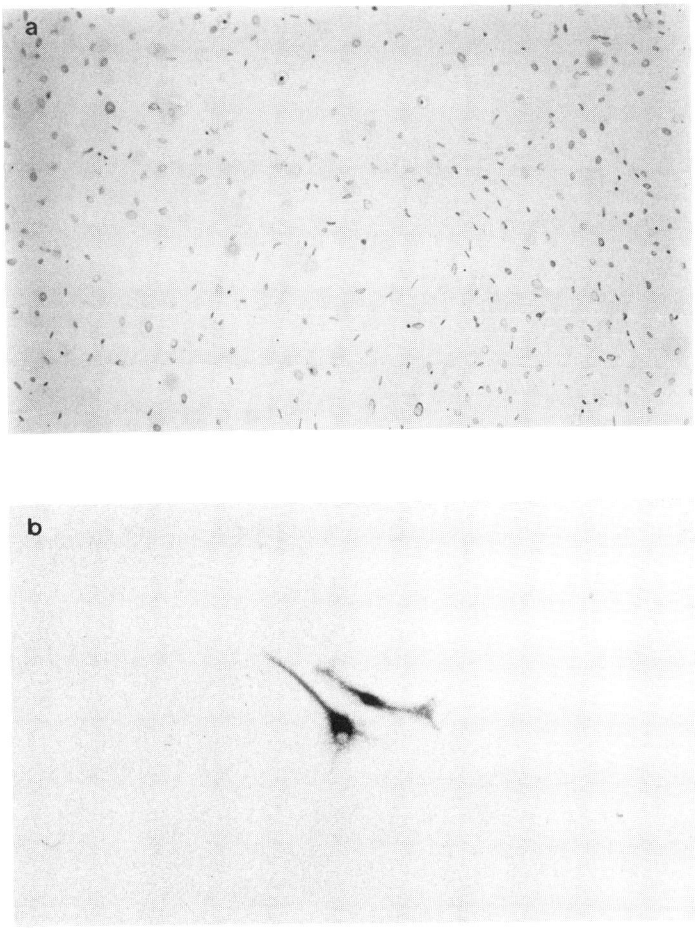

Figure 2

a) Control: Porcine insulin pre-absorbed antisera was incubated with neuron-enriched cultures. The cells were later, counter-stained with hematoxylin (95x).

b) Anti-insulin antibody (1:100) was incubated with neuron-enriched cultures yielding a positive insulin immunoreaction (330x).

a positive immunoreaction in ~3 to 5% of neurons. All glial cells were negative. Mouse serum and porcine insulin pre-absorbed antisera were used as controls. The reaction product for insulin in neurons was generally light, diffuse but more pronounced in the axonal processes than the cell body. Pre-treatment of cells with monensin, a K+ ionophore that prevents secretion of cellular proteins[17], resulted in an enhancement of the insulin immunoreaction but did not increase the percentage of positive cells (figure 2). The latter finding suggests that insulin is a secretory product of at least a subset of neurons[18].

Following the identification of the hormone in neurons, we attempted to establish whether these cells were the actual site of insulin synthesis by in situ hybridization. Rat insulin cDNA[19] was biotin-labeled and introduced into fixed, permeabilized neuronal cultures for a period of 18 hours at 37°C under low stringency conditions[20]. After thorough washing, the residual hybridized biotinylated cDNA was complexed to strepavidin-peroxidase and detected by using 3',5'-diaminobenzadine as a chromogen[14]. The biotinylated vector, pBR322 lacking the insulin insert, served as a control. As shown in figure 3, a subset of neurons (~3 to 5%) did exhibit a positive hybridization signal, confirming (i) that only a small fraction of cells is likely to be involved in insulin synthesis and (ii) that insulin synthesis does take place in the nervous system.

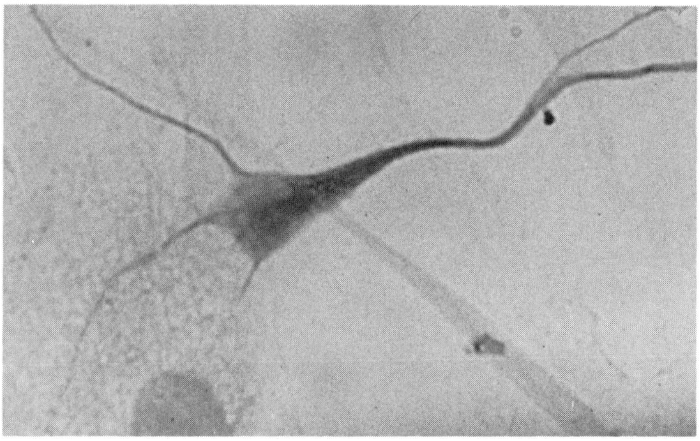

Figure 2

c) Higher magnification (750x) of a neuron demonstrating a positive insulin immunoreaction. Counter staining was with hematoxylin.

Recently, hybridizing ^{35}S-labeled oligodeoxyribonucleotide probe for insulin with frozen sections from the adult rat brain, Young observed the presence of labeled cells in the hypothalamic periventricular nucleus next to the ependymal lining of the third ventricle after 1 to 3 months of autoradiographic exposure, thereby demonstrating the presence of insulin mRNA. Specific structural localization of the peptide may be why we observed a certain subset of neurons alone to demonstrate the presence of both the insulin peptide and mRNA. Our data are consistent with the fact, that insulin is synthesized in the central nervous system but do not exclude other (additional) sources of insulin.

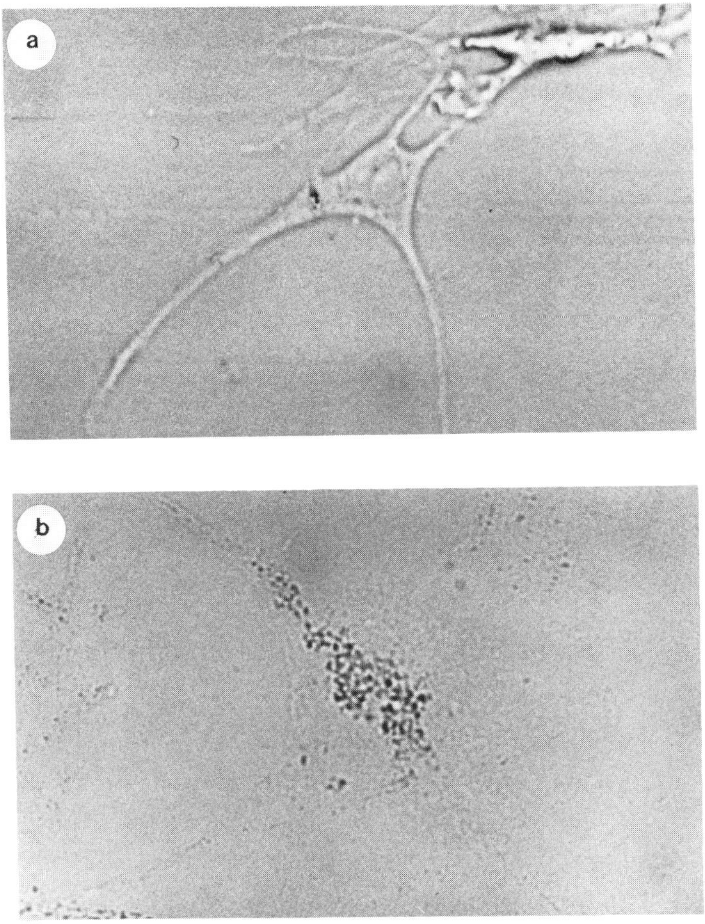

Figure 3

a) Control: Neurons hybridized with the biotinylated vector pBR322, lacking the insulin insert (750x).

b) Neurons hybridized with the biotinylated rat insulin cDNA (750x).

Acknowledgement:

The authors acknowledge the secretarial assistance of Ms. Vicki Shipp.

References:

1. D. LeRoith, S. A. Hendricks, M. A. Lesniak, S. Rishi, K. L. Becker, J. Havrankova, J. L. Rosenweig, M. J. Brownstein, and J. Roth, Insulin in brain and other extrapancreatic tissues of vertebrates and non-vertebrates. Adv. Metab. Disorders, Vol 10, p303-340 (1983).
2. A. Dorn, H. G. Bernstein, A. Rinne, H. J. Hahn and M. Ziegler, Insulin like immunoreactivity in the human brain. Histochem. 74:293 (1982).

3. D. W. Clarke, F. T. Boyd, M. S. Kappy and M. K. Raizada, Insulin stimulation macromolecular synthesis in cultured glial cells from rat brain. Am. J. Physiol. 249:C484-C489 (1985).
4. D. G. Puro and E. Agardh, Insulin-mediated regulation of neuronal maturation. Science 225:1170 1172 (1984).
5. F. T. Boyd Jr., D. W. Clarke, T. F. Muther and M. K. Raizada, Insulin receptors and insulin modulation of norepinephrine uptake in neuronal cultures from rat brain. J. Biol. Chem. 260:15880-15884 (1985).
6. J. Havrankova, D. Schmechel, J. Roth, M. Brownstein, Identification of insulin in rat brain. Proc. Natl. Acad. Sci. USA 75:5737-5741 (1978).
7. H. J. L. Frank, T. Jankovic-Vokes, W. M. Partridge and W. L. Morris, Enhanced insulin binding to blood brain barrier in vivo and to brain microvessels in vitro in newborn rabbits. Diabetes 34:728-733 (1985).
8. H. J. L. Frank, W. M. Partridge, W. L. Morris, R. G. Rosenfield and T. B. Choi, Binding and internalization of insulin and insulin-like growth factors by isolated brain microvessels. Diabetes 35:654-661 (1986).
9. D. G. Baskin, S. C. Woods, D. B. West, M. vanHouten, B. I. Posner, D. M. Dorsa and D. Porte Jr., Immunocytochemical detection of insulin in rat hypothalamus and its possible uptake from cerebrospinal fluid. Endocrinol. 113:1818-1825 (1983).
10. B. J. Wallum, G. J. Taborsky Jr., D. Porte, D. P. Figlewicz, L. Jacobson, J. C. Beard, W. K. Ward and D. Dorsa, Cerebrospinal fluid insulin levels increase during intravenous insulin infusions in man. J. Clin. Endocrinol. Metab. 64:190-194 (1987).
11. L. J. Stein, D. M. Dorsa, D. G. Baskin, D. P. Figlewicz, N. Ikeda, S. P. Frankmann, M. R. C. Greenwood, D. Porte Jr., S. C. Woods, Immunoreactive insulin levels are elevated in the cerebrospinal fluid of genetically obese Zucker rats. Endocrinol. 113:2299 (1983).
12. L. Villa-Komaroff, A. Gonzales, H. Y Song, B. Wentworth, P. Dobnes, Novel insulin related sequences in fetal brain. Adv. Exp. Med. Biol. 181:65 (1984).
13. S. U. Devaskar, L. Karycki and U. P. Devaskar, Varying brain insulin concentrations differently regulate the fetal brain insulin receptor. Biochem. Biophys. Res. Commun. 136:208-219 (1986).
14. L. A. Sternberger, P. M. Hardy Jr., J. J. Cuculis and H. G. Meyer, The unlabeled antibody enzyme method of immunohistochemistry. J. Histochem. Cytochem. 18:315-333 (1970).
15. R. Schechter, L. Karycki, A. Kahn and S. Devaskar, The identification of an insulin-like substance in the fetal rabbit brain (Abstr) Clin. Res. 34:982A (1986).
16. M. K. Raizada, Localization of insulin-like immunoreactivity in the neurons from primary cultures of rat brain. Exp. Cell Res. 143: 351-357 (1983).
17. R. M. Hembry, G. Murphy, T. E. Causton, J. T. Dingle, J. J. Reynolds, Characterization of a specific antiserum for mammalian collagenase from several species: Immunolocalization of collagenase in rabbit chrondrocytes and uterus. J. Cell Sci. 00:1-19 (1981).
18. R. Schechter, L. Karycki, F. Sadiq, T. Hilliard, A. Kahn and S. Devaskar, Antibody staining and in situ hybridization reveals that a subset of neurons in the rabbit neonatal brain produce insulin. (Abstr) Pediatric Research (1987) In Press.
19. A. Permutt, J. Chirgurin, S. Giddings, K. Kakita and P. Rothwein, Insulin Biosynthesis and Diabetes Mellitus. Clin. Biochem. 14(5): 230-236 (1981).

20. P. Liesi, J. P. Julein, P. Vilja, F. Grosveld and L. Rechardt, Specific detection of neuronal cell bodies: In situ hybridization with a biotin-labeled neurofilament cDNA probe. J. Histochem. Cytochem. 34:923-926 (1986).
21. W. S. Young, Periventricular hypothalamic cells in the rat brain contain insulin mRNA. Neuropeptides 8:93-97 (1986).

SYNTHESIS OF INSULIN OR A SIMILAR PEPTIDE IN THE PITUITARY GLAND AND IN RETINAL MULLER CELLS

G. Colin Budd and Ben Pansky

Departments of Physiology and Anatomy
Medical College of Ohio
Toledo, Ohio 43699

INTRODUCTION

Insulin or insulin-like peptides have been reported to be present in, and may be synthesized by, organisms that do not have pancreatic beta cells (LeRoith, et al., 1980, 1981, 1983; Falkner, et al., 1975; Meneses and Oritz, 1975; Duve and Thorpe, 1979; Yuri, et al., 1980)., Similar reports have appeared claiming localization and possible synthesis of insulin in the extrapancreatic tissues of vertebrates (Hendricks, et al.,1983). Proposed extrapancreatic sites of insulin synthesis in mammalian species have including the brain (Havrankova, et al., 1978; Raizada, et al., 1979; Bernstein, et al., 1980; Rosenzweig, et al.,1980; Stevenson, 1982; Raizada, et al., 1983; Lee, et al., 1984; Clarke, et al., 1986), rodent and human pituitary (Hatfield, et al., 1981; Budd, et al., 1986; Budd, et al., 1987), rodent and human retina (Das et al., 1984, 1985), human retinoblastoma cells (Pansky, et al., 1986), , yolk sac (Muglia and Locker, 1984), human placenta (Liu, et al., 1985) and mouse seminal vesicle (Stahler et al., 1986, 1987).

EXPERIMENTAL APPROACHES

A variety of experimental methods have been used by different investigators to evaluate the possible synthesis of insulin outside the pancreas. These investigators have not questioned the accepted evidence, acquired over 60 years ago, that the beta cells of the pancreatic islets synthesize insulin and release it into the circulation for distribution to target organs. However, there is now widespread interest in the possible synthesis of small amounts of insulin in extrapancreatic tissues for local activity in metabolism, growth promotion, neurohumoral modulation or possibly in neurotransmission.

One approach has been to chemically extract fresh tissue to obtain fractions that are enriched for peptides with the characteristics expected for insulin. These extracts are then investigated with sensitive radio-immunoassay methods to identify and quantitate insulin. This approach was used to determine the concentration of immunoreactive insulin in extracts of the mammalian brain. In some cases it has been shown that immuno-reactive insulin in the extracts corresponded to a tissue concentration that was higher than the plasma insulin concentration (Havrankova et al., 1978; Rosenzweig et al., 1980).

In other investigations, insulin-like immunoreactivity has been demonstrated by immunocytochemical techniques using tissue sections (frozen, paraffin- and epoxy-embedded tissues) and freshly isolated cell cultures. This technique has been used on brain, pituitary and retinal sections as well as on cell cultures of brain, pituitary and retinal Muller cells (Havrankova et al., 1978; Pansky & Hatfield, 1978; Hatfield et al., 1981; Dorn et al., 1981; Raizada 1983; Budd et al., 1986; Das et al., 1984; Pansky et al., 1986). The procedure involves the application of diluted anti-insulin antiserum followed by the detection of specific insulin antigen-antibody reactions within specific cells with one of a variety of specific histochemical reactions. The location of antigen-antibody reactions is detected by fluorescence, enzyme-labeling or autoradiography in conjunction with light or electron microscopy. To exclude the possibility of any uptake of exogenous insulin present in the medium, and to allow time for depletion of previously absorbed insulin, the cultured cells can be grown for 24 hours or more in serum-free medium before immunocytochemical staining.

Immunocytochemistry is a widely accepted technique for demonstrating the distribution of antigenic determinants, but it does not necessarily demonstrate sites of synthesis of the antigen. All cells, to some extent, incorporate molecules from their environment, and in some cells, including adrenergic neurons, the exogenous molecules are taken up and concentrated within secretory granules. Many cells also possess specific receptors to which antigens may be attached. Thus, the demonstration of insulin-like immunoreactivity in specific cells may be due to one or a number of possibilities including: a) the insulin-like activity may result from temporary binding of circulating pancreatic insulin to insulin receptors; b) uptake and storage in these cells; or c) the peptide may be locally synthesized in these cells.

A more direct approach is required, once a site of insulin accumulation or a potential synthesis site has been discovered, to determine if the cells are synthesizing insulin. All cells contain the gene for insulin in the chromosomal DNA but for the gene to be expressed, the DNA must be transcribed into messenger RNA (mRNA) which acts as the template for biosynthesis of insulin. If it can be shown that the cells contain insulin mRNA, it is reasonable to assume that they can synthesize insulin. Methods are available for isolation of poly A-mRNA (the form in which most eucaryotic mRNA is found) from tissues so that they can be used as templates for the production of complementary DNA (cDNA) fragments. The cDNA fragments can then be cloned and purified to be labeled and used as probes for the identification of specific mRNA species within mRNA extracts or intact cells by the procedure known as *in situ* hybridization. The *in situ* hybridization technique has been used in conjunction with a labeled rat or human insulin cDNA probe, to detect the presence of the intracellular insulin mRNA required for the *de novo* biosynthesis of insulin (Budd et al., 1986).

The *in situ* molecular hybridization method has been used, with labeled RNA or DNA probes, for the identification and localization of specific DNA nucleotide sequences in chromosomes (Gall & Pardue, 1971), viral RNA sequences in infected cells (Brahic & Haase, 1978), oncogenes in normal and transformed cells (Stoner et al., 1987) and for the localization of specific mRNA sequences within individual cells in tissue sections and monolayer cell cultures (Gee et al., 1983: Budd, et al., 1986; Das, et al., 1985).

It is important to employ appropriate positive and negative controls in both the immunocytochemical methods and the in situ hybridization technique. For immunocytochemistry, sections of pancreatic islets containing beta cells, or cultured beta cells serve as suitable positive controls. Negative controls include replacement of the insulin antiserum with antiserum against a different peptide, replacement with non-immune serum or bovine serum albumin or replacement with antigen-absorbed antiserum. Positive controls for in situ hybridization include pancreatic beta cells, which can confidently be expected to contain insulin mRNA. Negative controls include replacement of labeled insulin cDNA with a different specific cDNA (e.g. application of labeled growth hormone cDNA to pancreatic beta cells), replacement with a labeled non-specific oligonucleotide or plasmid DNA (e.g. labeled pBR322 plasmid DNA would not be expected to hybridize with specific mammalian cells) or pre-hybridization with unlabeled insulin cDNA to saturate the specific intracellular mRNA prior to hybridization with labeled insulin cDNA and thereby greatly reducing hybridization with the labeled probe.

RESULTS

We have studied whole brain tissue and tissue sections from rodents using radioimmunoassay and immunocytochemical techniques and pituitary and retinal tissues from rats, mice, hamsters and humans with immunocytochemical and in situ hybridization methods. The methods used to localize immunoreactivity to insulin antisera and hybridizable mRNA in situ have been described previously (Budd et al., 1986;). The pituitary and retinal studies were undertaken following initial studies in the CNS because of their close relationship to the CNS including their embryological origin, which endows them with neurons and glia that have been shown to contain a number of peptides. Human pituitary tissue was obtained during surgical removal of pituitary adenomas, or at autopsy, in appropriately selected cases (Budd et al., 1987). In addition, as it is difficult to grow human ocular tissue, especially retinal cells, in culture and no normal human retinal cell lines are available, we have investigated cells from a human retinoblastoma cell line (Y-79 cells) which have been maintained in continuous culture since 1971.

It was found with immunofluorescence staining of fresh frozen sections of brain and immunoperoxidase staining of sections of epoxy embedded fixed brain, that cell bodies and cytoplasmic processes of ependymal cells lining the ventricles were immunoreactive with insulin antisera. Ependymal cells of the ventricles (tanycytes) are known to have basal processes which branch and contact neurons, glia and periventricular capillaries. In addition, neurons and glia in the parenchyma lateral to the third ventricle in the hypothalamus were also immunoreactive.The choroid plexi of the third, lateral and fourth ventricles were also immunoreactive.

A significant finding that drew attention to the pituitary gland was the presence of immunoreactivity to insulin antisera in ependymal cell processes in the floor of the third ventricle, in the median eminence and occasionally in cell processes making contact with capillaries of the portal vasculature in the median eminence. Appropriate controls were carried out with these investigations.

A series of experiments using tissue sections of both paraffin and epoxy embedded material and also freshly isolated and cultured pituitary cells from several rodent species resulted in the demonstration of

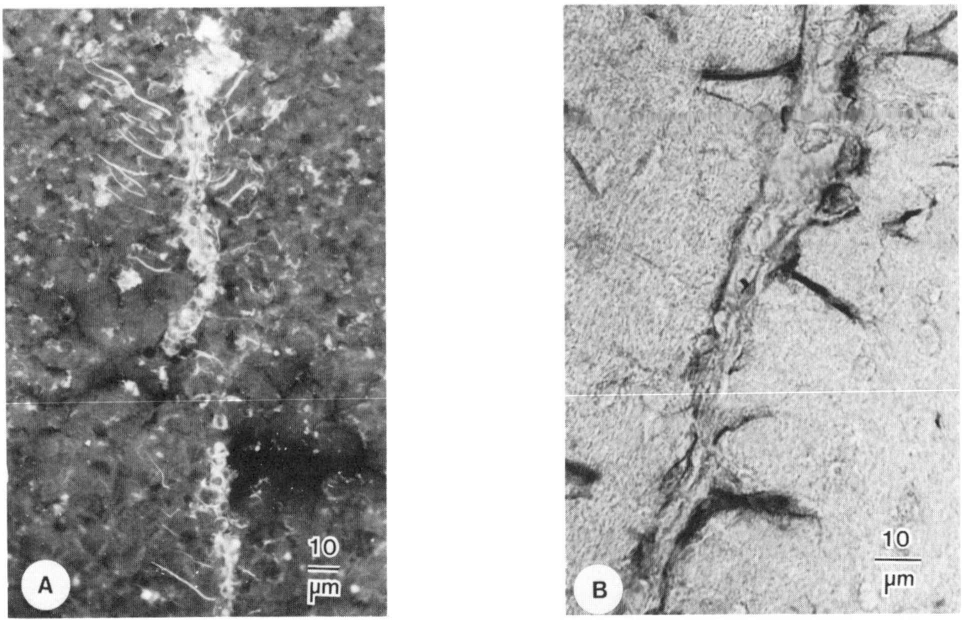

Fig. 1. A. Immunofluorescence localization of insulin, using guinea pig anti-insulin antiserum and fluoresceinated goat anti-guinea pig anti-IgG, in third ventricular tanycytes at the level of the hypothalamic ventromedial nucleus. B. Immunoreactive tanycyte processes of the third ventricle after using guinea pig anti-insulin antiserum followed by the PAP immunocytochemical procedure. Cytoplasm and processes are stained.

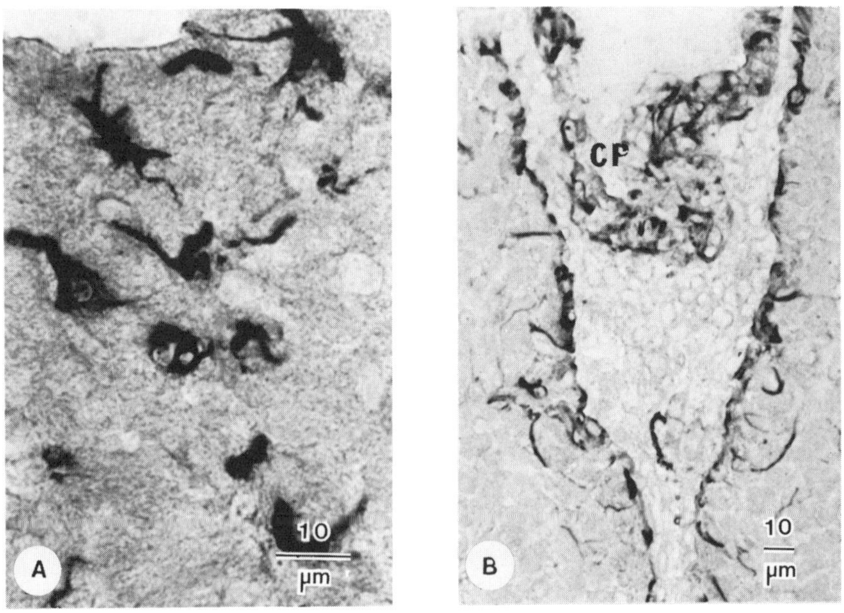

Fig. 2. Tissue sections of mouse brain adjacent to third ventricle treated with guinea pig anti-porcine insulin antiserum (PAP method). A. Cell bodies and processes of neuronal and glial elements show immunoreactivity. B. Tanycyte processes and choroid plexus (CP) in the third ventricle show immunoreactivity.

immunoreactivity to insulin antisera in anterior pituitary cells (Budd et al., 1986). Similar positive immunoreactivity has been observed in sections of human surgical and autopsy specimens (Budd, et al., 1987). Electron microscopic immunocytochemistry has revealed specifically stained cytoplasmic granules in some anterior pituitary cells. These studies are still in progress.

The presence of insulin-like immunoreactivity in pituitary cells may be due to uptake of circulating insulin released from the pancreas. Alternatively, there could be local synthesis within the pituitary cells themselves. Immunocytochemical staining alone is unable to distinguish between these possibilities. The detection of mRNA in the cytoplasm of cells by in situ DNA-RNA hybridization is a more definitive approach for demonstrating sites of synthesis of the specific peptide in question. Recently this technique, utilizing labeled insulin or proinsulin cDNA, has been carried out on cultured cells and extracted RNAs from tissues to demonstrate extrapancreatic insulin synthesis. Thus, extrapancreatic insulin gene expression has been shown to occur in cultured rat pituitary cells (Budd et al., 1986), rat yolk sac (Muglia & Locker, 1984), rat brain (Lee et al., 1984) and human placenta (Liu et al., 1985). Evidence is now accumulating in our laboratory from in situ RNA-DNA hybridization, that mouse, rat and hamster pituitary cells contain insulin messenger RNA (mRNA) which is a pre-requisite for the synthesis of insulin (Budd, et al 1986). Investigations are in progress to determine if insulin mRNA is also present in human anterior pituitary cells.

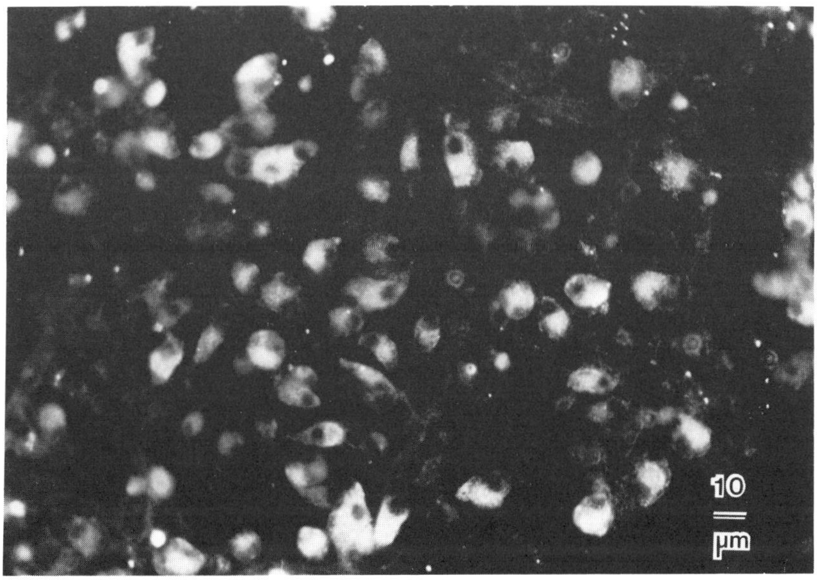

Fig. 3. Cultured mouse pituitary cells: immunofluorescent staining for insulin. Note cytoplasmic fluorescence as well as variable cell staining.

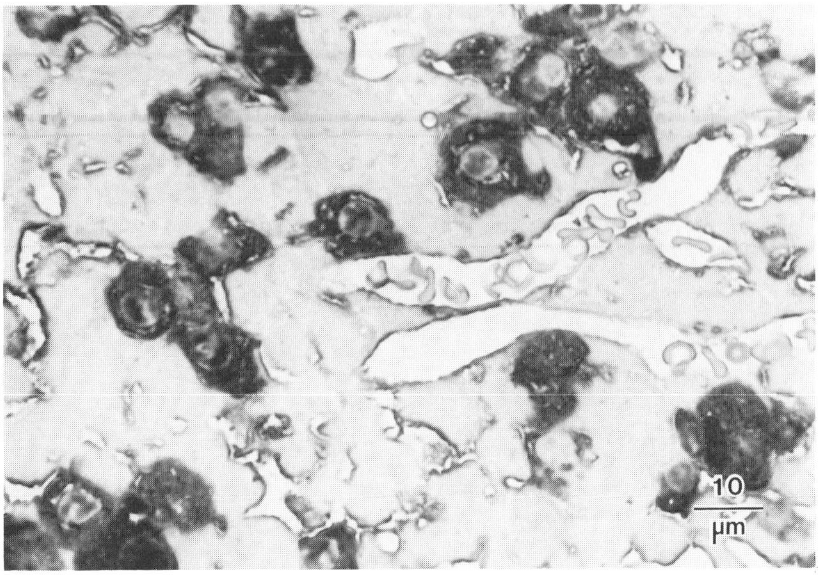

Fig. 4. Tissue section of mouse anterior pituitary using guinea pig anti-porcine insulin antiserum (1:400) and the peroxidase anti-peroxidase (PAP) staining procedure. Stained cells are seen with predominantly cytoplasmic staining among unstained cells, and vessels containing blood cells

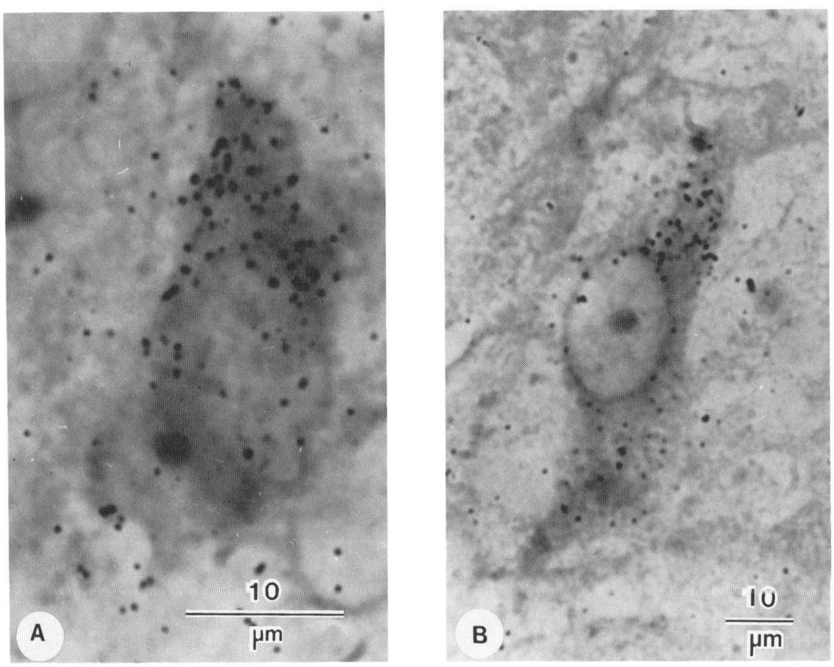

Fig. 5. A. Autoradiograph of cultured mouse anterior pituitary cells hybridized _in situ_ with P-32-labeled rat insulin cDNA. Autoradiographic grains are concentrated over the cytoplasm of a small fraction of epithelial cells. AR-10 emulsion, D-19 developer. B. _In situ_ hybridization of P-32-labeled insulin cDNA to cultured mouse anterior pituitary cells. Grains occur mainly over the cytoplasm of labeled cells. AR-10 emulsion

Immunoreactivity to insulin antisera has also been demonstrated in the cytoplasm of rat and human retinal Muller (glial) cells in both tissue sections and primary cultures of isolated rat retinal glial cells and human retinoblastoma cells. Similar glial cell immunoreactivity was observed in sections of the optic nerve and optic tract (Das et al., 1984). In addition, it was demonstrated that the rat Muller cells and human retinoblastoma cells contain a mRNA that specifies the synthesis of insulin or a closely homologous peptide (Das et al., 1985).

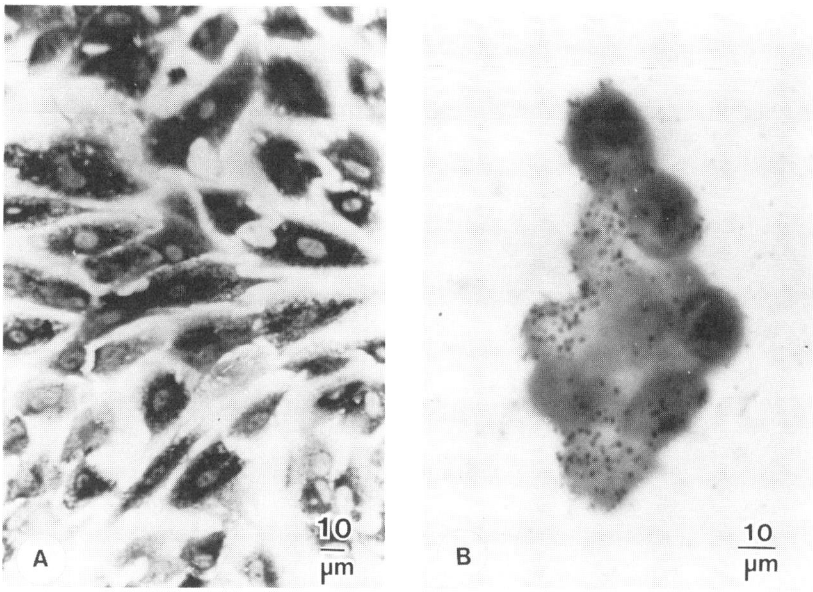

Fig. 6. A. Cultured rat retinal glial cells 24 days after plating, immunocytochemically stained with the PAP technique following the application of guinea pig anti-porcine insulin antiserum. B. Autoradiograph of cultured human retinoblastoma Y-79 cells hybridized <u>in situ</u> with tritium-labeled human insulin cDNA. Autoradiographic grains are seen to be heavily concentrated over the cytoplasm of the cells. AR-10 emulsion, D-19 developer.

DISCUSSION

The presence of immunoreactivity to insulin antisera has been observed in ependymal tanycytes in the rodent hypothalamus (Hatfield et al., 1978, 1981). Using a combination of immuno-cytochemistry and <u>in situ</u> DNA-mRNA hybridization it has also been demonstrated that rodent and human anterior pituitary cells and retinal glial cells contain, and possibly can synthesize, insulin or insulin-like transcripts (Budd et al., 1986).

The role that insulin or insulin-like peptides may play in pituitary or retinal functions is unknown. It may modulate cell metabolism and hormone secretion. Local synthesis within these sites could ensure continuous adequate local levels when circulating pancreatic levels fluctuate or are chronically reduced. If investigations continue to provide evidence for insulin or insulin-like peptide synthesis in these areas in human tissue, to correlate with that which has been obtained with rodents (Budd, et al 1986), it will be important to know if such cells exert an autocrine or paracrine influence on the synthesis and release of specific hormones or other substances, and what effect these may have on local cellular functions.

The physiological significance of the presence of insulin and other peptides in the CNS, pituitary and retina is controversial but their localization in these tissues implies that they may play a role in retinal function, possibly as neurotransmitters or neuromodulators (Varandani, et al., 1982; Karton & Brecha, 1983; Boyd, et al., 1985). In the CNS, it has been shown that insulin may play a role as a neuromodulator by stimulating the synaptosomal uptake of neurotransmitter amino acids (Rhoads, et al., 1984). The in vitro co-culture of cholinergic retinal neurons and muscle cells raises the possibility that insulin may serve as a developmental signal to regulate the emergence of effective neurotransmission across nascent synapses in the retina (Puro & Agardh, 1984). Insulin may also be important in modulating glucose or amino acid metabolism in these tissues. This is consistent, at least in the retina, with the fact that the Muller cell synthesizes and stores glycogen, and is active in glycolysis (Kuwabara & Cogan, 1961). Insulin in the retina may also serve a role in intercellular signalling (paracrine) as speculated in other extrapancreatic tissues (Rosenzweig et al., 1980).

Other investigative methods being used to identify the pituitary peptide retinal peptide(s) which may be very similar to insulin include: 1) isolation and identification of the specific labeled peptide from cell cultures of both tissues after providing them with labeled amino acid precursors in an insulin-free medium; 2) studying the effects of various peptides added to the cultured cells; 3) immuno-cytochemistry and in situ hybridization in conjunction with electron microscopic studies to more clearly identify the localization of intracellular sites; and 4) sequence identification of a specific clone in a cDNA library obtained by reverse transcription from RNA isolated from these cells

Our demonstration of insulin-like immunoreactivity and insulin-specific mRNA in anterior pituitary and retinal glial cells strengthens the concept that there may be extrapancreatic synthesis of insulin. The physiological role of extrapancreatic insulin or insulin-related peptide remains uncertain. However, it could be very significant for our further understanding of the pathogenesis of diabetes, especially as it involves the CNS, pituitary, retina and other interrelated systems.

ACKNOWLEDGEMENTS

The authors acknowledge the collaboration of Doctors James Hatfield, Barbara Cordell, Hardress Waller, Richard Lane, Carol Kollarits, Arup Das, Louis Glatzer, Michael Stahler, Ted Reid and Neilma Budd and the technical assistance of Angela Lineen in their investigations. This work was supported by grants AM 33761 and EY06886 from the National Institutes of Health of the United States of America and the Ohio Lions Eye Research Foundation.

BIBLIOGRAPHY

Bernstein, H.G., Dorn, A., Hahn, H-J., Kostmann, G., and Ziegler, M., 1980, Cellular localization of insulin-like immunoreactivity in the central nervous system of spiny mice, C56B16J and C57BlKsJ mice. Acta Histochem. Cytochem. 13:623-628

Boyd, F.T., Jr., Clarke, D.W., Muther, T.F. and Raizada, M.K., 1985, Insulin receptors and insulin modulation of norepinephrine uptake in neuronal cultures from rat brain. J. Biol. Chem. 15:15880-15884

Brahic, M. and Haase, A.T., 1978, Detection of viral sequences of low reiteration frequency by in situ hybridization. Proc. Natl. Acad. Sci. USA 75:6125-6129

Budd, G.C., Pansky, B., Cordell, B., 1986, Detection of insulin synthesis in mammalian anterior pituitary cells by immunocytochemistry and demonstration of insulin-related transcripts by in-situ RNA-DNA hybridization. J. of Histochem. Cytochem. 34:673-678

Budd, G.C., Pansky, B. and Budd, N.J., 1987, Insulin or insulin-like peptides in the human pituitary. Ann. Clin. Lab. Sci. (In Press)

Clarke, D.W., Mudd, L., Boyd, F.T., Jr., Fields, M. and Raizada, M.K., 1986, Insulin is released from rat brain neuronal cells in culture. J. Neurochem. 47:831-836

Das, A., Pansky, B., Budd, G.C. and Kollarits, C.R., 1984, Immunocytochemistry of mouse and human retina with antisera to insulin and S-100 protein. Curr. Eye Res. 3:1397-1403

Das, A., Budd, G.C., Pansky, B., Cordell, B., and Kollarits, C.R., 1985, Insulin-specific mRNA in rat retinal glial cells. Invest. Ophthalmol. Vis. Sci., Suppl. 26(3):337

Dorn A, Bernstein HG, Hahn HJ, Ziegler M, and Rummelfanger H., 1981, Insulin immunocytochemistry of the rodent's CNS: apparent species differences but good correlation with radioimmunological data. Histochemistry 71:609

Duve, H., Thorpe, A., 1979, Immunofluorescent localization of insulin-like material in the medial secretory cells of the blowfly Calliphora vomitoria. Cell Tissue Res. 200:187-191

Falkner, S., Emdin, S., Havu, N., Lundgren, G., Marques, M., Ostberg, Y., Steiner, D.F., and Thomas, N.W., 1975, Insulin in invertebrates and cyclostomes. Am Zool. 13:625-638

Gall, J.G., and Pardue, M.L., 1971, Nucleic acid hybridization in cytological preparations. In: "Methods in Enzymology," Vol. XXI. L. Grossman and K. Moldave, eds., Academic Press, New York.

Gee, C.E., Chen, C-L., Roberts, J.L., Thompson, R., Watson, S.J., 1983, Identification of the proopiomelanocortin neurones in rat hypothalamus by in situ cDNA-mRNA hybridization. Nature 306:374

Hatfield, J.S., Pansky, B., Waller, H. J. and Budd, G.C., 1981, Insulin-like immunoreactivity in cells of the mouse anterior pituitary. Micron 12:205-206

Hatfield, J.S., Pansky, B., Waller, H. J. and Budd, G. C., 1981, Immunoperoxidase-labeled insulin antibody localization in mouse hypothalamus and pituitary. J. Cell Biol. 83:138a

Havrankova J., Schmechel D., Roth J., and Brownstein M., 1978, Identification of insulin in the rat brain. Proc Natl Acad Sci USA 75:5737.

Hendricks S.A., Roth J., Rishi S., and Becker, K.L., 1983, Insulin in the nervous system. In "Brain Peptides," Krieger D.T., Martin J.B., and Brownstein J.J., editors. New York, John Wiley and Sons.

Karten H.J., and Brecha N., 1983, Localization of neuroactive substances in the vertebrate retina: evidence for lamination in the inner plexiform layer. Vision Res. 23:1197.

Kuwabara T., and Cogan D.G., 1961, Retinal glycogen. Arch Ophthalmol 66:680.

LeRoith D., Shiloach J., Roth J., and Lesniak, M.A., 1980, Evolutionary origins of vertebrate hormones: substances similar to insulins are native to unicellular enkaryotes. Proc Natl Acad Sci USA 77:6184.

LeRoith D., Shiloach J., Roth J., and Lesniak M.A., 1981, Insulin or a closely related molecule is native to Escherichia coli. J. Biol. Chem. 256:6533.

LeRoith D., Hendricks S.A., Lesniak M.A., Rishi S., Becker K.L., Havrankova J., Rosenzweig, J.L., Brownstein M.J., Roth J., 1983, Insulin in brain and other extrapancreatic tissues of vertebrates and nonvertebrates. In "Advances in Metabolic Diseases," Szabo A.J., Levine R., and Luft R., eds., Academic Press, New York, Vol.10.

Lee, C.H., Lin, B.C., Costa, E., and Chuang, D.M., 1984, Detection of mRNA species in the brain and other tissues of rat which hybridize with the pro-insulin gene. Fed. Proc. 43:2219A

Liu, K-S., Wang, C-Y., Mills, N., Gyves, M., and Ilan, J., 1985, Insulin genes expressed in human placenta from normal and diabetic pregnancies. Proc. Natl. Acad. Sci. USA 82: 3868-3870

Meneses, P., and Oritz, M.A., 1975, A protein extract from Drosophila melanogaster with insulin-like activity. Comp. Biochem. Physiol. 51A:483-485

Muglia, L., and Locker, J., 1984, Extrapancreatic insulin gene expression in the fetal rat. Proc. Natl. Acad. Sci. USA 81:3635-3639

Pansky, B., Das, A., Budd, G.C., and Reid, T.W., 1986, Insulin-like immunoreactivity in human retinoblastoma Y79 cell line. Neuroscience Lett. 68:187-191

Pansky B. and Hatfield J.S., 1978, Cerebral localization of insulin by immunofluorescence. Am. J. Anat. 153:459

Puro D.G. and Agardh E., 1984, Insulin-mediated regulation of neuronal maturation. Science 225:1170.

Raizada, M., 1983, Localization of insulin-like immunoreactivity in neurons from primary cultures of rat brain. Expl. Cell Res. 143:351-357

Raizada, M.K., Weyhenmeyer, J.A., Fellows, R.E., 1979, Cells cultured from rat brain synthesize immunoreactive insulin. In Vitro 15:185A

Raizada, M.K., 1983, Localization of insulin-like immunoreactivity in the neurons from primary cultures of rat brain. Exp. Cell Res. 143:351.

Rhoads, D.E., DiRocco, R.J., Osburn, L.D., Peterson, N.A., and Raghupathy, E., 1984, Stimulation of synaptosomal uptake of neurotransmitter amino acids by insulin: possible role of insulin as a neuromodulator. Biochem. Biophys. Res. Comm. 119:1198.

Rosenzweig, J.L., Havrankova, J., Lesniak, M.A., Brownstein, M., and Roth, J., 1980, Insulin is ubiquitous in exrapancreatic tissues of rats and humans. Proc. Natl. Acad. Sci. USA 77: 572-576

Stahler, M.S., Pansky, B., and Budd, G.C., 1986, Immuno-cytochemical localization of insulin-like immunoreactivity in mouse seminal vesicle. Biol. of Reprod. 35:1075-1080

Stahler, M.S., Budd, G.C., and Pansky, B., 1987, Evidence for insulin synthesis in normal mouse seminal vesicle based on in situ RNA-DNA hybridization. Biol. Reprod. (In Press)

Stevenson, R.W., 1983, Further evidence for non-pancreatic insulin immunoreactivity in guinea pig brain. Horm. Metabol. Res. 15:526-529

Stoner, G.D., You, M., Skouv, J., Budd, G.C., Pansky, B. and Wang, Y., 1987, Detection of oncogene mRNA sequences by in situ hybridization. Ann. Clin. Lab. Sci. (In Press)

Varandani, P.T., Organisciak, D.T., and Nafz, M.A., 1982, The occurrence of glutathione-insulin transhydrogenase in the retina. Invest. Ophthalmol. Vis. Sci. 22:715.

Yuri, R., Fujita, T., and Ito, A., 1980, Insulin-, glucagon-, gastrin-, pancreatic polypeptide-like immunoreactive neurons in the brain of the silkworm, Bombyx mori. Biomed. Res. 1: 42-46

INSULIN IN THE CENTRAL NERVOUS SYSTEM: A REGULATOR OF APPETITE AND BODY WEIGHT

Dianne P. Figlewicz, Stephen C. Woods, Denis G. Baskin, Daniel M. Dorsa, Barbara J. Wilcox, Leslie J. Stein, and Daniel Porte, Jr.

Depts. of Psychology, Medicine, Biological Structure
and Pharmacology
University of Washington
Seattle, WA 98195
and
Division of Metabolism and Endocrinology
VA Medical Center
1660 South Columbian Way
Seattle, WA 98108

I. THE HYPOTHESIS

Although numerous potentially physiologic actions of insulin in the central nervous system (CNS) have been identified at the cellular level, the consequences of these actions at the level of the organism have not been defined. In this chapter we advance the hypothesis that insulin may act as a regulator of body weight. In 1979, Woods and Porte suggested that insulin levels in the cerebrospinal fluid (CSF) may act as an indicator of body adiposity and provide a negative feedback signal to regulate body weight on a long term basis.[1,2] This hypothesis was based upon three lines of experimental evidence: First, basal plasma insulin levels are correlated with body adiposity. Second, CSF insulin levels represent a slow integral over time of plasma levels, with rapid fluctuations in plasma insulin levels being damped. Third, direct infusion of insulin into the CSF and into certain brain sites can result in a decrease of food intake and body weight. These three lines of evidence will be reviewed. Additionally, this chapter will provide some discussion of the possible regulation involved in generating and sensing this signal, as well as possible defects in the brain insulin system in a genetically obese rat model. Readers who wish specific discussion of issues surrounding the brain insulin system are referred to the chapters in this text by LeRoith, Heidenreich, and Raizada, and to a recent review.[3]

Basal plasma insulin levels are correlated with body adiposity

Clinical studies[4,5] have demonstrated that fat cell size, a major determinant of adipose mass, is positively and linearly correlated with body weight. Further, body weight is positively and linearly correlated with fasting plasma insulin levels. Together, these correlations suggest that adipose mass is correlated with fasting plasma insulin levels.

CSF insulin levels are a slow integral over time of plasma insulin levels

As discussed by Woods and Porte, the level of insulin in the plasma is not an ideal adiposity signal for the CNS. Plasma insulin levels fluctuate rapidly, depending on the metabolic status and needs of the organism. An alternative candidate for an adiposity signal is insulin in the cerebrospinal fluid. Reports of measureable insulin in the cerebrospinal fluid date back to the 1960's and such measurements have now been established for a number of species including rat,[6] rabbit,[7] subhuman primate,[7,8] human,[9,10] and dog.[11] However, the source of insulin in CSF has been somewhat controversial. CSF insulin may be derived from either peripheral sources or from within the CNS. It is possible that some CSF insulin is synthesized and released into the spinal fluid by the CNS. Young[12] recently reported that periventricular hypothalamic cells contain messenger RNA for insulin. However, data from a number of laboratories suggest that at least a portion of CSF insulin is derived from the periphery, and, further, that CSF insulin levels are sensitive to perturbations in peripheral insulin levels.

Studies in humans revealed that CSF insulin levels decreased following a body weight reduction diet regimen.[13] Consistent with this original human study, fasting for a number of hours results in lowered CSF insulin levels in other species, including rats[14] and baboons.[8] It has also been demonstrated that raising plasma insulin levels by feeding, glucose infusion, or insulin infusion results in significantly elevated CSF insulin levels in rats,[15] baboons,[8] dogs[16] and humans.[17] CSF insulin levels do not merely imitate plasma levels. Rather, there is a delay of 30-60 minutes before CSF insulin changes are detectable, and CSF insulin levels represent a very low percentage of plasma levels in every species examined. Experimental evidence shows that a sustained change of plasma insulin levels is needed to maintain an increase or decrease in CSF insulin levels. Since basal plasma insulin is related to adipose mass, and CSF insulin reflects steady state plasma insulin, it is reasonable to predict that CSF insulin is related to adiposity as well. Consistent with this, obese humans and rats have significantly higher CSF insulin levels than their lean controls.

The mechanism of transport of insulin from the plasma to the CSF is not understood

Although the mechanisms and anatomical sites of transport of insulin from the plasma to the CSF have not been elucidated, several independent lines of evidence suggest that transport is not simply diffusion, but rather involves a process which is saturable and may be regulated.

Insulin transport into the CSF from plasma may be receptor-mediated.[18,19] For example, it has been documented that macro-and microvessel endothelial cells are capable of internalizing receptor-bound insulin and releasing most of it in an intact state.[20,21,22,23] Further, in a system where endothelial cells were grown on a porous membrane, ^{125}I-insulin was transported from one side of the endothelial monolayer to the other.[24] The choroid plexus, a major site of CSF formation,[25] contains high numbers of insulin receptors,[26,27] which have been localized on the choroidal epithelium. It has not been elucidated whether these receptors are on the 'blood' or the 'CSF' side of the epithelial cells. CSF insulin is taken up into the hypothalamus[28] and may perhaps be transported to sites deeper further within the brain neuropil.

Data from our laboratory suggest that other factors besides plasma insulin levels may regulate the amount of insulin in the CSF.[29] We have obtained concomitant samples of plasma and CSF from rats and assayed these samples for insulin. To estimate the accessibility of plasma insulin to the CNS, we have compared the plasma to CSF ratio (PCR) of insulin values. We observed that the PCR increases between 4 and 8 mo. of age in both Wistar and heterozygous Zucker Fa/fa rats.[30] Additionally, female rats exhibit a higher PCR than male rats; this is due both to higher plasma levels and lower CSF levels of insulin. Finally, the PCR differs between strains of rat, when rats are matched for age and gender. One obvious caveat is that CSF insulin levels reflect not only the transport or entry of insulin, but also insulin degradation. Uptake of insulin from the CSF, and ultimately its degradation, may also be a receptor-mediated or regulated process, and may be independent of insulin transport into CSF. Nevertheless, it appears that CSF insulin levels are not a constant function of plasma levels for any given species.

Insulin receptors are located in CNS sites which participate in the regulation of ingestive behaviors

Specific insulin receptors have been identified and their concentrations measured throughout the CNS with the use of both classical membrane binding techniques and quantitative autoradiography. (See the chapter by Heidenreich for a discussion of the biochemistry of the CNS insulin receptor.) Besides the choroid plexus, high concentrations of insulin receptors have been measured in the rat olfactory bulb,[31,32] a structure which plays a role in the maintenance of normal feeding patterns.[33] Relatively high concentrations of insulin binding sites are also found in several of the hypothalamic nuclei, including the paraventricular and dorsomedial nuclei.[34] It should be noted that high concentrations of receptors are also localized in CNS areas which are not generally associated with regulation of appetite and energy balance, such as the molecular layer of the cerebellar cortex.[34] Thus, insulin presumably has other roles in CNS function besides the regulation of body weight. However, the critical issue is that insulin receptors are present at CNS sites involved with appetite and energy balance regulation. This supports the hypothesis that CNS insulin receptors may transduce an adiposity signal provided by CSF insulin levels.

The issue of CNS insulin receptor regulation remains controversial. Several studies have attempted to assess whether chronic changes of ambient insulin levels can alter CNS insulin binding in a similar manner to peripheral target tissue insulin binding. In vivo manipulations of plasma insulin levels for the most part have yielded negative results.[31,35,36,37] However, in these studies CSF or CNS insulin levels were not measured and it is not known whether CNS insulin receptors were exposed to the proportionately altered insulin concentrations as were peripheral insulin receptors. Short-term in vitro manipulation of ambient insulin levels did not alter insulin binding.[32] Alteration of nutritional status and energy balance[38,39,40] appears to be one in vivo situation which may influence the binding of insulin in the CNS, but the mechanism underlying this regulation has not been clarified. Hopefully, future studies pursued from a number of different approaches will provide insight into the potential, as well as physiologic, regulation of CNS insulin receptor number and affinity.

The precise cellular location of neuronal insulin receptors in the CNS is not known. One hypothesis is that the receptors are localized presynaptically, allowing insulin to modulate release of other neurotransmitters and synaptic transmission events. This hypothesis has recently been examined by Wilcox. Following administration of 6-hydroxydopamine to destroy noradrenergic axon terminals, insulin binding was measured in specific hypothalamic nuclei using quantitative autoradiography. For a lesion in which 65% depletion of norepinephrine was achieved, insulin binding was decreased 25% in the arcuate nucleus and 15% in the dorsomedial nucleus; no change of insulin binding was found in the ventromedial nucleus (manuscript in preparation). These results suggest that at least some neuronal insulin receptors are localized presynaptically. Alternatively, insulin receptors might be located postsynaptically: such a localization would imply a "traditional" neurotransmitter function for insulin. Anatomical delineation of pre- vs. postsynaptic localization of insulin receptors in different CNS sites should help to define insulin's actions at these sites, both cellularly and at a whole-systems level.

Direct chronic intraventricular administration of insulin can decrease food intake and body weight

Woods et al demonstrated that chronic intraventricular administration of small quantities of insulin (100 μU/kg x day) significantly depressed food intake, and ultimately the body weight of baboons.[1] This phenomenon has also been observed in rats, by several investigators and with a variety of experimental protocols.[41,42,43,44,45] The rat appears to be less sensitive to central insulin than the baboon; thus, species variability for sensitivity to this regulation may exist. Further, Plata-Salamán and Oomura have recently reported that intraventricular insulin only induces a decrease of food intake in non-food-deprived rats.[46] The efficacy of insulin to decrease food intake of rats varies depending upon time of day administered and nutritional status of the animals. These observations support the concept that metabolic and neuroendocrine status of an animal may interact with central insulin to modulate its efficacy. Calculation of the drop in caloric consumption by insulin-treated animals suggests that the major effect of CNS insulin is to decrease food intake, and not alter energy balance.

CNS insulin may modulate appetite by interacting with short-term satiety factors

One means whereby central insulin may decrease total food intake could be to alter sensitivity of an animal to presumptive satiety factors which are released physiologically upon initiation of a meal.[47] We recently tested this hypothesis in baboons trained to eat on a fixed meal schedule.[48] Dose response data were generated by administering increasing amounts of cholecystokinin octapeptide (CCK) prior to a 30 min. meal. A chronic intracisternal insulin infusion was begun, and the animals were then tested with a dose of CCK which had produced a submaximal suppression of meal size in the absence of insulin. Concomitant with insulin, the dose of CCK was 2-3 times as effective in reducing meal size. Thus, the efficacy of one putative short-term satiety factor can be enhanced by increased CSF levels of insulin. One limitation of this study was the restricted meal regimen on which these animals were maintained. That is, the efficacy of CCK was tested within a 30 min. period. Compensation for the effect of CCK might have occurred if the test mealtime were longer. Whether central insulin infusion can alter an animal's sensitivity to either exogenous or endogenous satiety signals in a free-feeding situation remains to be tested.

The cellular mechanisms underlying the central action of insulin to decrease body weight have not been identified. Cellular actions with relatively long-term consequences such as stimulation of RNA and protein synthesis[49,50] or stimulation of the growth of neurite connections,[51,52] which have been demonstrated in cell culture studies, may be good candidates. Alternatively, central insulin may modulate or interact with other neurotransmitter systems such as the catecholamines,[53,54] which contribute to appetite and body weight control.

II. THE OBESE ZUCKER RAT: A MODEL OF ALTERED BRAIN INSULIN ACTION

The obese (fa/fa) Zucker rat is an animal model of early-onset obesity and altered energy balance.[55] The rat exhibits numerous neuroendocrine disorders including impaired reproductive capacity. We became interested in this model because it demonstrates early hyperinsulinemia, with no corresponding hypoglycemia, yet it is also hyperphagic. Our hypothesis would suggest that elevated plasma insulin levels should lead to elevated CSF insulin levels and, in turn, to suppression of food intake. Thus, we investigated the brain insulin system of these animals. The studies described below were carried out using 4-month female rats provided by the colony at Vassar College.

The Zucker fa/fa rat has levels of CSF insulin which are elevated, but may not be appropriate for their plasma insulin levels

One potential pathology in the Zucker rat could be that insulin is not transported from the plasma to the CSF to provide a feedback signal for appetite. We tested this by obtaining simultaneous CSF and plasma samples, under both fasting and free-feeding conditions, from lean (Fa/Fa), heterozygous (Fa/fa), and obese (fa/fa) Zucker rats.[14] Assay of the samples for immunoreactive insulin (IRI) revealed that following an overnight fast, the fa/fa Zucker rats were significantly hyperinsulinemic, and the phenotypically lean Fa/fa Zucker rats had plasma insulin levels which were slightly but significantly elevated when compared with the lean Fa/Fa rats. Corresponding CSF insulin levels also revealed a 'fa' gene dose-effect: highest CSF insulin levels were observed in the fa/fa rats while Fa/fa rats had intermediate CSF insulin levels. Measurement of insulin in the same rats under free-feeding conditions revealed an increase over fasting levels in plasma and CSF IRI in all three genotypes.

These results demonstrate that the obese fa/fa Zucker rat is capable of transporting insulin into the CSF. However, the PCR of the obese fa/fa animals was much higher than that of the lean animals. This suggests that CSF insulin levels may be inappropriately low for the plasma IRI levels of the obese animals. Thus, they may receive an inadequate appetitive feedback signal.

To further test whether Zucker fa/fa rats have a defect in transport of insulin from plasma to the CSF, we infused lean (Fa/fa) and obese Zucker rats peripherally with insulin for six days,[56] at a dose which elevated the plasma IRI of the Fa/fa rats to match that of saline infused obese Zucker rats. While plasma insulin levels of insulin-infused obese rats were twice those of insulin-infused lean rats, CSF levels of obese rats did not increase accordingly; CSF IRI levels of insulin-infused obese rats were actually less than those of insulin-infused lean rats. Additionally, plasma IRI levels were comparable between insulin-infused Fa/fa rats and saline infused fa/fa rats, but the CSF IRI of the Fa/fa rats was twice that of the fa/fa rats.

The precise relationship between CSF and plasma IRI over a range of plasma IRI concentrations has not been established for thc normal rat. Nonetheless our data suggest that, if a saturable transport system mediates the transfer of insulin from plasma to CSF, the obese Zucker rat has a defective transport system. We conclude that fa/fa Zucker rats have inappropriately low CSF IRI levels for their plasma IRI levels which provide an inadequate CNS feedback signal. This, in turn, may contribute to their hyperphagia. As discussed above, our experiment did not allow us to distinguish between impaired transport of insulin into the CSF, or an enhanced degradation of CSF insulin.

Extractable brain insulin content is decreased in Zucker rats carrying the 'fa' gene for obesity

Potential sources of insulin which is extracted from the brain include receptor-bound insulin and insulin remaining in the interstitial fluid. We hypothesized that, as both plasma and CSF insulin levels are elevated in the fa/fa rat, their brain insulin content should be increased in comparison to age- and gender-matched Fa/Fa rats. In contrast to our hypothesis, measurement of brain insulin content revealed significant decreases in every brain area of the fa/fa rats which was measured.[57] In the olfactory bulb and hypothalamus, insulin content was below the limits of assay detectability. Insulin content in the brains of the Fa/fa Zucker rats was intermediate between that of the fa/fa and Fa/Fa rats.

Insulin binding is decreased in the olfactory bulb of Zucker rats carrying the 'fa' gene

Brain insulin content was found to be very low in the Zucker Fa/fa and fa/fa olfactory bulb and hypothalamus. These two regions are known to have higher densities of insulin receptors than other brain areas in normal rats. We therefore hypothesized that insulin binding might be reduced in the brains of Zucker rats carrying the 'fa' gene. Measurement and subsequent analysis of insulin binding to membranes from the olfactory bulb, medial and lateral hypothalamus, and cerebral cortex revealed a decrease in the number of high affinity insulin binding sites in the olfactory bulb of both the phenotypically lean Fa/fa and the obese fa/fa rats.[58] We have recently replicated this observation in the "Wistar fatty" rat,[59] a Wistar Kyoto rat into which the 'fa' gene has been bred. As the Fa/fa rat is not extremely hyperinsulinemic, the decreased binding we observed cannot be downregulation of the receptor by elevated ambient insulin levels. Rather, it appears that the expression of the 'fa' gene somehow results in altered regulation of insulin receptors.

As we did not observe decreased insulin binding in all brain regions measured, we conclude that the decrease in brain insulin content cannot be accounted for by a decrease in brain insulin receptors. Recent quantitative autoradiographic studies in our laboratory support the observation that decreases in CNS insulin binding are localized in anatomically discrete regions.[60] Decreased brain insulin content in the fa/fa animals may be due to an enhanced degradation of insulin.

Response to chronic intraventricular insulin is impaired in the obese Zucker fa/fa rat

To directly test whether the obese Zucker rat is capable of responding to exogenous insulin with a decrease of food intake and body weight, groups of fa/fa and Fa/fa Zucker rats were infused intraventricularly with 2 mU insulin/day for 14 days.[61] Fa/fa rats responded by decreasing their food intake and body weight relative to saline-infused controls. In contrast, fa/fa rats infused with insulin showed no differences in food intake and body weight compared with saline-infused fa/fa controls. Thus, the obese fa/fa rat has an impaired response to central insulin, even when it is provided directly to the CSF. As a decrease in CNS insulin receptors was not uniformly observed throughout the CNS, and was also observed in the Fa/fa rat, which responded to insulin infusion, we suggest that the Zucker fa/fa rat may have a post-receptor defect in insulin action at the cellular level.

III. CONCLUSIONS AND FUTURE DIRECTIONS

Evidence from our laboratory and others supports a potential role of plasma-derived insulin in the long-term regulation of body weight. This regulation may well be a dynamic process, changing with the age, gender, nutritional status, and developmental status of an animal.

Future directions for our work include further study of the relationship between plasma and CSF insulin levels and how this relationship is regulated. These studies are crucial for our understanding of how an adiposity signal to the CNS is generated and maintained. Quantitative receptor autoradiography will enable us to measure numbers of insulin receptors in very discrete brain regions, and assess changes of insulin binding in animals in which we also assess changes in CNS insulin actions, both at behavioral and cellular levels. Studies of the brain insulin system in other models of obesity, such as dietary-induced obesity, may provide new insights of clinical relevance. Finally, we hope to integrate our understanding of CNS insulin action with knowledge of other systems which can regulate appetite, energy balance, and body weight.

ACKNOWLEDGEMENTS

The authors extend thanks to Dr. M.R.C. Greenwood, for our continuing collaboration and on-going discussions. We acknowledge gratefully our colleagues who have contributed to this work: Elizabeth Lotter, L. David McKay, Jan Strubbe, David West, Hitoshi Ikeda, Anton Steffens, Brad Wallum, Eric Corp, and Al Sipols. Support for the authors' studies described herein was provided by the American Diabetes Association, PHS Grants AM-35816, AM-17844, AM-14047, AM-12829, NS-20311 and the Veterans Administration.

REFERENCES

1. S. C. Woods, E. C. Lotter, L. D. McKay, and D. Porte, Jr., Chronic intracerebroventricular infusion of insulin reduces food intake and body weight of baboons, Nature 282:503 (1979).
2. D. Porte, Jr., and S. C. Woods, Insulin effects on the central nervous system (CNS): evidence for a long term control system for body weight regulation, in: "Proc. 10th Congress of Int. Diabetes Federation," Excerpta Medica, Amsterdam (1980).
3. D. G. Baskin, D. P. Figlewicz, S. C. Woods, D. Porte, Jr., and D. M. Dorsa, Insulin in the brain, Ann. Rev. Physiol. 49:335 (1987).
4. J. D. Bagdade, E. L. Bierman, and D. Porte, Jr., The significance of basal insulin in the evaluation of the insulin response to glucose in diabetic and non-diabetic subjects, J. Clin. Invest. 46:1549 (1967).
5. S. C. Woods, E. Decke, and J. R. Vasselli, Metabolic hormones and regulation of body weight, Psych. Rev. 81:26 (1974).
6. T. Ono, A. B. Steffens, and K. Sasaki, Influence of peripheral and intracerebroventricular glucose and insulin infusions on peripheral and cerebrospinal fluid glucose and insulin levels, Physiol. Behav. 30:301 (1983).
7. P. M. Daniel and J. R. Henderson, Insulin in bile and other fluids, Lancet 1:1256 (1967).
8. S. C. Woods, D. B. West, L.J. Stein, D. P. Figlewicz, and D. Porte, Jr., Meals and intravenous glucose or insulin infusion increase cerebrospinal fluid insulin levels in the baboon, Submitted, Peptides, 1986.
9. W. A. Mahon, J. Steinke, G. M. McKhann, and M. L. Mitchell, Measurement of I^{131}-insulin and of insulinlike activity in cerebrospinal fluid of man, Metabolism 11:416 (1962).
10. R. U. Margolis and N. Altszuler, Insulin in the cerebrospinal fluid, Nature 215:1375 (1967).
11. S. C. Woods and D. Porte, Jr., Effect of intracisternal insulin on plasma glucose and insulin in the dog, Diabetes 24:905 (1975).
12. W. S. Young, III, Periventricular hypothalamic cells in the rat brain contain insulin mRNA, Neuropeptides 8:93 (1986).
13. O. E. Owen, G. A. Reichard, Jr., G. Boden, and C. R. Shuman, Comparative measurements of glucose, beta-hydroxybutyrate, acetoacetoate, and insulin in blood and cerebrospinal fluid during starvation, Metabolism 23:7 (1974).
14. L. J. Stein, D. M. Dorsa, D. G. Baskin, D. P. Figlewicz, H. Ikeda, S. P. Frankmann, M. R. C. Greenwood, D. Porte, Jr., and S. C. Woods, Immunoreactive insulin levels are elevated in the cerebrospinal fluid of genetically obese Zucker rats, Endocrinology 113:2299 (1983).
15. A. B. Steffens, A. J. W. Scheurink, D. Porte, Jr., and S. C. Woods, Effects of changes in peripheral glucose and insulin levels on cerebrospinal fluid glucose and insulin levels, manuscript in prepraration.

16. S. C. Woods and D. Porte, Jr., Relationship between plasma and cerebrospinal fluid insulin levels of dogs, Am. J. Physiol. 233:E331 (1977).

17. B. J. Wallum, G. J. Taborsky, Jr., D. Porte, Jr., D. P. Figlewicz, L. Jacobson, J. C. Beard, W. K. Ward, and D. Dorsa, Cerebrospinal fluid insulin levels increase during intravenous insulin infusions in man, J. Clin. Endo. Metab. 64:190 (1977).

18. H. J. L. Frank and W. M. Pardridge, Insulin binding to brain microvessels, Adv. Metab. Disorders 10:291 (1983).

19. W. M. Pardridge, J. Eisenberg, and J. Yang, Human blood-brain barrier insulin receptor, J. Neurochem. 44:1771 (1985).

20. I. Jialal, G. L. King, S. Buchwald, C. R. Kahn, and M. Crettaz, Processing of insulin by bovine endothelial cells in culture: internalization without degradation, Diabetes 33:794 (1984).

21. N. Kaiser, I. Vlodavsky, A. Tur-sinai, Z. Fuks, and E. Cerasi, Binding, internalization and degradation of insulin in vascular endothelial cells, Diabetes 31:1077 (1982).

22. K. Dernovsek, R. Bar, B. Ginsberg, and M. Lioubin, Processing of cell-bound insulin by capillary and macrovascular endothelial cells in culture, J. Clin. Endo. Metab. 58:761 (1984).

23. K. D. Dernovsek and B. S. Bar, Rapid transport of biologically intact insulin through cultured endothelial cells, Am. J. Physiol. 248:E244 (1985).

24. G. L. King and S. Johnson, Receptor-mediated transport of insulin across endothelial cells, Science 227:1583 (1985).

25. T. H. Milhorat and M. K. Hammock, Cerebrospinal fluid as reflection of internal milieu of brain, in: "Neurobiology of Cerebrospinal Fluid," J.H. Wood, ed., Plenum Press, New York (1983).

26. D. G. Baskin, B. Brewitt, D. A. Davidson, E. Corp, T. Paquette, D. P. Figlewicz, T. K. Lewellen, M. K. Graham, S. C. Woods, and D. M. Dorsa, Quantitative autoradiographic evidence for insulin receptors in the choroid plexus of the rat brain, Diabetes 35:246 (1986).

27. J. M. Hill, M. A. Lesniak, J. Roth, and C. B. Pert, Autoradiographic localization of insulin receptors in rat brain: prominence in olfactory and limbic areas, Soc. Neurosci. Abstr. 11:1053 (1985).

28. D. G. Baskin, S. C. Woods, D. B. West, M. van Houten, B. I. Posner, D. M. Dorsa, and D. Porte, Jr., Immunocytochemical detection of insulin in rat hypothalamus and its possible uptake from cerebrospinal fluid, Endocrinology 113:1818 (1983).

29. D. Porte, Jr., D. G. Baskin, D. M. Dorsa, D. P. Figlewicz, D. B. West, L. J. Stein, H. Ikeda, and S. C. Woods, Regulation of CSF insulin, in: "Abstracts, VIII, International Conference of the Physiology of Food and Fluid Intake" (1983).

30. L. J. Stein, M. R. C. Greenwood, D. Porte, Jr., and S. C. Woods, Decreased plasma/CSF IRI ratio (PCR) in genetically obese and aged lean rats, Proc. Fourth Int. Congress Obesity: 54A (1983).

31. J. Havrankova, J. Roth, and M. Brownstein, Concentrations of insulin and of insulin receptors in the brain are independent of peripheral insulin levels: studies of obese and streptozotocin-treated rodents, J. Clin. Invest. 64:636 (1979).

32. N. R. Zahniser, M. B. Goens, P. J. Hathaway, and J. V. Vinych, Characterization and regulation of insulin receptors in rat brain, J. Neurochem. 42:1345 (1984).

33. C. Larue, Prandial drinking and the disruption of meal patterns in olfactory bulbectomized rats, Physiol. Behav. 15:491 (1975).

34. E. S. Corp, S.C. Woods, D. Porte, Jr., D. M. Dorsa, D. P. Figlewicz, and D. G. Baskin, Localization of ^{125}I-insulin binding sites in the rat hypothalamus by quantitative autoradiography, Neurosci. Letters 70:17 (1986).

35. S. T. Pacold and W. G. Blackard, Central nervous system insulin receptors in normal and diabetic rats, Endocrinology 105:1452 (1979).

36. Y. Sakamoto, Y. Oomura, H. Kita, S. Shibata, S. Suzuki, T. Kuzuya, and S. Yoshida, Insulin content and insulin receptors in the rat brain. Effect of fasting and streptozotocin treatment, Biomed. Research 1:334 (1980).

37. R. B. Melnyk and J. M. Martin, Failure of chronic experimental hyperinsulinism to alter insulin binding to hypothalamic receptors in the rat, Acta Endocrinol. 107:86 (1984).
38. R. B. Melnyk and J. M. Martin, Starvation-induced changes in insulin binding to hypothalamic receptors in the rat, Acta Endocrinol. 107:78 (1984).
39. S. Duran Garcia, J. Gomez Nieto, E. Romero Bobillo, F. Padron Rivas, and A. Maranon Cabello, Characterization of insulin receptors in rat hypothalamus: effect of obesity and starvation, in: "Diabetes and Obesity," J. Vague and Ph. Vague, eds., Excerpta Medica, Amsterdam-Oxford (1979).
40. E. S. Corp, N. J. Bohannon, B. J. Wilcox, S. C. Woods, D. M. Dorsa, D. Porte, Jr., and D. G. Baskin, Increased insulin binding in the paraventricular nucleus of rats after chronic caloric restriction: in vitro quantitative autoradiography, Soc. Neurosci. Abstr. 12:612 (1986).
41. D. J. Brief and J. D. Davis, Reduciton of food intake and body weight by chronic intraventricular insulin infusion, Brain Res. Bull. 12:571 (1984).
42. J. H. Strubbe and C. G. Mein, Increased feeding in response to bilateral injection of insulin antibodies in the VMH, Physiol. Behav. 19:309 (1977).
43. J. Panksepp and D. M. Nance, Insulin, glucose and hypothalamic regulation of feeding, Physiol. Behav. 9:447 (1972).
44. S. Nicolaidis, Lateral hypothalamic control of metabolic factors related to feeding, Diabetologia 20:426 (1981).
45. C. R. Plata-Salamån, Y. Oomura, and N. Shimizu, Dependence of food intake on acute and chronic ventricular administration of insulin, Physiol. Behav. 37:717 (1986).
46. C. R. Plata-Salamån and Y. Oomura, Effect of intra-third ventricular administration of insulin on food intake after food deprivation, Physiol. Behav. 37:735 (1986).
47. D. P. Figlewicz, F. Lacour, A. Sipols, D. Porte, Jr., and S. C. Woods, Gastroenteropancreatic peptides and the central nervous system, Ann. Rev. Physiol. 49:383 (1987).
48. D. P. Figlewicz, D. West, L. J. Stein, S. C. Woods, and D. Porte, Jr., Insulin alters the sensitivity of baboons to CCK-induced single meal suppression, Am. J Physiol. 250:R856 (1986).
49. J. W. Yang and R. E. Fellows, Characterization of insulin stimulation of the incorporation of radioactive precursors into macromolecules in cultured rat brain cells, Endocrinology 107:1717 (1980).
50. M. K. Raizada, J. W. Yang, and R. E. Fellows, Binding of ^{125}I-insulin to specific receptors and stimulation of nucleotide incorporation in cells cultured from rat brain, Brain Res. 200:389 (1980).
51. E. Recio-Pinto and D. N. Ishii, Effects of insulin, insulin-like growth factor-II and nerve growth factor on neurite outgrowth in cultured human neuroblastoma cells, Brain Res. 302:323 (1984).
52. E. Y. Snyder and S. U. Kim, Insulin: is it a nerve survival factor, Brain Res. 196:565 (1980).
53. D. E. Rhoads, R. J. DiRocco, L. D. Osburn, N. A. Peterson, and E. Raghupathy, Stimulation of synaptosomal uptake of neurotransmitter amino acids by insulin: possible role of insulin as a neuromodulator, Biochem. Biophys. Res. Comm. 119:1198 (1984).
54. F. T. Boyd, Jr., D. W. Clarke, T. F. Muther, and M. K. Raizada, Insulin receptors and insulin modulation of norepinephrine uptake in neuronal cultures from rat brain, J. Biol. Chem. 260:15880 (1985).
55. G. A. Bray, The Zucker fatty rat: a review, Fed. Proc. 36:148 (1977).
56. L. J. Stein, D. P. Figlewicz, D. M. Dorsa, D. G. Baskin, D. Reed, D. Braget, M. Midkiff, D. Porte, Jr., and S. C. Woods, Effect of insulin concentrations on cerebrospinal fluid insulin concentrations in heterozygous lean and obese Zucker rats, Int. J. Obesity 9:A145 (1985).
57. D. G. Baskin, L. J. Stein, H. Ikeda, S. C. Woods, D. P. Figlewicz, D. Porte, Jr., M. R. C. Greenwood, and D. M. Dorsa, Genetically obese Zucker rats have abnormally low brain insulin content, Life Sciences 36:627 (1985).

58. D. P. Figlewicz, D. M. Dorsa, L. J. Stein, D. G. Baskin, T. Paquette, M. R. C. Greenwood, S. C. Woods, and D. Porte, Jr., Brain and liver insulin binding is decreased in Zucker rats carrying the 'fa' gene, Endocrinology 117:1537 (1985).
59. D. P. Figlewicz, H. Ikeda, L. J. Stein, D. M. Dorsa, S. C. Woods, and D. Porte, Jr., Brain insulin binding is decreased in Wistar Kyoto rats carrying the 'fa' gene, Peptides 7:61 (1986).
60. B. J. Wilcox, E. S. Corp, D.P. Figlewicz, D. M. Dorsa, M. R. C. Greenwood, D. Porte, Jr., and D. G. Baskin, Characterization of insulin binding in hypothalamus of three genotypes of Zucker rat by *in vitro* quantitative autoradiography, Soc. Neurosci. Abstr. 12:1488 (1986).
61. H. Ikeda, D. B. West, J. J. Pustek, D. P. Figlewicz, M. R. C. Greenwood, D. Porte, Jr., and S. C. Woods, Intraventricular insulin reduces food intake and body weight of lean but not obese Zucker rats, Appetite 7:381 (1986).

INSULIN IN THE BRAIN: A FEEDBACK LOOP INVOLVING BRAIN INSULIN AND CIRCUMVENTRICULAR ORGANS

M. Ian Phillips

Department of Physiology
University of Florida
Gainesville, FL. 32610

INTRODUCTION

Until fairly recently, insulin has been considered a purely peripheral hormone secreted exclusively by the beta cells of the pancreas and one which did not influence the brain. The independence of the central nervous system (CNS) from peripheral insulin has always had a certain teleological logic to it. The brain, being so important physiologically, must be preserved from having to require insulin to control its glucose metabolism. Since insulin is a 51-amino acid peptide, it does not have access to the brain because of the blood brain barrier. Thus, there were two good reasons to suppose that insulin was not involved in the glucose metabolism of the brain. In addition, glucose levels in the blood could take care of the metabolic signals for the brain's information. However, in the past few years, several lines of evidence indicate that insulin and its receptors are present in the central nervous system. This new body of evidence has arisen at the same time as evidence for other peptides being found in the brain which were also thought to be excluded from the CNS and only available to peripheral tissues. The list of such peptides has grown as it has become clear that peptides are produced not only in the gut and pancreas, but in many other tissues including the CNS. Nevertheless, the function of these peptides in the brain is unknown and the interrelationship between the peripheral peptide levels and the central presence of the same peptides has not been satisfactorily explained. In this brief review, we shall propose that insulin, like many others peptides produced in the periphery, is involved in a feedback loop. Most hormones under hypothalamic or pituitary control have a long feedback loop or a short feedback loop to the hypothalamus. This is easy to understand when it involves steroids such as testosterone or estrogen because these steroids are lipid soluble and can pass through the blood brain barrier with ease. The peptides, however, are lipophobic and large enough to be excluded by the blood brain barrier. We shall hypothesize that the key to understanding feedback of peptides lies in the role of the circumventricular organs and that the central peptides maintain the "set-point" of the feedback system.

THE CIRCUMVENTRICULAR ORGANS

The circumventricular organs close to the hypothalamus include the SFO (subfornical organ), OVLT (organum vasculosum lamina terminalis) and ME (median eminence). All have an incomplete, or absent, blood brain barrier.

Peptides, such as insulin, arrive from plasma at these circumventricular organs and appear to be sequestered in these organs (Van Houten and Posner, 1983). The CVOs are rich in glial cells which appear to limit the diffusion of peptides into the surrounding brain tissue. This is important because if the circumventricular organs freely allowed access to all parts of the brain, there would be little point in having a blood brain barrier.

We suggest that peptide levels in the circumventricular organs excite specific receptors of CVO neurons but do not diffuse into the brain parenchyma or CSF. Those reports where insulin is said to cross the BBB into the CSF (Baskin et al., 1983; Woods and Porte, 1975) have used supraphysiological levels of insulin i.v. The CVO input is transmitted via axonal action potentials to neurons containing the same peptides within the brain. It is the one-to-one communication of external peptide to the same peptide internally that maintains specificity of response. Thus, the hypothalamus and other parts of the brain contain peptidergic cells to duplicate those in the periphery whose secretions cannot reach the brain areas. The response to peptides in the circumventricular organs will define the response of the feedback loop (Fig. 1). It is proposed that the levels of the brain peptide released by peripheral CVO stimulation act as the reference ("set-point") for the feedback response. In the case of insulin, therefore, the critical control of glucose in the brain may be regulated by a level of brain insulin activity.

THE INSULIN FEEDBACK HYPOTHESIS

It is hypothesized that insulin levels in the plasma are detected by circumventricular organs such as the OVLT, ME and SFO. Receptors on neurons in the CVOs are stimulated and the effect of this stimulation relayed to hypothalamic and/or hypothalamic controlling sites. These sites contain insulin synthesizing cells and the action potentials from the CVOs stimulate the release of insulin. The effect of insulin is relayed to the hypothalamus. This triggers a descending inhibitory influence, possibly by the sympathetic nervous system, onto the pancreas to inhibit the further secretion of insulin from beta cells. The effect of this circuit is to reduce plasma insulin. The reduction in plasma insulin would attenuate the stimulation of the cells in the CVO and the release of brain insulin, thereby completing the loop (Fig. 1).

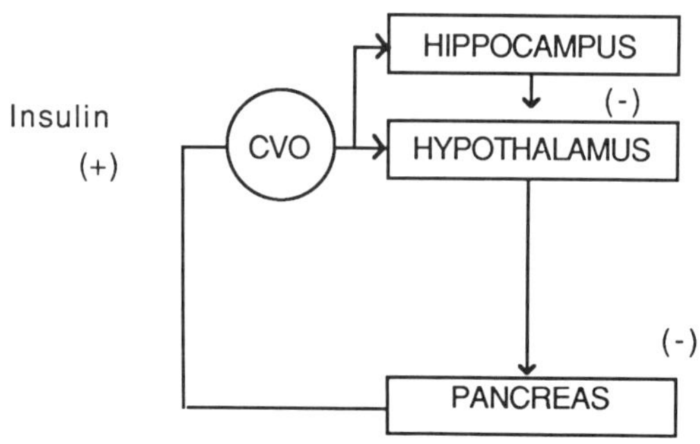

Figure 1. Proposed model of peptide feedback. In this case, insulin is the peptide. Plasma insulin cannot cross the blood brain barrier but can stimulate neurons in the circumventricular organs (CVO).

For this hypothesis to be valid, certain requirements would be necessary: 1) The CVOs must limit the spread or diffusion of plasma insulin, 2) there must be specific receptors for insulin in the CVOs, 3) the signals have to be transmitted from the CVOs to the hypothalamus and other parts of the brain, 4) the peptide must be synthesized in the brain, 5) the neurons that synthesize the peptide, in this case insulin, must be released from the neurons which synthesized it, 6) there must be specific receptors on the next order neurons for the insulin to bind, 7) there must be a biological response to insulin by the cells with binding sites to show that they are receptors and 8) the output from these cells must have connections to nuclei known to control plasma insulin levels.

Although the evidence is still fragmentary, putting together those fragments gives a picture which is consistent with this hypothesis although a long way from proving that it exists.

THE PRESENCE OF INSULIN IN THE CIRCUMVENTRICAL ORGANS

When labeled insulin is injected into the plasma, it is found to be concentrated in the circumventricular organs, particularly the median eminence, but also the SFO, OVLT and area postrema (Van Houten and Posner, 1979, 1983). This finding is true of several other peptides including angiotensin II, ACTH, calcitonin and ANF. What is interesting and overlooked in many studies where these data are cited is that the accumulation of labelled peptide is restricted to the CVO. This indicates the CVO does not permit diffusion of the peptide into adjacent parts of the brain. If there were diffusion then the autoradiography would instantly reveal the spread of peptide. By the use of glial fibrillary protein antibody we have found that the CVOs are filled with glial cells or, in the case of the area postrema, bordered by glial cells. Injecting dye on either side of this glial border prevents diffusion into the CVO and injecting dye into the plasma demonstrates that it is limited to the CVO (Fig. 2). High concentrations of peptide or a rapid change in blood pressure can overcome this diffusional barrier. Under physiological conditions, however, the glia appear to play a role in limiting diffusion. Clarke et al. (1984) have demonstrated high affinity binding to insulin by glial cells in culture. This could be by uptake of the peptide or physically limiting diffusion. Thus, accounts of high plasma insulin getting into CSF (Baskin et al., 1982) may result from a breakdown of this barrier or reaching a concentration which is beyond the capacity of the glial cells to bind.

INSULIN RECEPTORS IN THE CVOs

The presence of labeled insulin, shown by autoradiography in the circumventricular organs, implies that there is receptor binding (Van Houten and Posner, 1979). However, these organs are of such a small size that they have not been thoroughly investigated. We do not have Scatchard data on the CVOs. Other areas of the brain have been subjected to Scatchard analysis and also studies in cell culture (Palovcik et al., 1984; Kappy and Raizada, 1982). The specificity of the insulin receptor in the brain is similar to that in peripheral tissue but the neural receptor does not show negative cooperativity (Gammeltoft et al., 1987) although it does show a nonlinear Scatchard plot indicating a high affinity and low affinity subset of receptors. The receptors appear to be independent of plasma insulin (Havrankova et al., 1983) but the studies in neuronal culture clearly show down regulation with exposure to high levels of insulin in the medium. In their studies of glial insulin receptors, Clarke et al. (1984) demonstrated that glial insulin receptors down regulate in the presence of high insulin whereas neuronal cell insulin receptors do not respond. As mentioned above, the CVOs are rich in glial cells.

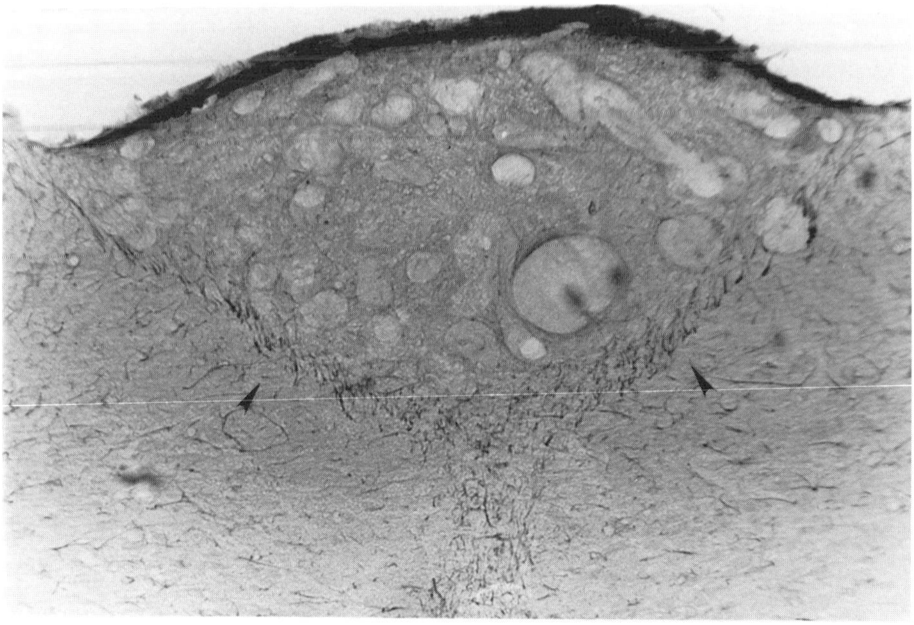

Figure 2. Glial border surrounding the area postrema (AP). The figure shows glial cells stained by GFAP antibody with the Sternberger immunocytochemistry technique. The glia inhibit diffusion of dye from CVO to brain parenchyma or CSF.

CONNECTIONS OF THE CVOs TO OTHER PARTS OF THE BRAIN

The stimulation of insulin receptors in the CVOs could lead to the stimulation (or inhibition) of several nuclei within the brain. This is based on horseradish peroxidase and labeled amino acid transport studies to and from the CVOs. The SFO has efferents to the paraventricular nucleus, the supraoptic nucleus, the septal region and the anterior hypothalamus (Miselis et al., 1979). The OVLT has efferents to the supraoptic nucleus, the paraventricular nucleus and also to the hippocampus (Phillips and Camacho, 1987).

PRESENCE OF INSULIN IN THE BRAIN

It was the difference between plasma levels of insulin and acid-ethanol extracts of whole rat brain by Havrankova et al. in 1978 which provided the first evidence for brain producing insulin independently of the pancreas. Havrankova et al. in 1979 found an authentic 6,000 dalton insulin with full biologic activity in the rat brain. The quantities varied from 10 ng/gm in the brainstem and cerebral cortex to 80 ng/gm in hypothalamus. On average, rat brains contain 8 ng/gm but in rats treated with streptozotocin to make them diabetic, the average levels were doubled to 16 ng/gm. These data showed that the source of insulin in the brain was not derived from plasma insulin. These results, however, did not go unchallenged when other groups (Eng and Yallow, 1980; Rosenzweig et al., 1980) reported levels in the extracts of dog brains, rabbit brains and rat brains (Baskin et al., 1983) to be very low and quite close to the limits of detectability. However, plasma levels, which are expressed as about 1 ng/ml, are still much lower than that found in brain tissue because a gram of brain tissue does not contain NML of plasma. It could be argued that even with lower levels in the plasma, the amounts found in the brain represent an accumulation derived from plasma insulin. Several reports of insulin in the cerebrospinal fluid indicate that as plasma levels increase, so do CSF levels (Margolis and Altszuler, 1967; Woods and Porte, 1975). Unfortunately, this does not resolve the question since the levels used were above physiological levels and these concentrations may overcome the CVO-brain barrier. Also, alterations in plasma levels make cause a corresponding alteration in brain synthesis. So far, in the species in which insulin has been measured in the brain which includes the rat, dog, monkey and pig brain, levels have been higher than in the plasma.

To visualize the localization of peptide hormones, immunocytochemistry has been applied in the brain. While this technique depends on the quality of the antibody, it can be used in conjunction with the measurement and characterization of peptides if properly controlled. These controls include absorption controls, presence and absence of the antibody and the use of a variety of antibodies. Havrankova et al. (1978) reported that insulin-like staining was found in neurons in both the olfactory bulb and cortex of rats. Dorn et al. (1983) and Bernstein et al. (1984), using immunofluorescence, demonstrated insulin in several areas of rat and mouse brain including pyramid cells, hippocampus and hypothalamus. They have also demonstrated insulin in the human brain (Dorn et al., 1983). They found co-localization of the C-peptide with insulin in the hippocampus, cortex, amygdala, cerebellum and hypothalamus. The presence of the precursor C-peptide with insulin is stronger evidence for the immunoreactive insulin being synthesized in these cells. Again, these results have not gone unchallenged. Baskin et al. (1982) were not able to identify insulin staining in neurons. The staining that they observed was intercellular or bound to cell surfaces. It is possible that in their study where they used paraffin sections, the antigenicity of the antibody was ineffective. However, they were unable to confirm the report of Le Roith et al. (1983) that immunocytochemical was found in neurons even using the same antibodies as Le Roith et al. The antibody was used in high concentration (1:20-1:200). Unfortunately, this can mean either that the antibody is weak or there is low antigen present but the consequence is that high concentrations of antibody lead to non-specific staining. Thus, the immunocytochemistry data has not yet been definitive for either the presence or absence of insulin in the brain. Taking a different approach, Raizada (1983) applied immunohistochemistry to neuronal cells in culture. These cells, which are derived from one-day-old fetal rat brains, are independent of plasma insulin. Raizada found distinct staining of the soma and neurites of neurons to insulin antibody but no staining in the glial cells. This has been confirmed and extended by Devaskar et al. (1987). Thus, the presence of brain insulin in neurons can be demonstrated in culture but it remains to be definitively shown in different localizations of the brain. One reason for the success of identification of insulin in brain cells in culture is that insulin may play a role in the developing fetal brain as a growth factor to stimulate neurons and/or glial cells.

Characterization of insulin found in the brain indicates that it is authentic insulin. The immunoactive insulin from brain extracts has an elution pattern on gel filtration which is similar to insulin in binding to insulin receptors. The biological activity of extracted insulin is inhibited by insulin antibodies. However, pro-insulin has not been determined in the extracts and further work needs to be carried out on mRNA. Theoretically, if brain tissue produces its own insulin, there should be mRNA for insulin in the rat brain. So far, this has not been demonstrated in brain tissue (Giddings et al., 1981). In practice, however, this is difficult to demonstrate. The ideal method is the in situ hybridization of a cloned DNA complimentary to rat insulin mRNA. Since the message is for the pro-insulin, the clone would have to be to pro-insulin mRNA. Again, the cell culture of brain cells has provided evidence for the presence of this message (Cooper and Clarke, 1985).

Clarke et al. (1987) found a 2.4 kB mRNA which hybridizes with a genomic insulin DNA probe. Since it is considerably larger than the 550 base pro-insulin, the 2.4 kB mRNA probably represents pre-pro-insulin mRNA. Recently, W.S. Young (1986) has reported that cells in the rat hypothalamus contain insulin mRNA. A ^{35}S-labeled oligodeoxyribonucleotide probe for insulin was hybridized on rat brain frozen sections and autoradiography showed staining in the periventricular region. Support of this finding comes from Budd and Pansky (1987) who have found immunofluorescence of insulin antisera in cells lining the third ventricle. Also, Budd and Pansky (1987) have used a cDNA probe for rat or human insulin and detect the presence of intracellular insulin mRNA in rat pituitary cells. However, the probes have not been applied to the brain and in each case in which mRNA has been recognized, the mRNA has not been sequenced to prove that insulin is encoded.

In summary, there is sufficient evidence to indicate that insulin is synthesized in brain tissue de novo but exactly where, when and how much remains to be finalized.

INSULIN RELEASE

Although no studies have demonstrated insulin is released by brain stimulation, Clarke et al. in 1986 have demonstrated that insulin can be released from neuronal cells in culture. The neurons were depolarized with high potassium (60 mm) in the medium. This resulted in a 3-fold increase of insulin in the medium. The effect could be blocked by removing calcium ions from the medium. Under the same conditions, glial cells did not release insulin into the medium, implying that the release is a property of the neurons. The released insulin was characterized by reverse phase HPLC and two peaks were found corresponding to insulin standard peaks of rat one and rat two insulin. While this study is the only one of its kind, the data indicates that there is insulin released from neural tissue upon depolorization and this insulin is not derived from insulin in the horse serum medium in which the cells are grown.

INSULIN IN THE HIPPOCAMPUS

The study of Dorn et al. (1983) demonstrated that both insulin and C-peptide immunoreactivity exist in the cell soma and dendrites of all the areas they investigated in the human brain. One of these areas was the hippocampus. The hippocampus has a unique structure in which most of the synapses are laid out in transverse layers. Therefore, a transverse slice of hippocampus in vitro retains synaptic function and spontaneous activity. The hippocampal slice is widely used for electrophysiological studies in vertebrate brains because of its stability in vivo and large pyramid cells. Since these cells were shown to contain the C-peptide and the insulin immunoreactivity, it is a tissue in which central electrophysiological responses to insulin can be studied. We have found that insulin has binding sites in hippocampus and that these are probably receptors because they lead to a biological response (Palovcik et al., 1984). Hippocampal slices have also been used to show that insulin causes a dose-dependent stimulation of Na^+/K^+-ATPase activity (Bernstein et al., 1981).

The effect of insulin on spontaneous firing of hippocampal pyramidal cells was measured in isolated brain slices. Male adult Sprague-Dawley rats (180-200 g) were used throughout as subjects. The rats were decapitated and the brains were rapidly removed and placed in artificial cerebrospinal fluid (ACSF) consisting of 124 mM NaCl, 5 mM KCl, 1.25 mM KH_2PO_4, 1.3 mM $MGSO_4$, 26 mM NaH-CO_3, 2.5 mM $CaCl_2$ and 10 mM glucose. The hippocampus was carefully dissected out and 400 μ thick slices were sectioned as described

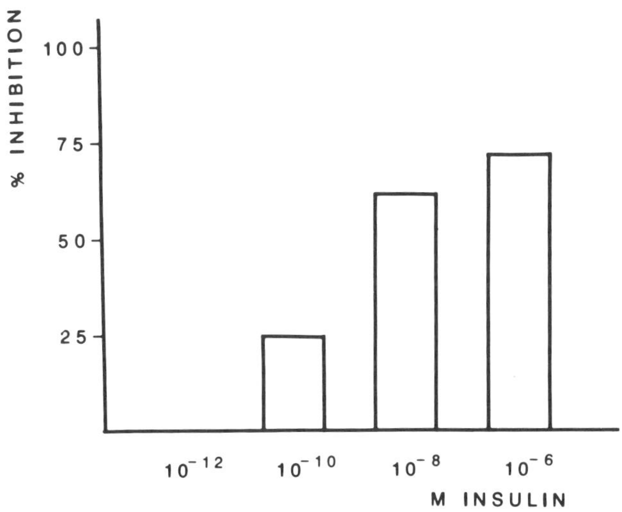

Figure 3. Result of recording 35 cells in 35 hippocampal slices in vivo.

previously (Palovcik and Phillips, 1986). Slices were transferred to a nylon mesh screen in a continuous perfusion chamber which contained ACSF. Hippocampal slices were perfused with freshly prepared buffer for up to 100 h at the rate of 30 ml/h. Various insulins, including desoctapeptide, or pro-insulin, were injected into the perfusion medium and took one minute to reach the slices. Extracellular recordings were obtained with 10 μ tip electrodes filled with perfusion medium and lowered into the CA1 pyramidal cell layer. Spikes were displayed on a digital memory oscilloscope. Single pyramidal cell spikes were selected by triggering on the largest spike (3-5 mV), that followed a characteristic hippocampal pyramidal bursting pattern, using a window discriminator. Output pulses from the discriminator were accumulated on a resetting scope raster-stepper to provide a 1/s output of "rate of firing" and permanently recorded on a Brush 2-channel recorder. After a stable pattern of spontaneous firing was established in the cell, insulin was injected into the chamber. Insulin caused a prominent decrease in the frequency of spontaneous spikes over a wide dose range. This effect of insulin was maintained for up to 30 minutes depending on the dose. Insulin had a robust inhibitory effect above 10^{-9} M. This inhibitory effect of insulin is not likely to be due to the presence of zinc found complexed with insulin because pro-insulin, which did not contain this metal, also showed a dose-dependent inhibitory effect. In addition, the concentrations of zinc present in these studies (10^{-10}-10^{-8} M) are 3-6 orders of magnitude lower than shown for most physiological or pharmacological effects of zinc (Itoh and Ebadi, 1982; May and Contoreggi, 1982). Figure 3 shows that the inhibitory effect of insulin was dose-dependent and IC_{50} was in the nanomolar range, indicating that a half maximum inhibitory response to insulin was similar to the affinity constant of [^{125}I]insulin binding to its receptors (Kappy et al., 1984). Inhibitory response of pro-insulin was about 10% and that of desoctapeptide insulin was 0%. These observations indicate that potencies of these insulins to inhibit spontaneous firing of hippocampal neurons are similar to their ability to compete for insulin binding to its receptors. This suggests that insulin-induced electrophysiological responses may be insulin receptor-mediated. The majority of cells (63%) were inhibited by insulin, 9% showed excitation, 13% showed consistent patterns of excitation and inhibition and 15% showed no response (n = 35).

INSULIN BINDING

Membranes from hippocampus of Sprague-Dawley rat brains were prepared as described previously (Kappy et al., 1984) in order to determine if hippocampus contains specific insulin receptors. The high-speed pellet obtained by centrifugation of the homogenate at 25,000 g was suspended in 1 mM sodium bicarbonate buffer to a protein concentration of 3.0 mg/ml and used for binding studies immediately. Protein content was determined by the method of Lowry et al. (1951), with 1% sodium dodecylsuflate added to the alkaline reagent, and with bovine serum albumin (BSA) as the standard. Porcine insulin was iodinated to 150-180 μCi/μg specific activity with chloramine T and separated from sodium iodide on coarse cellulose (Whatman) by the method of Lesniak (1978).

For [^{125}I]insulin binding, 50 μl membranes were incubated in triplicate, with 50 μl HEPES buffer, pH 8.0 in 1% BSA and 50 μl [^{125}I]insulin (20,000 cpm, 0.1 nM) in a final volume of 150 μl. Fifty μl of unlabeled insulin (3.4 μM) was used to determine non-specific binding. Incubation was carried out in 400 μl microfuge tubes for 90 minutes at 15°C at which time a plateau of specific binding had been reached. All tubes were centrifuged for 2 minutes in a Beckman microfuge to separate free [^{125}I]insulin from the bound hormone. Supernatants were aspirated from the membrane pellets, which were washed once with ice-cold HEPES buffer containing 1% BSA. The pellets were excised and placed in 12 x 75 mm test-tubes for counting. Specific [^{125}I]insulin binding was determined by subtracting the amount of insulin bound in the presence of 3.4 μM unlabeled insulin from the total binding and was expressed per mg protein. The intra-assay variability of this binding assay procedure was 6.2% and the degradation of [^{125}I]insulin was minimal (<5%).

[^{125}I]Insulin binding to membranes prepared from various anatomical regions of the brain has been shown to be rapid, reversible, highly specific for insulin and thus resembles insulin binding to known insulin target tissues (Kappy and Raizada, 1982; Kappy et al., 1984). Unlabeled porcine insulin competed for [^{125}I]insulin binding to hippocampal membranes in a dose dependent manner and 50% inhibition of the binding was observed with 1.6 nM insulin. Pro-insulin and desoctapeptide insulin competed for the binding according to their known physiological potencies. Scatchard analysis of the binding data (Fig. 4) for hippocampal membranes resulted in a curvilinear plot similar to that obtained for whole brain, hypothalamic and olfactory bulb membranes (Kappy et al., 1984). Analysis of the data according to a negative cooperativitiy model (DeMeyts et al., 1976) provided affinities of empty (K_e) and filled (K_f) sites to be 1.0 x 10^8 M^{-1} and 0.5 x 10^8 M^{-1}, respectively. The total number of binding sites (R_o) for these membranes was calculated to be 3.3 x 10^{-11} M per milligram protein. These observations indicated that binding of [^{125}I]insulin to hippocampal membranes is specific and fulfills criteria of a hormone-receptor interaction.

The results demonstrated that there was a consistent response of brain cells in the hippocampus to a wide range of doses of insulin. The response was consistently one of inhibition. Electrophysiological responsiveness matched the presence of high affinity binding sites for [^{125}I]insulin with demonstrable specificity. The output of the hippocampus is multiple but a major pathway is the descending fornix which distributes fibers to the hypothalamic nuclei including the ventromedial nucleus.

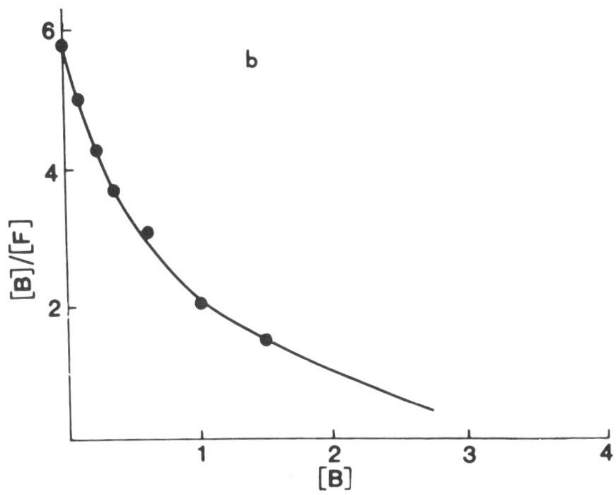

Figure 4. Scatchard analysis of binding of ^{125}I-insulin to membranes of hippocampal slices. Membranes were incubated for 90 minutes at 15°C in the presence of increasing concentrations of unlabeled insulin. The bound and free ^{125}I-insulin was determined in triplicates.

THE HYPOTHALAMIC NUCLEI

Stimulating the lateral hypothalamus (LH) has been reported to induce changes in glucose level and insulin secretion. In some cases, the reports have demonstrated that glucose levels and insulin secretion are facilitated by LH stimulation (Berthoud et al., 1980; Booth et al., 1969). However, LH stimulation also releases glucagon which inhibits hyperinsulinemia (Helman et al., 1980). Others have found no effect of LH stimulation (Frohman and Bernardis, 1971). Stimulating the ventral medial hypothalamic nucleus (VMH) produced hyperglycemia (Frohman and Bernardis, 1971; Shimazu et al., 1966) and had a reciprocal influence on the lateral hypothalamic nuclei on blood glucose levels and liver glycogen content (Shimazu et al., 1966). It is generally agreed, however, that lesions of the VMH produce hyperinsulinemia (Berthoud and Jeanrenaud, 1979; Frohman and Bernardis, 1968; Hales and Kennedy, 1964; Steffens et al., 1972). Stimulation of the LH increases single unit activity in the pancreatic vagus nerve (Oomura, 1983). Although these studies have not proved that there is a direct effect on the pancreas, stimulating the hypothalamus or the imbalance caused by lesioning one area may lead to activation of the sympathetic nerves innervating the pancreas and inhibit insulin secretion. Several studies have shown that LH stimulation induces catecholamine secretion (Katafuchi et al., 1986).

A considerable number of studies have emphasized the role of hypothalamic nuclei in the detection of glucose and the "glucostat" hypothesis (Oomura, 1983). The role of insulin feedback is not inconsistent with those studies. Such an essential function as glucose metabolism probably has parallel control systems and the notion that insulin in the brain establishes the "set-point" of glucose metabolism brings both sets of data together.

In summary, the two nuclei, the VMH and the LH, which have been shown by lesioning studies to play a role in feeding and appetite, also alter insulin and metabolism. The results with the VMH are clear, namely that the same lesion which induces obesity in rats also induces hyperinsulinemia. Inhibition of the VMH elevates insulin, whereas inhibition of the LH (ventral) decreases insulin. This may be by inhibition of sympathetic nerves.

SUMMARY

The effect of elevated plasma insulin is to act on the brain as part of a negative feedback loop. The plasma insulin reaches the circumventricular organs where it is sequestered by the high binding capacity of glial cells. It does not cross the blood brain barrier, however. It also binds to neurons and stimulates circuits emanating from the CVOs. One of many efferents is to the hippocampus. The hippocampus contains insulin in pyramid cells as shown by immunocytochemistry and there are receptors as shown by receptor binding analysis. The major response of the hippocampus to insulin is inhibition. The output of this inhibition can travel via the fornix to the hypothalamus and in the hypothalamus to the lateral hypothalamic nucleus. Inhibition of the lateral hypothalamic nucleus in turn leads to an inhibition of pancreatic beta cell secretion by sympathetic activation or parasympathetic inhibition. In the case of negative feedback, the beta cells respond by lowering secretion of insulin which would then be detected by the CVO (Fig. 5).

In this way insulin, and other peptide hormones, released from target glands and the pituitary can feed back onto the brain without crossing the blood brain barrier. The CVOs in this model are the essential transducers of peptides, such as insulin, from plasma to brain. Stimulation of the appropriate

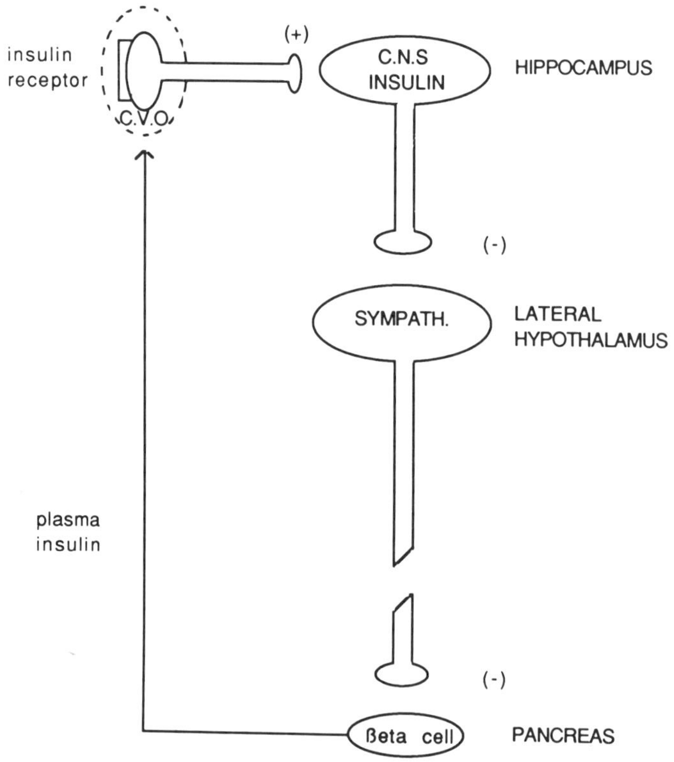

Figure 5. The feedback circuit of insulin, from the pancreatic source of synthesis to the CVO receptors, and the input into the brain by axons from CVO stimulated cells to insulin containing cells in the hippocampus. The negative output resulting from insulin stimulation inhibits β-cell insulin release via hypothalamic sympathetic efferents (disinhibition).

peptide containing neuron might be a way of maintaining high specificity of the response for a given peripheral hormone in the CVO. The brain peptide is the representative of the peripheral peptide and its release may set the level of response, i.e., the "set-point" of a feedback loop is determined by the amount of brain peptide release. This would lead to predictions concerning the levels of brain insulin in obesity, where levels would be low and in fasting, where levels would increase.

ACKNOWLEDGEMENTS

Supported by NIH grant 1-RO1-HL27334 to M. Ian Phillips. I am grateful to Mrs. C. Gabbard for her patient typing of this manuscript.

REFERENCES

Baskin, D.G., Porte, D., Jr., Guest, K., and Dorsa, D.M., 1983, Regional concentrations of insulin in the rat brain. Neuroendocrinology 112:898-903.

Baskin, D.G., Woods, S.C., West, D.B., Van Houten, M., Posner, B.I., Dorsa, D. and Porte, D., Jr., 1982, Immunocytochemical detection of insulin in rat hypothalamus and its possible uptake from cerebrospinal fluid. Endocrinology 113:1818-1825.

Bernstein, H.G., Dorn, A., Reiser, M. and Ziegler, M., 1984, Cerebral insulin-like immunoreactivity in rats and mice. Acta Histochem., 74:33-36.

Bernstein, H.G., Poeggel, G., Dorn, A., Luppa, H., and Ziegler, M., 1981, Insulin stimulates sodium-potassium activated ATPase from rat hippocampus. Experientia 37:434-435.

Berthoud, H.R., Bereiter, D.A. and Jeanrenaud, B., 1980, Role of the autonomic nervous system in the mediation of LHA electrical stimulation-induced effects on insulinemia and glycemia. J. Auton. Nerv. Syst., 2:183-1980.

Berthoud, H.R. and Jeanrenaud, B., 1979, Actue hyperinsulinemia and its reversal by vagotomy after lesions of the ventromedial hypothalamus in anesthetized rats. Endocrinology 105:146-1511.

Booth, C.A., Coons, E.E. and Miller, N.E., 1969, Blood glucose response to electrical stimulation of the hypothalamic feeding area. Physiol. Behav., 4:991-1001.

Budd, G.C. and Pansky, B., 1987, Synthesis of insulin or a similar peptide in the pituitary gland and in retinal muller cells, in: "Insulin and Related Peptides in the Central Nervous System", M.K. Raizada, M.I. Phillips and D. Le Roith, eds., Plenum Press, New York.

Clarke, D.W., Boyd, F.T., Jr., Kappy, M.S. and Raizada, M.K., 1984, Insulin binds to specific receptors and stimulates 2-deoxy-d-glucose uptake in cultured glial cells from rat brain. J. Biol. Chem., 259:11672-11675.

Cooper, D.L. and Clarke, D.W., 1985, Transcription of the insulin gene in the brain and submandibular gland of the rat. Pediatr. Res., 19:311A.

DeMeyts, P., Bianco, A.H. and Roth, J., 1976, Site-site interaction among insulin receptors: Characterization of negative cooperativity. J. Biol. Chem., 251:1877-1888.

Devaskar, S.U. and Holekamp. N., 1984, Insulin downregulates neonatal brain insulin receptors. Biochem. and Biophy. Res. Commun., 120:359-367.

Devaskar, S.U., Schechter, R. and Kahn, A., 1987, Localization of insulin to neuronal cells, in "Insulin and Related Peptides in the Central Nervous System", M.K. Raizada, M.I. Phillips and D. Le Roith, eds., Plenum Press, New York.

Dorn, A., Rinne, A., Bernstein, H.G., Hahn, H.J. and Ziegler, M., 1983, Insulin and C-peptide in human brain neurons (insulin/C-peptide/brain peptides/immunohistochemistry/radioimmunoassay). J. Hirnforsch., 24:495-499.

Eng, J. and Yalow, R.S., 1980, Insulin recoverable from tissues. Diabetes 29:105-109.

Frohman, L.A. and Bernardis, L.L., 1968, Growth hormone and insulin levels in weanling rats with ventromedial hypothalamic lesions. Endocrinology 82:1125-1132.

Frohman, L.A. and Bernardis, L.L., 1971, Effects of hypothalamic stimulation on plasma glucose, insulin and glucagon levels. Am. J. Physiol., 221:1596-1603.

Gammeltoft, S., Ballotti, R., Finn, C., Nielsen, A., Kowalski, A., Haselbacher, G., Humbel, R., Westermark, B. and Van Osberghan, E., 1987, Two types of receptors for insulin-like growth factors are expressed on normal and malignant cells from mamallian brain, in: "Insulin and Related Peptides in the Central Nervous System", M.K. Raizada, M.I. Phillips and D. Le Roith, eds., Plenum Press, New York.

Giddings, S.J., Chirgwin, J. and Permutt, M.A., 1981, The effects of fasting and feeding on preproinsulin messenger RNA in rats. Endocrinology, Suppl. A-624, 238.

Hales, C.N. and Kennedy, G.C., 1964, Plasma glucose, non-esterified fatty acid and insulin concentrations in hypothalamic-hyperphagic rats. Biochem. J., 90:620-624.

Havrankova, J., Roth, J. and Brownstein, M., 1978, Insulin receptors are widely distributed in the central nervous system of the rat. Nature (Lond.), 272:827-829.

Havrankova, J., Roth, J. and Brownstein, M., 1979, Concentrations of insulin and of insulin receptors in the brain are independent of peripheral insulin levels. J. Clin. Invest., 64:636-642.

Havrankova, J., Schmechel, D., Roth, J. and Brownstein, M.J., 1978, Identification of insulin in rat brain (brain peptides/insulin receptors). Proc. Natl. Acad. Sci., U.S.A. 75:5737-5741.

Helman, A.M., Amira, A., Nocolaidis, S. and Assan, R., 1980, Glucagon release induced by ventrolateral hypothalamic stimulation in the rat. Endocrinology 106:1612-1619.

Itoh, M. and Ebadi, M., 1982, The selective inhibition of hippocampal glutamic acid decarboxylase in zinc-induced epileptic seizures. Neurochem. Res., 7:1287-1298.

Kappy, M.S. and Raizada, M.K., 1982, Adult-level insulin binding is present in term fetal rat CNS membranes. Brain Res., 249:390-392.

Kappy, M.S., Sellinger, S. and Raizada, M.K., 1984, Insulin binding in four regions of the developing rat brain. J. Neurochem., 42:198-203.

Katafuchi, T., Yoshimatsu, H., Oomura, Y. and Sato, A., 1986, Responses of adrenal catecholamine secretion to lateral hypothalamic stimulation and lesion in rats. Brain Res., 363:141-144.

Le Roith, D., Hendricks, S.A., Lesniak, M.A., Rishi, S., Becker, K.L., Havrankova, J., Rosenzweig, J.L., Brownstein, M.J. and Roth, J., 1983, Insulin in brain and other extrapancreatic tissues of vertebrateand nonvertebrates, in: CNS Regulation of Carbohydrate Metabolism, A.J. Szabo, ed., Academic Press, New York.

Lesniak, M., 1978, Iodination of insulin, in: "Seventh Training Course in Radioligand Assay Technique", The Endocrine Society, Bethesda, MD., pp. 57-58.

Lowry, O.H., Rosebrough, N.J., Farr, A.L. and Randall, R.J., 1951, Protein measurement with Folin phenol reagent. J. Biol. Chem., 193:265-275.

Margolis, R.U. and Altszuler, N., 1967, Insulin in the cerebrospinal fluid. Nature (London) 215:1375-1376.

May, J.M. and Contoreggi, C.S., 1982, The mechanism of the insulin-like effects of ionic zinc. J. Biol. Chem., 257:4362-4368.

Miselis, R.R., 1981, The efferent projections of the subfornical organ of the rat: A circumventricular organ within a neural network subserving water balance. Brain Res., 230:1.

Oomura, Y., 1983, Glucose as a regulator of neuronal activity, in "CNS Regulation of Carbohydrate Metabolism", A.J. Szabo, ed., Academic Press, New York.

Palovcik, R. and Phillips, M.I., 1986, A constant perfusion slice chamber for stable recording during the addition of drugs. J. Neurosci. Meth., 17:129-139.

Palovcik, R., Phillips, M.I., Kappy, M.S. and Raizada, M.K., 1984, Insulin inhibits pyramidal neurons in hippocampal slices. Brain Res., 309:187-191.

Phillips, M.I., 1987, The function of glia in the CVOs. Brain Res., Submitted.

Phillips, M.I. and Camacho, A., 1987, The organum vasculosum of the lamina terminalis and median preoptic nucleus: Anatomical connections and physiological functions, in: Circumventricular Organs and Body Fluids, P. Gross, ed., CRC Press, Boca Raton, Fl.

Raizada, M.K., 1983, Localization of insulin-like immunoreactivity in the neurons from primary cultures of rat brain. Exp. Cell Res., 143:351-357.

Raizada, M.K., Yang, J.W. and Fellows, R.E., 1980, Binding of [^{125}I]insulin to specific receptors and stimulation of nucleotide incorporation in cells cultured from rat brain. Brain Res., 200:389-400.

Rosenzweig, J.L., Havrankova, J., Lesniak, M.A., Brownstein, M. and Roth, J., 1980, Insulin is ubiquitous in extrapancreatic tissues of rats and humans. Proc. Natl. Acad. Sci., U.S.A. 77:572-576.

Roth, R.A., Morgan, D.O., Beaudoin, J. and Sara, V., 1986, Purification and characterization of the human brain insulin receptor. J. Biol. Chem., 3753-3757.

Shimazu, T., Fukuda, A. and Ban, T., 1966, Reciprocal influences of the ventromedial and lateral hypothalamic nuclei on blood glucose level and liver glycogen content. Nature 210:1178-1179.

Van Houten, M., Nance, D.M., Gauthier, S. and Posner, B.I., 1983, Origin of insulin-receptive nerve terminals in rat median eminence. Endocrinology 113:1393-1399.

Van Houten, M., Posner, B.I., Kopriwa, B.M. and Brawer, J.R., 1979, Insulin binding sites in the rat brain: In vivo localization to the circumventricular organs by quantiative radioautography. Endocrinology, 105:666-673.

Woods, S.C. and Porte, D., Jr., 1975, Effect of intracisternal insulin on plasma glucose and insulin in the dog. Diabetes 24:905-909.

Young, W.S., III, 1986, Periventricular hypothalamic cells in the rat brain contain insulin mRNA. Neuropeptides, 8:93-97.

STRUCTURAL EVIDENCE FOR A SUBTYPE OF INSULIN RECEPTOR IN THE CENTRAL NERVOUS SYSTEM

Kim A. Heidenreich

University of California, San Diego
Department of Medicine; M-023E
La Jolla, CA 92093

Introduction

Since the discovery of insulin[1] and insulin receptors[2] in the brain in 1978, there has been an increasing number of investigations into the physiological role of insulin in the central nervous system (CNS). One area of CNS physiology affected by insulin is the regulation of feeding behavior and body weight. Chronic intracerebral ventricular infusion of insulin reduces food intake and body weight[3], suggesting that insulin acts as a satiety factor in the CNS. Consistent with this notion is the report that Zucker rats carrying the fa gene have fewer brain insulin receptors[4]. Furthermore, insulin has been shown to directly alter the firing rate of glucose-sensitive neurons in the ventromedial and lateral hypothalamus[5].

Another apparent role for insulin in the CNS is regulation of growth and differentiation of nervous tissue. Insulin and insulin receptors are present throughout the brain[1,2] and appear very early in development[6]. The number of insulin receptors is highest in areas of the brain capable of regeneration[2,7] and peaks at stages of development associated with rapid brain growth[8]. Intracisternal injection of insulin in neonatal rats increases the activity of the rate-limiting enzyme in the biosynthesis of polyamines which promote growth in many tissues[9]. Insulin supports the survival of neurons grown in tissue culture[10] and increases process formation in neurons[11]. Additionally, insulin has been implicated as a developmental signal in the emergence of neurotransmission across nascent synapses in tissue culture[12].

The presence of various growth-promoting and differentiation effects of insulin in the CNS can be contrasted to the absence of any documented short-term metabolic effects of insulin in brain. Regulation of glucose transport and metabolism is a major role of insulin in peripheral tissues, particularly muscle, adipose tissue, and liver; however, this action of insulin appears to be absent in brain. Thus, the activation of insulin receptors in the CNS leads to a different set of biologic responses compared to those in peripheral tissues. The differential response to insulin could result from differences in the insulin receptor molecules, differences in the post-receptor pathways, or both of these factors.

The intent of this chapter is to summarize studies from our laboratory indicating that insulin receptors in the CNS are structurally distinct from insulin receptors in other tissues. Differences occur in the carbohydrate side chains of the receptors, with the most prominent variations occuring in terminal sialylation of the chains. Identification of the structural features of insulin receptors in brain has allowed us to identify tissues and cells that express this subtype of insulin receptor and may provide insight into tissue-specific differences in insulin action.

Size discrepancy of insulin receptors in brain and adipocytes

Our current concepts regarding the structural and functional domains of the insulin receptor have come from purification studies[13,14], affinity-labeling experiments[15,16], and knowledge of the predicted amino acid sequence derived from insulin receptor cDNA[17,18]. Insulin receptors are plasma membrane glycoproteins consisting of 4 disulfide-linked subunits arranged in a B-α-α-B complex[19,20]. The α-subunits are extracellular and contain the insulin binding site[15,16]. The B-subunits traverse the membrane and have tyrosine kinase activity located at their cytoplasmic domains[21-24]. Both subunits are glycosylated[25,26] and on SDS gels, the α-subunit has an apparent molecular weight of 125-130,000, whereas, the B-subunit has an apparent molecular weight of 90-95,000.

In the experiments described in this chapter, we have used photoaffinity labeling procedures to analyze and compare the structure of insulin receptors in rat adipocytes and rat brain. With these procedures, an iodinated, photoreactive analog of insulin (^{125}I-B2(2-nitro-4-azidophenylacetyl)-des-Phe^{B1}-insulin) is covalently coupled to the α-subunit as the result of a photochemical reaction. The details of the preparation of the photoreactive insulin analog[27] and the photoaffinity labeling procedures[28] have been described elsewhere. Following photoaffinity labeling, the tissues are solubilized and analyzed by SDS gel electrophoresis and autoradiography.

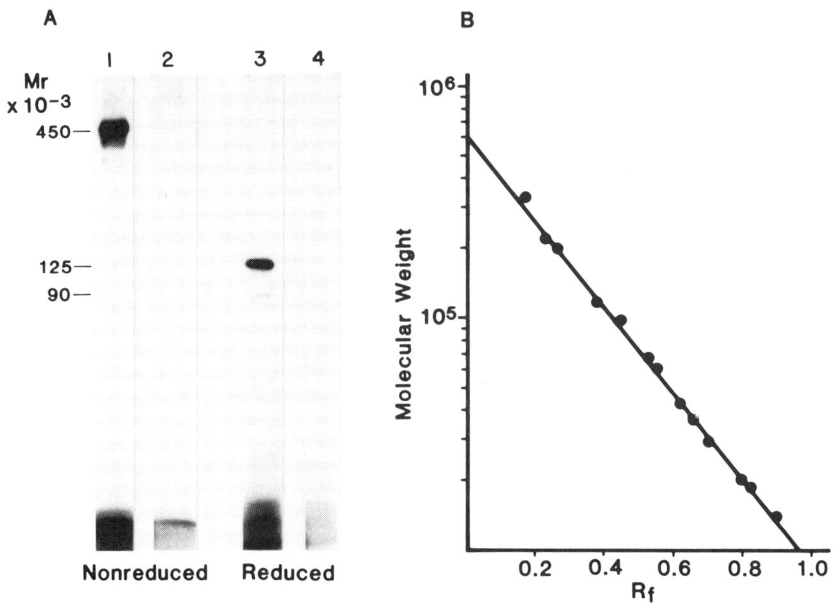

Fig. 1: Autoradiogram of photoaffinity labeled insulin receptors in rat adipocytes.

Figure 1 shows an autoradiogram obtained from rat adipocytes. In the absence of reducing agents, radioactivity was associated with the intact insulin receptor which on our gel system had an apparent molecular weight of 450,000 (lane 1). Upon reduction, radioactivity was almost exclusively found in the 125 kDa α-subunit with only a very small amount of labeling associated with the 90 kDa B-subunit (lane 3). This labeling pattern is representive of all the non-neural tissues that we've examined including placenta, cultured muscle cells, adrenal medulla, and fibroblasts, and can be contrasted to results obtained in brain.

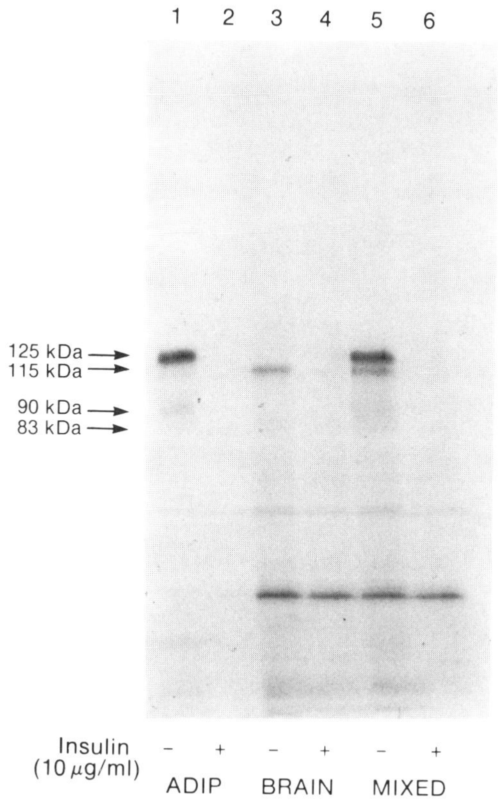

Fig. 2: Autoradiogram of photoaffinity labeled insulin receptors in adipocytes and brain.

Figure 2 shows an autoradiogram of photoaffinity labeled insulin receptors analyzed under reducing conditions from rat adipocyte and rat brain. As shown in Figure 1, the α-subunit in adipocytes had an apparent molecular weight of 125,000 (lane 1). However, in brain the subunit labeled by insulin had an apparent molecular weight of 115,000 (lane 3). The smaller size of the binding subunit in brain was not due to proteolysis occuring during preparation of brain membranes since mixing adipocytes with brain homogenates prior to labeling did not decrease the amount of 125 kDa subunits (lane 5). That is, there was no degrading activity in brain homogenates capable of converting the 125 kDa subunit to the 115 kDa.

When photoaffinity labeled receptors from brain were analyzed on SDS gels in the absence of reducing agents, radioactivity was associated with a 430 kDa protein which was approximately 20kDa smaller than the intact insulin receptor in other tissues indicating that the size discrepancy is apparent for intact insulin receptors as well as for the α-subunits. Labeling of the 430 kDa and 115 kDa proteins was completely blocked by 1 ug/ml unlabeled insulin but not by 1 ug/ml IGF-I. Additionally, the receptor labeled by the insulin analog in brain was immunoprecipitated by anti-insulin receptor antibodies from an insulin resistant patient provided by Dr. Lawrence Mandarino at UCSD. Thus, the proteins labeled by the photoactive analog of insulin in brain have the general characteristics typical of other insulin receptors.

Comparison of the glycosylation properties of insulin receptors in brain and adipocytes

In the following experiments, we examined whether differences in N-linked glycosylation could account for the size discrepancy of the α-subunits in brain and adipocytes. Earlier work had shown that insulin receptors contain N-linked oligosaccharides[29]. The general pathway for the biosynthesis of N-linked glycosylated proteins is thought to begin with the assembly of the oligosaccharide chain on a lipid donor, dolichol, located on the inner face of the endoplasmic reticulum membrane. The intact chains are then transferred cotranslationally onto asparagine residues in the nascent polypeptide chain. The N-linked carbohydrate chains are then processed in the endoplasmic reticulum and Golgi to high mannose chains and, in some cases, the high mannose chains are further modified to form complex chains. The complex oligosaccharide chains are frequently capped with sialic acid.

To probe for possible differences in N-linked glycosylation of insulin receptors in brain and adipocytes we used the following enzymes: endo-B-N-acetylglucosaminidase F (Endo F), endo-B-N-acetylglucosaminidase H (Endo H), and neuraminidase. Endo F removes both high mannose and complex type oligosaccharide chains intact from glycoproteins by hydrolyzing the dichitobiose bond between the first and second N-acetylglucosamine residues at the core. Endo H is more selective than Endo F, in that, it cleaves only high mannose residues. Neuraminidase cleaves terminal sialic acid residues from complex type oligosaccharide chains.

The general protocol was to treat photoaffinity labeled membranes with the various glycosidases and then analyze the intact receptors and their enzymatic products by SDS gel electrophoresis and autoradiography[28]. Results obtained with Endo F are seen in Figures 3 and 4. Endo F treatment of photoaffinity labeled membranes from brain (lanes 1-6) and adipocytes (lanes 7-12) resulted in a concentration-dependent shift in the mobilities of the 115 kDa subunit and the 125 kDa subunit, respectively (Figure 3). The enzyme preparation did not appear to contain contaminating proteases since the cleavage of the proteins was very selective. For example, none of the nonspecifically labeled proteins in brain was affected by the enzyme. Furthermore, inclusion of a cocktail of protease inhibitors during Endo F treatment had no effect on the electrophoretic pattern. Using a maximally effective concentration of Endo F, the brain α-subunit was reduced from 115 kDa to 100 kDa and the adipocyte α-subunit was reduced from 125 kDa to 100 kDa (Fig. 4). Thus, after removal of all the carbohydrate chains, the α-subunit from both tissues had the same apparent molecular weight indicating that the size discrepancy is due to differences in N-linked glycosylation.

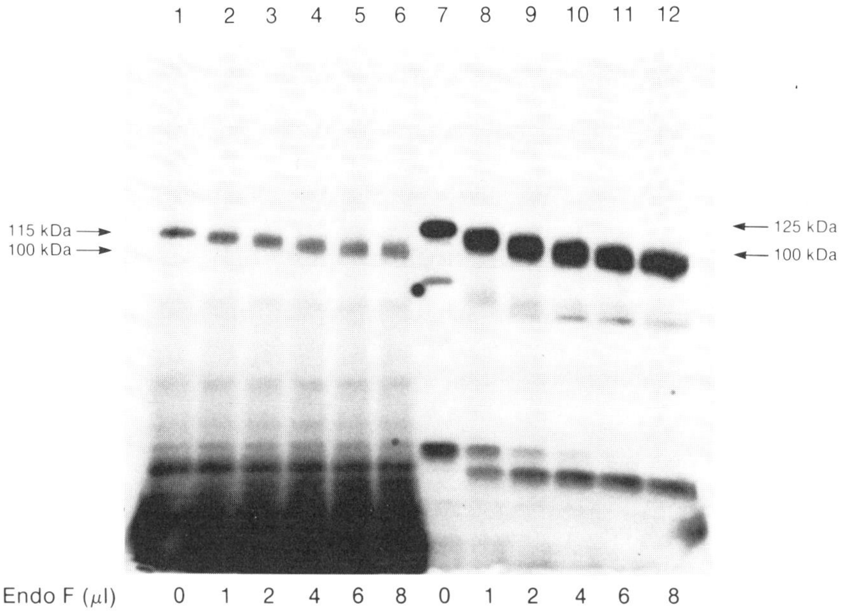

Fig. 3: Treatment of photoaffinity labeled insulin receptors with Endo F.

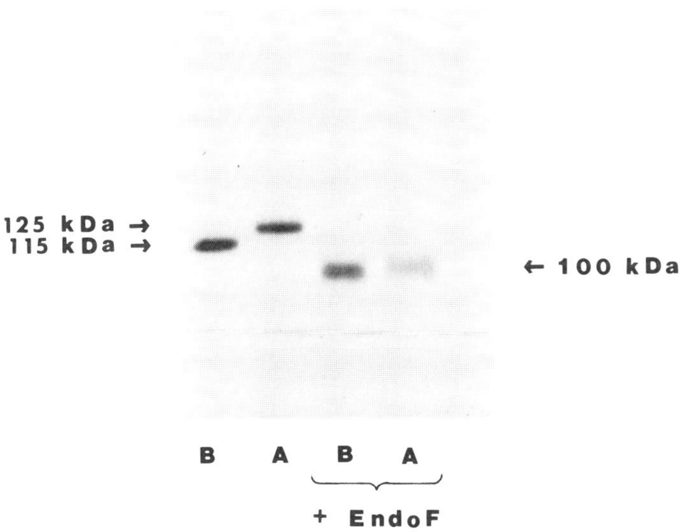

Fig. 4: Comparison of the molecular weights of the α-subunits after deglycosylation.

Differences in the glycosylation of the α-subunits could involve the number of glycosylation sites, the composition of oligosaccharide chains, or both of these factors. Based on the predicted amino acid sequence derived from the nucleotide sequence of the insulin receptor cDNA[17,18], there are 15 possible N-linked glycosylation sites on the α-subunit. To date, there is no information about the actual number of sites that are glycosylated. So, whether this differs in brain and adipocytes remains an open question. With regards to the composition of oligosaccharides, we have found evidence indicating that it differs between the two α-subunits. The most striking difference is in the terminal processing of the complex carbohydrate chains. Treatment of the adipocyte α-subunit with neuraminidase increased the mobility of this protein on SDS gel (Fig. 5, compare lane 6 to lane 1). Whereas, treatment of the brain α-subunit with neuraminidase has no apparent effect (Fig. 5, compare lane 12 to lane 7). Also, shown in Figure 5 are the results obtained with Endo H which selectively cleaves high mannose oligosaccharide chains. Treatment of adipocyte receptors with Endo H resulted in a shift in the mobility of the 125 kDa subunit (lanes 3-5). A similar shift was observed for the 115 kDa subunit following Endo F treatment (lanes 9-11). Therefore, both α-subunits contain high mannose chains.

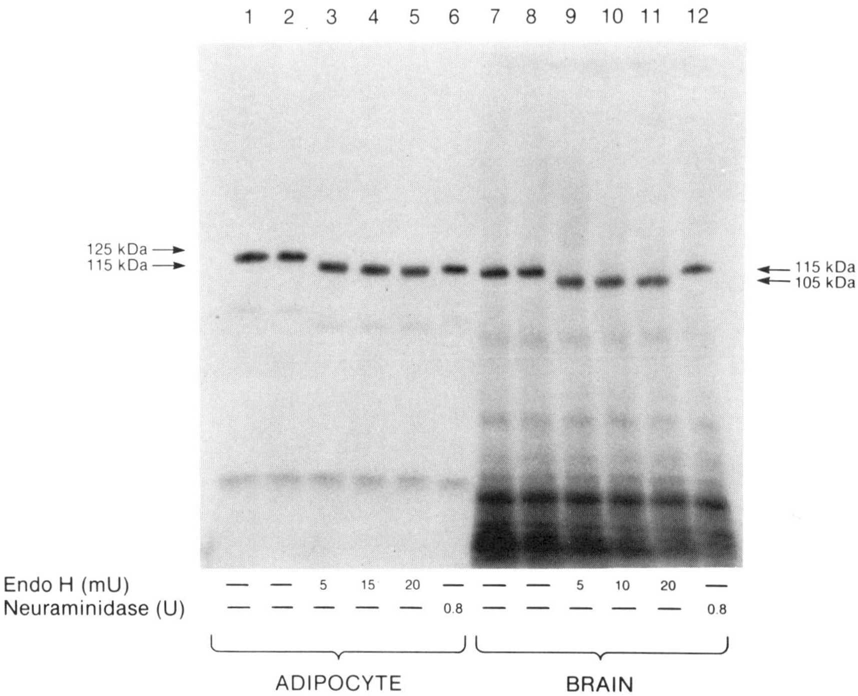

Fig. 5: Treatment of insulin receptors with Endo H and neuraminidase.

The presence of high mannose chains in the brain α-subunit taken together with the insensitivity of this subunit to neuraminidase raised the possibility that the 115kDa contained all high mannose chains. To examine this possibility, we compared the activities of Endo H and Endo F. One would predict that if all of the chains were of the high mannose type than Endo H would cleave to the same extent as Endo F. The results showed that for the 125 kDa subunits and the 115 kDa subunits, the degree of shift obtained with Endo H was less than that observed for Endo F, indicating the presence of complex chains in addition to high mannose chains in both subunits (Fig. 6). One can, therefore, conclude that the complex chains present in brain are either devoid of sialic acid (perhaps they are capped with fucose) or are capped with a type of sialic acid resistant to the neuraminidases used in our studies.

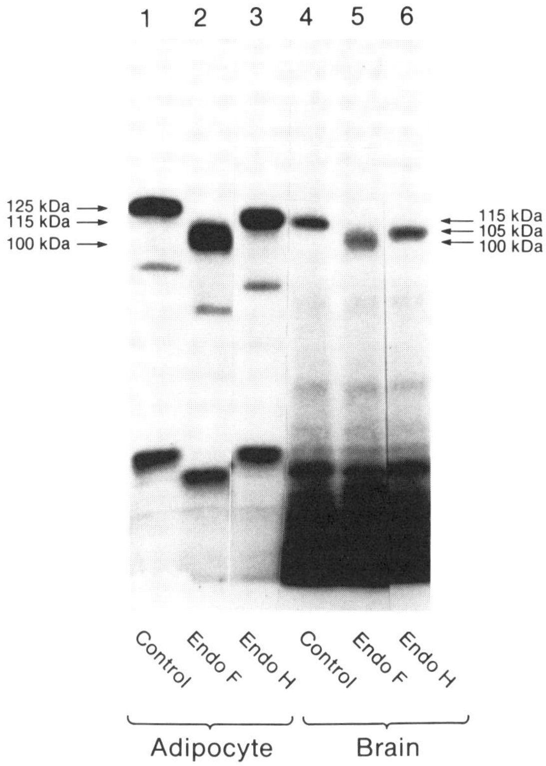

Fig. 6: Comparison of the activities of Endo H and Endo F.

Peptide mapping of the deglycosylated insulin receptors from brain and adipocytes

The similar size of the deglycosylated α-subunits in brain and adipocytes suggested that variations in glycosylation of the subunits resulted from differential processing of the same translation product. To further investigate this hypothesis, we assessed the degree of homology in the protein backbones of the subunits by peptide mapping. In these experiments, insulin receptors from both tissues were photoaffinity labeled, analyzed on SDS gels, and then removed from the gels by electroelution. The eluted insulin receptors were subjected to Endo F to remove the N-linked oligosaccharides. The deglycosylated receptors were then partially digested with various proteases including trypsin, chymotrypsin, papain, elastase, and staph V8 protease, and analyzed by electrophoresis and autoradiography. With this protocol, one has the limitation of detecting only those peptides labeled by the photoaffinity analog of insulin. One might argue that the number of labeled peptides would be

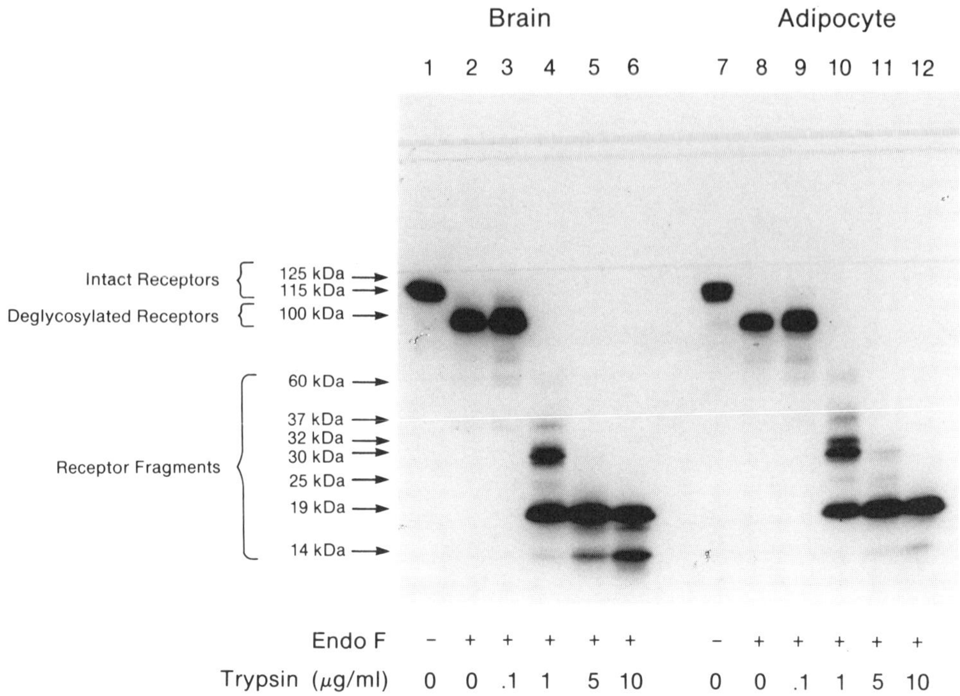

Fig. 7: Peptide maps of the deglycosylated α-subunits.

two few for an adequate comparison. However, preliminary results showed that quite a few peptides were generated from each enzyme, possibly indicating that there are several sequences in the α-subunit involved in insulin binding. Furthermore, we used five different enzymes with varying substrate specificities in order to increase the number of peptides generated.

Figure 7 is an autoradiogram of the peptide maps obtained using trypsin. Lane 1 shows the intact 115 kDa subunit from brain. Lane 2 shows the deglycosylated 115kDa subunit and lanes 3-6 show the proteolytic fragments generated from the deglycosylated subunit with increasing concentrations of trypsin. At 0.1 ug/ml trypsin little detectable proteolysis had occurred (lane 3). However, at concentrations of trypsin of 1 ug/ml to 10 ug/ml, degradation proceeded in a sequential manner with the accumulation of smaller molecular weight fragments (lanes 4-6). There were at least eight fragments generated ranging from 60 kDa to 14 kDa. The right side of the autoradiogram (lanes 7-12) shows results obtained with the adipocyte 125 kDa subunit. One can readily see that the pattern of proteolytic fragments generated from the deglycosylated 125 kDa subunit was distinguishable from those generated from the deglycosylated 115 kDa subunit. Using similar procedures, we've obtained peptide maps for the four other enzymes mentioned. Each enzyme yielded a different set of fragments from those obtained with trypsin. In all cases, the fragments generated by partial digestion were identical for both α-subunits. We've concluded from these experiments that the protein backbones of the two subunits are similar and that the variations in glycosylation are due to differences in post-translational processing.

Distribution of the "brain subtype" of insulin receptor

"In vitro" binding assays[2,7,30] and autoradiographic studies[7,31] indicate that insulin receptors are distributed throughout the brain. Regions showing the highest density of insulin receptors include olfactory bulb, choroid plexus, hippocampus, cerebral cortex, and hypothalamus. With photoaffinity labeling procedures, we examined the structure of insulin receptors in these regions, with the exception of choroid plexus, and found that all regions contained the 115 kDa receptor[32]. Consistent with these data is the finding that membrane fractions prepared from whole brain homogenates contained only the 115 kDa subunit. Thus, it appears that the structure of insulin receptors is uniform throughout the brain. In contrast to nervous tissue in the brain, blood vessels in brain do not have the brain subtype of insulin receptor, but rather have the peripheral insulin receptor. This has been demonstrated in purified microvessels from rat brain using photoaffinity labeling (K.A. Heidenreich, unpublished data) and affinity cross-linking[33,34] procedures.

In areas outside of the brain, we have detected the 115 kDa subunit in rat spinal cord and human retina. However, in rat superior cervical ganglion, part of the peripheral nervous system, and in adrenal medulla, derived from neural crest, we have detected only the 125kDa subunit. A summary of these data are shown in Table 1. The common features of tissues containing the brain subtype of insulin receptor are that they are contained within the blood-brain barrier and are embryologically derived from the same tissue, the neural tube.

TABLE 1: INSULIN RECEPTORS IN DIFFERENT NERVOUS TISSUES

Tissue	α-subunit	
	115 kDa	125 kDa
Rat brain	++	0
Human brain	++	0
Human retina	++	0
Rat spinal cord	++	0
Rat superior cervical ganglia	0	++
Rat adrenal medulla	0	++

Membranes from the various tissues were photoaffinity labeled with ^{125}I-NAPA-DP-insulin, solubilized, and analyzed by SDS-polyacrylamide gel electrophoresis under reducing conditions.

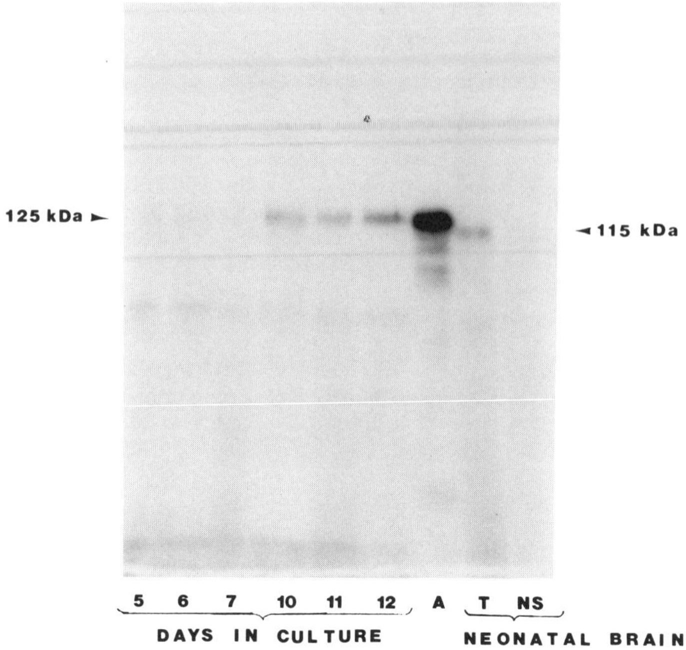

Fig. 8: Autoradiogram of photoaffinity labeled insulin receptors in primary astrocyte cultures.

Insulin receptors in cells cultured from CNS

In order to study the functional properties of the "brain subtype" of insulin receptor, we needed to establish cells in culture that express the 115 kDa subunit. In preliminary experiments, we screened a number of established neuroblastoma and glioma cell lines for the presence of insulin receptors[35]. The cell lines examined had been previously defined as neuronal on the basis of their ability to generate action potentials, by measurements of veratridine-induced influx, and by the presence of neuronal-specific antigens[36,37]. Cell lines were defined as glial based on their inability to generate action potentials, failure to respond to Na^+ uptake studies, and the expression of glial-specific antigens[36,37]. "In vitro" binding assays showed that three neuroblastoma (B103, B65, and XKM) and two glioma (B92, C6) cell lines had detectable insulin receptor binding at trace concentrations of ^{125}I-insulin. Examination of insulin receptor structure in two of the clonal cell lines revealed that the neuroblastoma (B103) and glioma (B92) cells expressed the 125 kDa subunit rather than the 115 kDa subunit[35]. The 125 kDa subunits in both cell lines had increased mobilities on SDS gels after neuraminidase treatment, similar to that seen for the adipocyte insulin receptor.

The reason for the apparent expression of the peripheral type of insulin receptor in clonal cell lines derived from rat CNS is unclear but may be related to the transformation state of the cells. For example, transformed cells frequently express glycoproteins with abnormally high sialic acid content[38]. The expression of the 125 kDa subunit rather than the 115 kDa subunit could result from nonspecific increases in sialyltransferase activity in transformed cells. Alternatively, the difference may be related to the differentiation state of the cells. This point will be emphasized later in this chapter.

We next examined primary cultures derived from either neonatal or fetal brain. By varying a number of conditions including tissue source, developmental age, seeding density, cellular adhesiveness, and culture medium, we were able to obtain cultures containing primarily astrocytes or neurons. The astroglial cultures were prepared from neonatal rat cerebral cortex using methods previously described[39]. The cultures were examined on days 4 through 12 by morphologic criteria and by photoaffinity labeling with the photoactive analog of insulin. On day 4 the cultures consisted of two categories of cells: large, flat, phase-light cells with irregular contours and small, round, phase-dark cells with one or more processes. Both of these cell types stained for glial fibrillary acidic protein, a specific marker for astrocytes[40]. By day 12, the cultures were confluent and greater than 95% of the cells were the flat type. Photoaffinity labeling cultures on day 5 revealed a faint band of 125 kDa and the labeling of this band increased from day 5 to 12 as the astroglial cells proliferated (Fig. 8). There was no labeling of a 115 kDa protein in the astroglial cultures at any time in culture even though the original neonatal brain tissue had only the 115 kDa labeled. Thus, the astroglial cultures represent another example of a tissue derived from the CNS that expresses the peripheral type of insulin receptor.

Different results were obtained when neuronal cultures were examined. Neuronal cultures were prepared by a modification of methods described by Varon et. al.[41] from embryonic rats (day 17) or chicks (day 7). The cells were dissociated with trypsin and plated at a low density on a laminin substratum. On day 5, greater than 90% of the cells were neuronal based on their ability to bind anti-neurafilament, a neuronal-specific antibody. In cultures from both species, photoaffinity labeling with the insulin analog revealed a 115 kDa protein that was indistinguishable from the α-subunit labeled in adult rat brain. The time course of the appearance of the 115 kDa subunit in neuronal cultures prepared from day 7 embryonic chick forebrain is seen in Figure 9. The number of insulin receptors in the cultures increased from day 1 to day 4, a time period during which cell number remained constant and the amount of cellular processes increased dramatically. Insulin receptor affinity remained constant during this time.

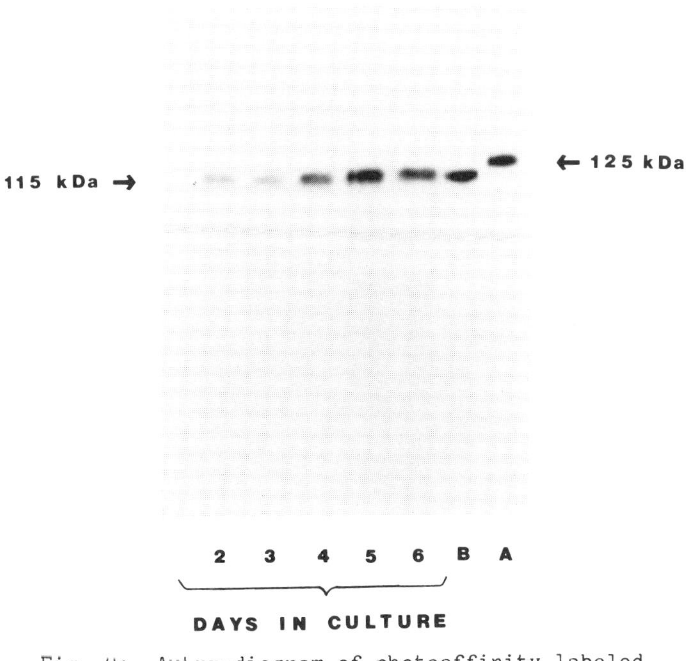

Fig. 9: Autoradiogram of photoaffinity labeled insulin receptors in primary neuronal cultures.

The presence of the CNS subtype of insulin receptor in primary cultures of neurons, but not astrocytes, suggests that the 115kDa subunit is restricted to neurons "in vivo". Since the 125kDa subunit is not detected in adult rat brain, it follows that glial cells express very few insulin receptors "in vivo". However, it is also possible that glial cells "in vivo" express the 115kDa subunit but loose this capacity in culture. The presence of the 115kDa subunit in primary neurons and the changes in the concentration of 115kDa subunits with differentiation support a role for insulin in neuronal development.

Summary and Conclusions

Insulin receptors in the central nervous system are structurally distinct from insulin receptors in other tissues. The α-subunits of insulin receptors in the CNS have smaller apparent molecular weights than the α-subunits of insulin receptors in adipocytes. The difference in molecular weights of the subunits appears to be due to variations in N-linked glycosylation since the size discrepancy of the α-subunits is no longer apparent after removing N-linked oligosaccharides with Endoglycosidase F. Although both the 125kDa subunit and the 115kDa subunit contain oligosaccharide chains of the high mannose type and complex type, the 125kDa subunit has increased mobility on SDS gels after neuraminidase treatment, the 115kDa subunit does not. Therefore, the terminal processing of the complex chains in the subunits differs. The protein backbones of the α-subunits are very similar since peptide maps generated from the deglycosylated 115 kDa subunit are identical to those generated from the deglycosylated 125 kDa subunit. Distribution studies show that the 115 kDa subunit is found in central nervous system tissues including brain, retina, and spinal cord, and is expressed in differentiated neurons in culture. We conclude that the post-translational processing of insulin receptors in the central nervous system differs from that in other tissues and speculate that the altered structure of insulin receptors may contribute to specialized actions of insulin in neurons.

Acknowledgements

This work was supported by grants from the Juvenile Diabetes Foundation and the National Science Foundation. The author would like to acknowledge the contributions of Dr. Dietrich Brandenburg, Dr. Marstin Manthorpe, and Patricia Gilmore to these studies and thank Elizabeth Martinez and Cleon Tate for the preparation of this manuscript.

References

1. J. Havrankova, D. Schmechel, J. Roth, and M. Brownstein, Identification of insulin in rat brain, Proc. Natl. Acad. Sci. 75:5732-5741 (1978).
2. J. Havrankova and J. Roth, Insulin receptors are widely distributed in the central nervous sytem of the rat, Nature 272:827-829 (1978).
3. S.C. Woods, E.C. Looter, L.D. McKay, and D. Porte, Jr., Chronic intracerebraventricular infusion of insulin reduces food intake and body weight in baboons, Nature 282:503-505 (1979).
4. D.P. Figlewicz, D.M. Dorsa, L.J. Stein, D.G. Baskin, T. Paquette, M.R.C. Greenwood, S.C. Woods, and D. Porte, Jr., Brain and liver insulin binding is decreased in Zucker rats carrying the "fa" gene, Endocrinology 117:1537-1543 (1985).
5. Y. Oomura and H. Kita, Insulin acting as a modulator of feeding through the hypothalamus, Diabetologia 20:290-298 (1981)

6. L. Bassas, F. DePablo, M.A. Lesniak, and J. Roth, Ontogeny of receptors for insulin-like peptides in chick embryo tissues: Early dominance of insulin-like growth factor over insulin receptors in brain, Endocrinology 117:2321-2329 (1985).
7. J.M. Hill, M.A. Lesniak, C.B. Pert, and J. Roth, Autoradiographic localization of insulin receptors in rat brain: Prominence in olfactory and limbic areas, Neuroscience 17:1127-1138 (1986).
8. M. Kappy, S. Sellinger and M. Raizada, Insulin binding in four regions of the developing rat brain, J. Neurochem. 42:198-203 (1984).
9. J.W. Yang, M.K. Raizada and R.E. Fellows, Effects of insulin on cultured rat brain cells: Stimulation of ornithine decarboxylase activity, J. Neurochem. 36:1050-1057 (1981).
10. J.R. Bottenstein and G.H. Sato, Growth of a rat neuroblastoma cell line in serum-free supplemented medium, Proc. Natl. Acad. Sci. 76:514-517 (1979).
11. E. Recio-Pinto, F.F. Lang, and D.N. Ishii, Insulin and insulin-like growth factor II permit nerve growth factor binding and the neurite formation response in cultured human neuroblastoma cells. Proc. Natl. Acad. Sci. 81:2562-2566 (1984).
12. D. Puro and E. Agardh, Insulin-mediated regulation of neuronal maturation, Science 225:1170-1172 (1984).
13. S. Jacobs, Y. Shechter, K. Bissell, and P. Cuatrecasas, Purification and properties of insulin receptors from rat liver membranes, Biochem. Biophys. Res. Commun. 77:981-988 (1977).
14. T.W. Siegal, S. Ganguly, S. Jacobs, O.M. Rosen, and C.S. Rubin, Purification and properties of the human placental insulin receptor, J. Biol. Chem. 256:9266-9273 (1981).
15. C.C. Yip, C.W.T. Yeung, and M.L. Moule, Photoaffinity labeling insulin receptors of rat adipocyte membrane, J. Biol. Chem. 253:1743-1745 (1978).
16. P.F. Pilch, and M.P. Czech, Interaction of cross-linking agents with the insulin effector system of isolated fat cells, J. Biol. Chem. 254:3375-3381 (1979).
17. A. Ullrich, J.R. Bell, E.Y. Chen, R. Herrera, L.M. Petruzzelli, T.J. Dull, A. Gray, L. Coussens, Y.C. Liao, M. Tsubokawa, A. Mason, P.H. Seeburg, C. Grunfeld, O.M. Rosen, and J. Ramachandran, Human insulin receptor and its relationship to the tyrosine kinase family of oncogenes, Nature 313:756-761 (1985).
18. Y. Ebina, L. Ellis, K. Jarnagin, M. Edery, L. Graf, E. Clauser, J. Ou, F. Masiarz, Y.W. Kan, I.D. Goldfine, R.A. Roth, and W.J. Rutter, The human insulin receptor cDNA: The structure basis for hormone-activated transmembrane signalling, Cell 40:747-758 (1985).
19. J. Massague, P.F. Pilch, and M.P. Czech, Electrophoretic resolution of three major insulin receptor structures with unique subunit stoichiometries, Proc. Natl. Acad. Sci. 77:7137-7141 (1980).
20. S. Jacobs, E. Hazum, and P. Cuatrecasas, The subunit structure of rat liver insulin receptor, J. Biol. Chem. 255:6937-6940 (1980).
21. M. Kasuga, F.A. Karlson, and C.R. Kahn, Insulin stimulates the phosphorylation of the 95,000-dalton subunit of its own receptor, Science 215:185-187 (1982).
22. E. Van Obberghen and A. Kowalski, Phosphorylation of the hepatic insulin receptor, FEBS Lett. 143:179-182 (1982).
23. L.M. Petruzzelli, S. Ganguly, C.J. Smith, M.H. Cobb, C.S. Rubin, and O.M. Rosen, Insulin activates a tyrosine specific protein kinase in extracts of 3T3-L1 adipocytes and human placenta, Proc. Natl. Acad. Sci. 79:6792-6796 (1982).
24. J. Avruch, R.A. Nemenoff, P.J. Blackshear, M.W. Pierce, and R. Osthanondh, Insulin-stimulated tyrosine phosphorylation of the insulin receptor in detergent extracts of human placental membranes, J. Biol. Chem. 257:15162-15166 (1982).

25. S. Jacobs, E. Hazum, and P. Cuatrecasas, Digestion of insulin receptors with proteolytic and glycosidic enzymes: Effects on purified and membrane-associated receptor subunits, Biochem. Biophys. Res. Commun. 94:1066-1073 (1980).
26. J.A. Hedo, L.C. Harrison, and J. Roth, Binding of insulin receptors to lectins: Evidence for common carbohydrate determinants on several membrane receptors, Biochemistry 20:3385-3393 (1981).
27. M.H. Wisher, M.D. Baron, R.H. Jones, P.H. Sonksen, D.J. Saunders, P. Thamm, and D. Brandenburg, Photoreactive insulin analogues used to characterize the insulin receptor, Biochem. Biophys. Res. Commun. 92:492-498 (1980).
28. K.A. Heidenreich and D. Brandenburg, Oligosaccharide heterogeneity of insulin receptors. Commparison of N-linked glycosylation of insulin recepttors in adipocytes and brain, Endocrinology 118:1835-1842 (1986).
29. J.A. Hedo, M. Kasuga, E. Van Obberghen, J. Roth, and C.R. Kahn, Direct demonstration of glycosylation of insulin receptor subunits by biosynthetic and external labeling: Evidence for heterogeneity, Proc. Natl. Acad. Sci. 78:4791-4795 (1981).
30. S. Gammeltoft, P. Staun-Olsen, B. Ottensen, and J. Fahrenkrug, Insulin receptors in rat brain cortex. Kinetic evidence for a receptor subtype in the central nervous system, Peptides 5:937-944 (1984).
31. W.S. Young, III, M.J. Kuhar, J. Roth, and M.J. Brownstein, Radiohistochemical localization of insulin receptors in the adult and developing rat brain, Neuropeptides 1:15-22 (1980).
32. K.A. Heidenreich, N.R. Zahniser, P. Berhanu, D. Brandenburg, and J.M. Olefsky, Structural differences between insulin receptors in the brain and peripheral target tissues, J. Biol. Chem. 258:8527-8530 (1983).
33. J.F. Haskell, E. Meezan, and D.J. Pillon, Identification of the insulin receptor of cerebral microvessels, Am. J. Physiol. 248:E115-E125 (1985).
34. W.M. Pardridge, J. Eisenberg, and J. Yang, Human blood-brain barrier insulin receptor, J. Neurochem. 44:1771-1778 (1985).
35. K.A. Heidenreich, and P.R. Gilmore, Structural and functional characteristics of insulin receptors in rat neurobalstoma cells, J. Neurochem. 45:1642-1648 (1985).
36. D. Schubert, S. Heinemann, W. Carlisle, H. Tarikas, B. Kimes, J. Patrick, J.H. Steinbach, W. Culp, and B.L. Brandt, Clonal cell lines from rat central nervous system, Nature 249:224-227 (1974).
37. W.B. Stallcup, and m. Cohn, Correlation of surface antigens and cell type in clonal cell lines from the rat central nervous sytem, Exp. Cell Res. 98:2858-297 (1976).
38. L. Warren, J.P. Fuhrer, and C.A. Buck, Surface glycoproteins of normal and transformed cells: A difference determined by sialic acid and growth-dependent sialyltransferase, Proc. Natl. Acad. Sci. 69:1838-1846 (1972).
39. M. Manthorpe, R. Adler, and S. Varon, Development, reactivity, and GFA immunofluorescence of astroglia-containing monolayer cultures from rat cerebrum, J. Neurocytol. 8:605-621 (1979).
40. A. Bignami, L.F. Eng, D. Dahl, and C.T. Uyeda, Localization of the glial fibrillary acidic protein in astrocytes by immunofluorescence, Brain Res. 43:429-435 (1972).
41. S. Varon, S.D. Skaper, G. Barbin, I. Selak, and M. Manthorpe, Low molecular weight agents support survival of cultured neurons from the central nervous system, J. Neuroscience 4:654-658 (1984)

PHYSIOLOGICALLY UNIQUE INSULIN RECEPTORS ON NEURONAL CELLS

Mohan K. Raizada[1], Frederick T. Boyd, Derrel W. Clarke[1] and Derek Le Roith[2]

[1]Department of Physiology, University of Florida, Gainesville, FL 32610, and [2]Diabetes Branch, National Institute of Arthritis, Diabetes, Digestive and Kidney Diseases, National Institute of Health, Bethesda, MD 20205

ABSTRACT

Neuronal cells in primary culture from the brain have been utilized in the present study to determine the physiological and biochemical roles of neuronal insulin receptors. Kinetic characteristics of ^{125}I-insulin binding to neuronal cells were similar to those for glial and peripheral cells although the α and β subunits of the neuronal receptor were significantly smaller in size. Insulin inhibited [^{3}H]-norepinephrine uptake and stimulated [^{3}H]-serotonin uptake in neuronal cells, the effect most likely mediated by insulin receptors. In addition, insulin upregulated, while tunicamycin failed to exert any effects on, neuronal insulin receptors. These observations indicate that the neuronal insulin receptor is physiologically distinct from the glial and peripheral receptors and suggest that insulin may have a neuromodulatory role in the brain function.

INTRODUCTION

Substantial evidence exists in the literature which demonstrates that the brain contains insulin-sensitive areas, suggesting that insulin may have significant physiological and biochemical effects on the brain. This contention is further strengthened by the observations documenting the presence of insulin-specific receptors in the brain (1-5). In addition, insulin has been shown to stimulate the release of catecholamines (6,7) and influence firing rate of nigrostriatal and hippocampal neurons (8,9). These actions of insulin are in contrast with the conflicting reports of its effect on sugar uptake. We postulated that some of these conflicting observations on the effects of insulin in the brain may be the result of complexities of the CNS and the presence of heterogenous cell types in the brain which may respond differently. This led us to develop differential *in vitro* cell culture procedures in order to investigate the functional role of insulin in the relatively homogenous cell populations from the brain. For example: studies have shown that astrocytic glial cells in primary culture from neonatal rat brain possess specific insulin receptors which are kinetically, physiologically and biochemically indistinguishable from the insulin receptors on peripheral target tissue (10,11). The presence of insulin-specific receptors has also been demonstrated in neuronal cells in primary culture (12,13). These neuronal cultures have been utilized further to study the structural, physiological and biochemical properties of insulin receptors on the neurons and to compare them with their peripheral non-neuronal and glial counterparts. The observations suggest that the neuronal insulin receptor is physiologically and biochemically distinct from the peripheral non-neuronal and glial insulin receptors.

MATERIALS

One-day-old Sprague-Dawley rats were obtained from our breeding colony. Dulbecco's modified Eagle's medium and fetal bovine serum (FBS) were purchased from GIBCO, Grand Island, NY. Deoxyribonuclease I, trypsin 1 × crystalline were from Worthington. Plasma-derived horse serum (PDHS) was obtained from Hyclone Laboratories, Logan UT. Bovine serum albumin (BSA), poly-L-lysine, cytosine arabinoside, pargyline HCl, L-ascorbic acid, and (-)-norepinephrine (NE) were from Sigman Chemical Co., St. Louis, MO. (-)-[7-^{3}H]-norepinephrine (specific activity 16.9 - 24 Ci/mmol), D[6-^{3}H-(N)]-glucosamine hydrochloride (specific activity 56.8 Ci/mmol), (-)-[^{3}H]-serotonin (specific activity 16.9 - 24 Ci/mmol) were obtained from New England Nuclear, Boston, MA. Crystalline porcine insulin was purchased from Elanco Products Co., Indianapolis, IN, and B26 labelled ^{125}I-porcine insulin was kindly provided by Dr. Bruce Frank of Eli Lilly Laboratories, Indianapolis, IN.

METHODS

Preparation of neuronal and glial cells in primary culture

Neuronal cells in primary cultures were prepared from one-day-old rat brains essentially as described previously (14). Briefly, brains were removed, cleaned free of blood vessels and pia mater, chopped into small pieces and subjected to trypsin and DNase I treatment to dissociate cells. Dissociated brain cells were washed free of hydrolytic enzymes by the growth medium containing 10% PDHS and plated in poly-L-lysine-precoated tissue culture dishes in the same medium. After maintenance of cultures for 3 days at 37°C in 5% CO_2:95% air, they were treated with 10 μM cytosine arabinoside in DMEM containing 10% PDHS for 48 hr. The medium containing the drug was replaced with DMEM containing PDHS and cultures were allowed to establish for an additional 10 - 15 days before being used for experiments. Previous studies have demonstrated that the above-described culture procedure yields 70 - 85% neuronal cell types and the remaining cells are of the astrocytic glial type.

Primary cultures of astrocytic glial cells from one-day-old rat brain were prepared as described previously (10,11). Brain cells were established in culture for the first three days as described above for neuronal cultures. On day 3, cultures were fed with DMEM containing 10% FBS and allowed to grow for an additional 4 - 6 days. Cells were dissociated by trypsin treatment, resuspended in the DMEM-FBS medium, plated in culture dishes of the appropriate sizes and allowed to grow for 6 - 10 days before being used for experiments.

Insulin binding assays

Binding of ^{125}I-insulin to intact neuronal and glial cells attached to tissue culture dishes was measured essentially as described previously (10,12,13). Quantitation of ^{125}I-insulin binding to membranes prepared from neuronal and glial cultures was carried out by the procedure described previously (15).

Crosslinking of ^{125}I-insulin to insulin receptors

Neuronal membranes were labelled with ^{125}I-insulin followed by crosslinking of the hormone receptor complex with 0.1 mM disuccinimidyl suberate (15). The crosslinked receptor complex was solubilized with 1% Triton X-100 in the presence of 2 mM PMSF followed by the analysis on the SDS-PAGE under reducing conditions essentially as described previously (15).

Table 1: Kinetic characteristics of ^{125}I-insulin binding to neuronal cultures

Parameters	
Association, $t_{\frac{1}{2}}$	35 min
Dissociation, $t_{\frac{1}{2}}$	15 min
IC_{50} -- Porcine Insulin	16 nM
K_d (High affinity site)	11 nM
K_d (Low affinity site)	65 nM
B_0 (Binding capacity)	1.8 pmol/mg protein

Insulin receptor autophosphorylation and phosphorylation of artificial substrates

Insulin receptor autophosphorylation was performed as described previously (15). WGA-purified receptor preparations were incubated in the absence and presence of 10^{-7} M insulin in a final volume of 350 μl 50 mM HEPES buffer, pH 7.6, with 2 mM PMSF and 0.5 U/ml α_2-macroglobulin. Phosphorylation was initiated by the addition of 100 μl of reaction mixture containing 5 μM [γ^{32}P]ATP, 1 mM CTP, 3 mM manganese acetate, 1 mM sodium vanadate and 20 mM $MgCl_2$. The reaction was stopped, receptor immunoprecipitated and analyzed on SDS-PAGE as described previously (15).

Phosphorylation of artificial substrates by WGA-purified receptor was performed essentially as described previously (15).

Measurement of [^{3}H]-monoamine uptake

Uptake of [^{3}H]-monoamines into neuronal cells in primary culture was determined in cells attached to 60 mm culture dishes. Growth medium was removed, cultures washed once with PBS containing 0.75 mM $CaCl_2$, 0.75 mM $MgCl_2$ and 30 mM glucose. Uptake was determined by incubating cultures with 1.0 ml of PBS containing 100 μM pargyline, 200 μM ascorbate and 0.1 μM of the appropriate (-)-[^{3}H]-monoamine for 2 min. In certain experiments cultures were preincubated at 37°C for 10 min with insulin. Following uptake, reaction mixture was removed and cultures were rinsed twice with ice-cold PBS. Cells were dissolved in 0.2 N NaOH and radioactivity counted as described previously (14). Use of selective monoamine uptake inhibitors (maprotiline for norepinephrine and fluvoxamine for serotonin) was made to determine the effect of insulin on specific uptake of monoamines via NE or serotonin uptake systems.

RESULTS

Characterization of insulin receptors on neuronal cells

Binding of ^{125}I-insulin to neuronal cultures fulfills all the major criteria for it to be termed a true hormone-receptor interaction. This binding is rapid, reversible and specific (Table 1). Scatchard analysis shows a typical curvilinear plot characteristic of insulin binding to other target tissues.

^{125}I-Insulin was crosslinked to its neuronal receptor to determine the MW of the α-subunit of the receptor by SDS-PAGE under reducing conditions. Figure 1 shows that the molecular weight (MW) of the α-subunit was 124,000 which was similar to that reported from the neonatal and adult rat brain and was significantly lower than the MW of the α-subunit from the liver (15). Insulin receptors were solubilized and purified on WGA as described previously (15). Purified insulin receptors were then utilized to characterize the β-subunit by determining the autophosphorylation of the receptor and comparing the MW of the phosphorylated β-subunit with the same from the liver receptor. Solubilized and lectin-purified insulin receptors of neuronal cells stimulated the autophosphorylation of a protein with a MW of 90,000 as seen on the SDS-PAGE (Figure 2). This phosphoprotein has been identified as the β-subunit of the insulin receptor because of its ability to be quantitatively precipitated by anti-insulin receptor antiserum. The MW of the β-subunit of the receptors from neuronal culture was similar to that from the brain but was significantly smaller than the MW of the β-subunit of the liver insulin receptor.

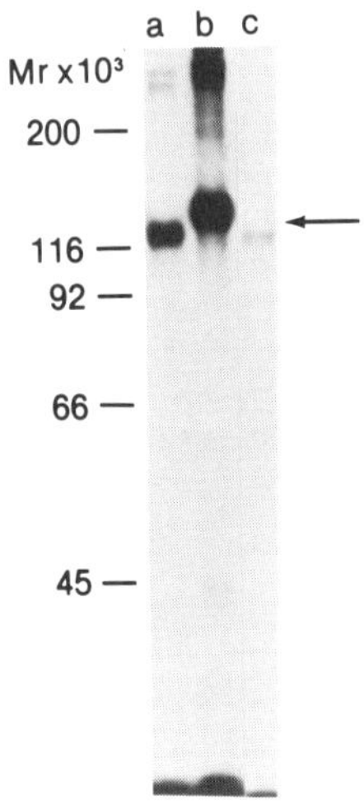

Fig. 1. Autoradiogram of ^{125}I-insulin crosslinked insulin receptors from neuronal cultures. Crude membranes from one-day-old neonatal rat brain, liver and neuronal cells were incubated with ^{125}I-insulin (10 ng/ml) and crosslinked using 0.1 mM disuccinimidyl suberate. The membranes were solubilized in 1% Triton X-100, centrifuged at 180,000 x g for 30 min and anti-insulin receptor antiserum used to immunoprecipitate the insulin receptor. The crosslinked receptors were applied to SDS-PAGE under reducing conditions. Lane (a) = brain, lane (b) = liver and lane (c) = neuronal cells. The arrow indicates the M_r of the glial cell insulin receptors (~M_r 130 kDa) whereas the M_r of the liver receptors was ~ 135 kDa and that of brain ~ 118 kDa.

Lectin-purified insulin receptors showed the ability to stimulate the phosphorylation of ^{32}P into the exogenous substrate poly(Glu,Tyr) (4:1) where tyrosine is the only phosphorylable amino acid. Insulin caused a concentration-dependent stimulation of ^{32}P from ATP into the exogenous substrate with an IC_{50} of 2.5 nM. Human proinsulin, in contrast, was significantly less potent in the stimulation of phosphorylation with an IC_{50} of 79 nM (Figure 3).

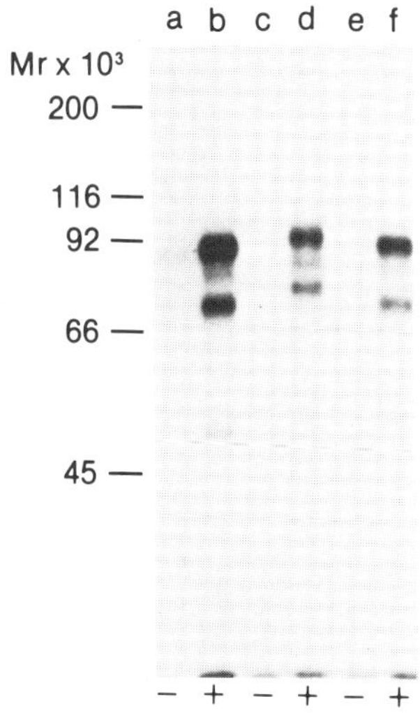

Fig. 2. Insulin-stimulated autophosphorylation of lectin-purified neuronal insulin receptors. WGA-purified membranes from neonatal rat brain liver and neuronal cells were incubated with (+) or without (-) insulin (10^{-7} M). After 30 min at 22°C, phosphorylation was initiated by the addition of 5 μM [γ-^{32}P]ATP, 1 mM CTP, 1 mM sodium vanadate, 20 mM $MgCl_2$ and 3 mM manganese acetate. After 7 min the reaction was stopped and anti-insulin receptor antiserum was used to immunoprecipitate the insulin receptor which was applied to SDS-PAGE. Lanes a,b = brain, lanes c,d = liver, and lanes e,f = neuronal cell cultures.

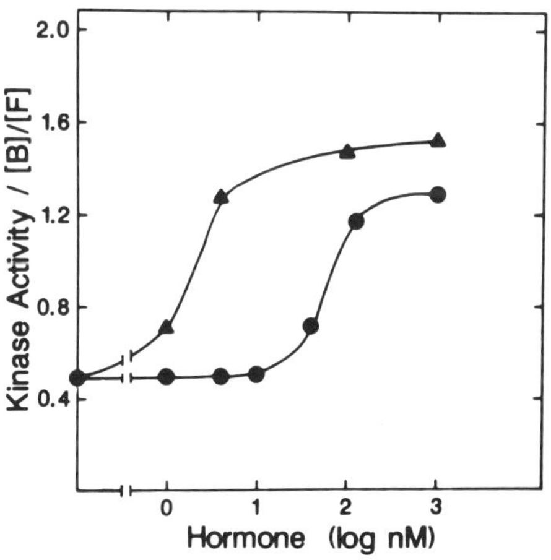

Fig. 3. The effect of insulin and proinsulin on phosphorylation of exogenous substrate poly(Glu,Tyr) (4:1) by lectin-purified insulin receptors. Lectin-purified neuronal insulin receptors were incubated with poly(Glu,Tyr) (4:1) in the presence of increasing concentrations of insulin (O) or proinsulin (Δ) for 30 min at 24°C. This was followed by phosphorylation reaction as described in the "Methods".

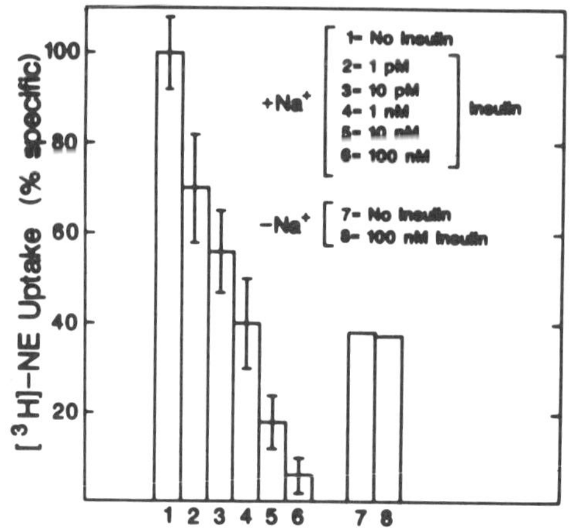

Fig. 4. The effect of insulin on [^{3}H]-norepinephrine uptake by neuronal cells in culture. Neuronal cultures were incubated in the Na^+-containing PBS (1-6) or in the PBS where Na^+ was replaced by choline chloride (7,8) with indicated concentrations of insulin with or without 100 μM maprotiline, an inhibitor of specific NE uptake. Specific NE uptake was determined by subtracting the nonspecific uptake (in the presence of maprotiline) from total uptake (in the absence of maprotiline).

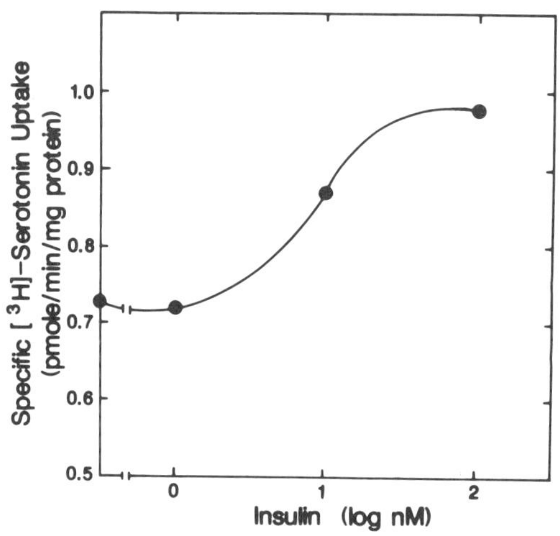

Fig. 5. Effect of insulin on specific [^{3}H]-serotonin uptake in neuronal cultures. Neuronal cultures were preincubated with indicated concentrations of insulin for 10 min at 37°C. This was followed by measurement of [^{3}H]-serotonin uptake in the absence and presence of 100 μl fluvoxamine. Specific uptake was determined by subtracting nonspecific uptake (in the presence of fluvoxamine) from total uptake.

Cellular effects of insulin on neuronal cells

Incubation of neuronal cultures with insulin resulted in a concentration-dependent inhibition of specific [^{3}H]-norepinephrine uptake (Figure 4). As low as 1 pM insulin produced a significant inhibition, and a maximum inhibition of >90% of specific [^{3}H]-NE uptake was observed with 100 nM insulin. This inhibitory effect

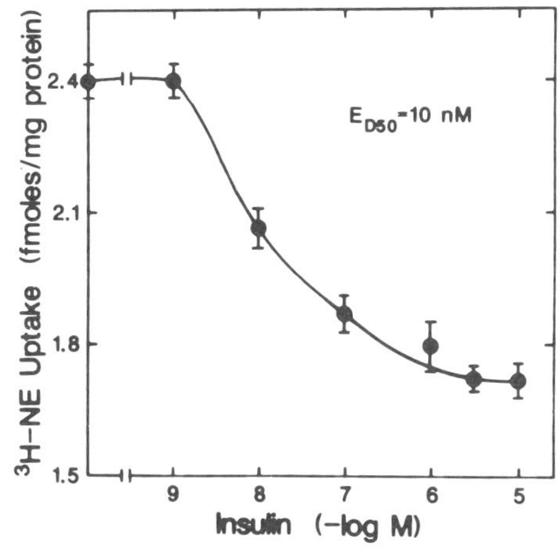

Fig. 6. The effect of insulin on total [^{3}H]-norepinephrine uptake in synaptosomes from adult rat brain. Synaptosomes were prepared as described previously (18). They were preincubated with indicated concentrations of insulin for 2 min at 37°C. This was followed by the measurement of [^{3}H]-NE uptake essentially as described for neuronal cultures under "Methods".

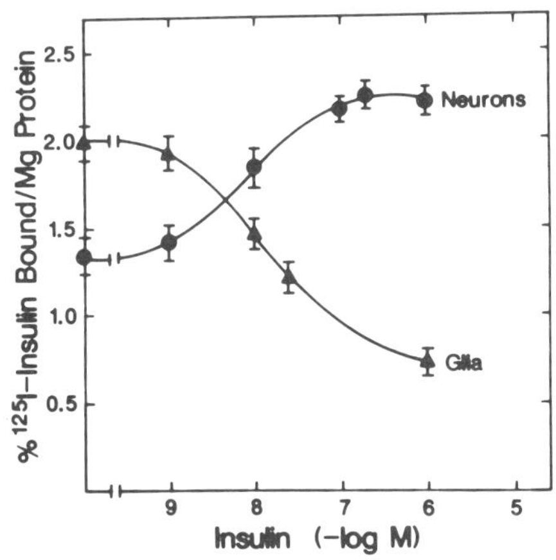

Fig. 7. The effect of insulin on insulin receptors in neuronal cultures. Neuronal cultures were incubated with varying concentrations of insulin for 24 hr at 37°C. Cultures were rinsed over a period of 15 min to remove unlabelled insulin and were used for quantitation of ^{125}I-insulin binding as described under "Methods". Data for glial cultures are provided for comparison.

of insulin was sodium ion-dependent, since insulin failed to inhibit the uptake when Na^+ was replaced with choline chloride (Figure 4). In contrast with the inhibitory effect on [^{3}H]-NE, insulin caused a dose-dependent stimulation of [^{3}H]-serotonin uptake (Figure 5). Maximum stimulation of 38 - 50% of [^{3}H]-serotonin uptake was observed with 9 nM insulin.

The effect of insulin on the specific uptake of [^{3}H]-NE by the synaptosomes prepared from the adult rat brain was studied to eliminate the possibilities that this unique influence of insulin on neuronal cells in culture is not induced by <u>in vitro</u>

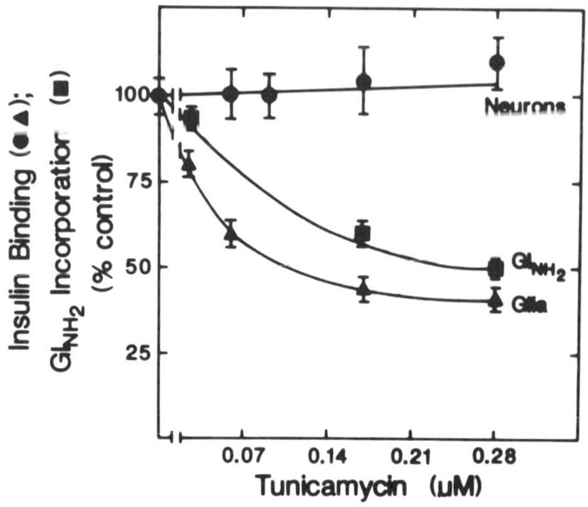

Fig. 8. The effect of tunicamycin on neuronal insulin receptors and [^{3}H]-glucosamine incorporation. Neuronal cultures were incubated with indicated concentrations of tunicamycin. ^{125}I-Insulin binding and [^{3}H]-glucosamine incorporation were measured as described previously (12). Data for glial cultures under similar experimental conditions are provided for comparison.

cell culture or that it is not unique to neonatal brain. Figure 6 shows that incubation of synaptosomes prepared from the brains of adult rat with insulin resulted in a concentration-dependent inhibition of Na^+-sensitive uptake of [^{3}H]-NE. A maximum inhibition of 34% of total uptake was observed with 1 μM insulin with an IC_{50} of ~ 10 nM.

Regulation of neuronal insulin receptors

Incubation of peripheral target cells with insulin has been shown to induce downregulation of insulin receptors. Neuronal cultures were incubated with insulin for 24 hr in order to determine if similar downregulatory effects could be seen in the brain tissue. Figure 7 shows that, in contrast to peripheral tissue and glial cells in culture, insulin caused a dose-dependent increase in the specific binding of ^{125}I-insulin in neuronal culture. A 60 - 70% increase in the binding was observed with 1 μM insulin.

The effect of tunicamycin on neuronal insulin receptors was studied to compare its influence on the receptors from peripheral tissue and from the cultured glial cells. Figure 8 shows that although tunicamycin caused a concentration-dependent decrease in the binding of insulin to glial cells, it failed to have such an effect on the neuronal insulin receptor. This lack of an effect by tunicamycin on the binding was not due to the inability of tunicamycin to inhibit protein glycosylation, since it inhibited incorporation of [^{3}H]-glucosamine into both neuronal and glial cultures to the same extent.

DISCUSSION

The observations presented here support our hypothesis that neuronal cells possess a unique population of insulin receptors which may be involved in the neuromodulatory actions of insulin in the brain.

The neuronal insulin receptor is similar to the peripheral and glial receptors insofar as the kinetics of ^{125}I-insulin binding is concerned. In contrast, the neuronal insulin receptor expresses significantly different biochemical and physiological properties. The α and β subunits of the neuronal receptor are significantly smaller in size compared with those of the liver or other peripheral counterparts and compared with the α-subunit of the cultured glial insulin receptor from the neonatal brain, although the receptors from all tissues express comparable insulin-stimulated autophosphorylation and phosphorylation of exogenous substrate. The molecular weight of the neuronal α-subunit is similar to that reported from the neonatal and adult rat brains (3,15-17), indicating that the expression of a smaller MW subunit is probably preserved and could be expressed in primary cultures from one-day-old rat brain neurons. The precise significance or physiological consequence of such a decrease in the size of the α-subunit is not clearly understood at the present time, although it has been suggested that this difference may be the result of the extent of glycosylation of insulin receptors in the brain receptor (15-17). However, preliminary observations suggest that this decrease in the MW and the extent of glycosylation of insulin receptors from neuronal cells may not have any implication in the differential biological and physiological effects of insulin on neuronal, glial and peripheral cells.

Comparison of the physiological effects of insulin on neurons with those on the glial cells and other peripheral tissue also revealed significant differences. For example, insulin has been shown to stimulate sugar uptake in glial cells (10) and other peripheral tissue, whereas such an effect of insulin is not seen in neuronal cells. In contrast, insulin induced profound changes in the uptake of monoamines in neurons and not in the glial cells. Insulin inhibited NE uptake with as low as a 1 - 10 pM concentration, which occupies fewer than 5% neuronal insulin receptors. The inhibitory effect of insulin on neuronal NE uptake was similar to maprotiline's effect, a selective NE uptake inhibitor. Comparison of dose response of insulin's and maprotiline's inhibition on the uptake revealed that insulin was 600 times more potent on a molar basis. Insulin also caused a concentration-dependent stimulation of specific serotonin uptake. These observations, taken together, clearly suggest that insulin produces profound physiological effects on sugar uptake, DNA and protein synthesis in glial cells (10,11), whereas it influences the monoamine uptake system in the neuronal cells. These effects of insulin on neuronal cells are in accordance with previous findings (6-9) which support a neuromodulatory action of insulin in the CNS.

Significant differences in the effects of insulin and tunicamycin on the expression of insulin receptors on neuronal cells with those of glial and other peripheral target cells have been observed. Insulin, which classically downregulates its receptors in peripheral tissue as well as in glial cells, failed to do so in neuronal cells. In fact, insulin caused a significant increase in insulin binding in these cells. The significance of this upregulatory effect of insulin on its neuronal receptors is not understood at the present time, but may have implications on the developmental aspects of the brain. This suggestion is supported by the unpublished observations of Dr. Brennman (personal communication) who demonstrated superimposable, transient changes in the plasma insulin levels and the brain insulin receptors during fetal development. It is implied that the lack of a blood-brain barrier during early stages of brain development enables the plasma insulin to influence upregulation of the brain insulin receptors.

Tunicamycin, which inhibits the expression of insulin receptors at the cell surface of peripheral and glial cells, failed to do so in neuronal cells. This effect was not due to tunicamycin's lack of influence on glycosylation. Failure of tunicamycin to inhibit the expression of insulin receptors at the neuronal cell surface could be explained either by tunicamycin's inability to inhibit receptor glycosylation or by a very slow turnover rate of these receptors on neurons.

In summary, these observations indicate that insulin receptors on neurons significantly differ from their glial and peripheral counterparts and suggest that they may mediate a neuromodulatory type of action of insulin in the brain

ACKNOWLEDGMENTS

This work is supported by NIH grant HD-16722. Mohan K. Raizada is an Established Investigator of the American Heart Association.

REFERENCES

1. Havrankova, J., Roth, J., and Brownstein, M. (1978). Nature 272:827.
2. Young III, W.S., Kuhar, M.J., Roth, J., and Brownstein, M.J. (1980). Neuropeptides 1:15.
3. Gammeltoft, S. (1984). Physiol. Rev. 64:1321-1378.
4. Hendricks, S.A., Agardh, C.-D., Taylor, S.I., and Roth, J. (1984). J. Neurochem. 43:1302.
5. Hill, J.M., Lesniak, M.A., Pert, C.P., and Roth, J. (1986). Neurosci. 17:1127-1138.
6. Barbaccia, M., Chuang, D., and Costa, E. (1982). Adv. Biochem. Psychopharmacol. 33:511-518.
7. Sauter, A., Goldstein, M., Engel, J., and Ueta, K. (1983). Brain Res. 260:330-333.
8. Saller, C.F., and Chiodo, L.A. (1980). Science 210:1269-1271.
9. Palovcik, R.A., Phillips, M.I., Kappy, M.S., and Raizada, M.K. (1984). Brain Res. 309:187-191.
10. Clarke, D.W., Boyd, F.T., Kappy, M.S., and Raizada, M.K. (1984). J. Biol. Chem. 259:11672-11675.
11. Clarke, D.W., Boyd, F.T., Kappy, M.S., and Raizada, M.K. (1985). Am. J. Physiol. 249:C481-C489.
12. Boyd, F.T., and Raizada, M.K. (1983). Am. J. Physiol. 245:C283-C287.
13. Boyd, F.T., Clarke, D.W., Muther, T.F., and Raizada, M.K. (1985). J. Biol. Chem. 260:15880-15884.
14. Raizada, M.K. (1983). Exp. Cell Res. 143:351-357.
15. Lowe, W.L., Boyd, F.T., Clarke, D.W., Raizada, M.K., Hart, C., and Le Roith, D. (1986). Endocrinology 119:25-35.
16. Yip, C.C., Moule, M.L., and Yeung, C.W.T. (1980). Biochem. Biophys. Res. Commun. 96:1671-1678.
17. Heidenreich, K.A., Zahniser, R.N., Berhanu, P., Brandenburg, D., and Olefsky, J.M. (1983). J. Biol. Chem. 258:8527-8530.
18. Bottiglieri, D.F., Sumners, C., and Raizada, M.K. (1987). Brain Res., In Press.

INSULIN RECEPTORS IN BRAIN DEVELOPMENT

William A. Brennan Jr.

Department of Biochemistry and Molecular Biology
Harvard University
Cambridge, Massachusetts

INTRODUCTION

The presence of insulin in the nervous system has generated considerable interest since its discovery in insects less than a decade ago (for a review, see Hendricks et al., 1983). Since then, insulin or insulin-like material has been detected in numerous species, both vertebrate and invertebrate, as well as in bacteria and fungi (LeRoith et al., 1980; LeRoith et al., 1981). Accordingly, this has prompted the search in these tissues and cells for an insulin specific cellular target, namely the insulin receptor. Insulin receptors appear on nearly all vertebrate and many invertebrate cells, most of which have not previously been considered insulin-responsive. This has raised the possibility that insulin may elicit unique actions in these cells, distinct from its known effects on liver, muscle and fat. For example, insulin is essential for the *in vitro* growth and maintenance of all cell lines examined to date (Barnes and Sato, 1980). This may be particularly relevant when considering the role of insulin in the nervous system, since few of insulin's classical effects have been demonstrated in this tissue. Current thinking has led to the suggestion that insulin may have neuromodulatory actions in the central nervous system (CNS) (Boyd et al., 1985). Alternatively, insulin might play two different but not mutually exclusive roles in the nervous system: 1.) neuromodulatory, and 2.) promotion of growth and differentiation in the embryo and newborn brain. Few studies have examined the ontogeny of insulin receptors in the embryonic brain and little is known concerning the importance of insulin in the central nervous system. This chapter will therefore attempt to summarize current findings about the presence of insulin and insulin receptors in the developing brain.

COMPARISON BETWEEN INSULIN RECEPTORS IN THE NERVOUS SYSTEM AND PERIPHERAL TARGET TISSUES

The existence of insulin receptors in nervous tissue was first demonstrated by Posner (Posner et al., 1974), who showed specific binding of ^{125}I-insulin to membranes prepared from the brains of various vertebrate species. Havrankova et al. (1978) reported the presence of insulin receptors throughout the rat CNS, with the most prominent specific binding seen in the olfactory bulb, cerebral cortex and hippocampus.

With the advent of affinity labeling techniques, several studies examined the structure of the CNS insulin receptor. Yip et al. (1980), using the photoaffinity probe monoazidobenzoyl-insulin, showed that rat brain insulin receptor α-subunits travel faster on SDS-PAGE than similarly labeled α-chains from other tissues. Using a similar approach, Heidenreich et al. (1983) demonstrated that although insulin receptors are structurally indistinguishable throughout the brain, differences in molecular weight, carbohydrate composition and antigenicity exist between brain insulin receptors and receptors in peripheral target tissues. It is now generally accepted that a difference in the extent of glycosylation of CNS insulin receptors is responsible for their lower apparent molecular weight (Heidenreich et al., 1983; Hendricks et al., 1984; Heidenreich and Brandenburg, 1986; Lowe and LeRoith, 1986).

In addition to having structural differences, brain insulin receptors are in many ways functionally distinct from their counterparts in the more classical insulin-sensitive tissues. Brain receptors fail to exhibit down regulation and are not internalized after exposure to insulin as in other tissues (Zahniser et al., 1984; Van Schravendijk et al., 1984; Gammeltoft et al., 1984b). Despite these differences, it is clear from several studies that the brain insulin receptor functions as a tyrosine kinase (Rees-Jones et al., 1984; Gammeltoft et al., 1984; Lowe and LeRoith, 1986; Lowe et al., 1986), suggesting that one aspect of the mechanism for insulin-stimulated signal transduction may be the same in brain as in other tissues.

Whether the structural peculiarities of the brain insulin receptor described above have any bearing on insulin's role in the CNS is not known. One system which may be useful in answering this question is the developing brain, since at this stage the CNS is in direct communication with the peripheral circulation and therefore plasma insulin. The remainder of this chapter will focus on what is known about insulin and insulin receptors in brain development.

INSULIN IN BRAIN DEVELOPMENT

The presence of insulin has been demonstrated in nervous tissue from both vertebrate and invertebrate animals (Hendricks et al., 1983). While there is some controversy concerning the concentration and site of synthesis of brain insulin (Eng and Yalow, 1981), the ubiquity of this hormone in a wide variety of animal species argues for an extra-pancreatic origin of insulin in many cells and tissues (LeRoith et al., 1980; LeRoith et al., 1981).

It is not clear as yet which cell type(s) in the CNS are responsible for insulin synthesis, although fetal mouse brain cells which produce insulin in culture have been characterized as neuronal (Birch et al., 1984).

The situation regarding brain insulin levels in vivo during fetal life is complicated by the fact that in many species, the immature blood brain barrier is not intact (Carey, 1982). Nevertheless, insulin levels in fetal plasma should be a good approximation of the total insulin concentration in the brain if we assume that these two compartments are in equilibrium during embryonic development. Accordingly, Cohen and Turner (1972) have shown that plasma insulin levels in fetal rats are higher than those found in adult animals and rise markedly from the 18th to 21st day of gestation. The levels remain high on the 22nd day, then fall rapidly after birth. This suggests that in rat the embryonic brain is exposed to high levels of insulin during the latter third of gestation. The functional significance of elevated plasma insulin levels in utero with regard to brain development, however, remains unclear.

INSULIN RECEPTORS IN THE DEVELOPING BRAIN

a.) Insulin Binding

Young et al. (1980) were the first to examine the localization of insulin receptors in the fetal rat brain. Using autoradiography of ^{125}I-insulin, they demonstrated that insulin receptors in embryonic brain exhibit a spatial as well as temporal pattern of expression. Kappy and Raizada (1982) and Kappy et al. (1984) measured regional insulin binding in the newborn rat brain and found maximum levels of binding at 15 days of postnatal life with olfactory bulb showing the greatest level at all ages studied. Sara et al. (1983) studied the ontogenesis of insulin receptors in the human fetus showing that insulin receptor number and affinity changed during embryonic life although no obvious pattern was apparent. Finally, Brennan (1987) has measured insulin binding in rat brain membranes during fetal and early postnatal development (Fig. 1). The fluctuation in binding apparently reflects an increase in receptor protein since binding affinities for insulin remained constant. In addition, the level of insulin binding above correlates well with fetal plasma insulin levels (Cohen and Turner, 1972). In general, however, with the exception of the peak of insulin binding prior to birth in the rat, brain membranes bind 5-20 fold less insulin per mg of membrane protein than do membranes of liver cells or adipocytes (Hendricks et al., 1984; Kappy et al., 1982).

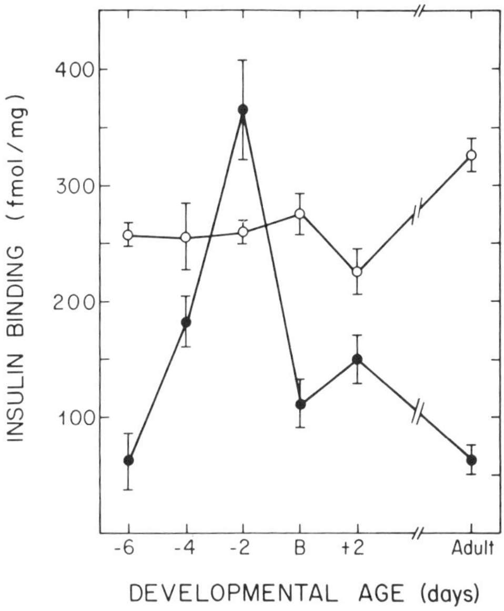

Figure 1. Insulin Binding in Brain and Liver Membranes During Development. Maximum insulin binding was calculated by Scatchard analysis. Closed circles represent data from brain membranes, open circles are data from liver membranes. The points are the mean ± S.E.

In addition to the lower density of brain receptors, there are apparent differences in the regulation of embryonic and adult insulin receptors compared with receptors in peripheral target tissues. Van Schravendijk et al. (1984) have shown that fetal mouse brain receptors fail to exhibit internalization and down regulation following exposure to insulin. This is also the case with insulin receptors in neonatal rat brain with physiological concentrations of insulin (Boyd and Raizada, 1983), although some down regulation is observed in neonatal rabbit brain receptors using pharmacological insulin concentrations (Devaskar and Holekamp, 1984). Moreover, several studies with adult rat brain insulin receptors indicate that insulin does not induce receptor internalization or down regulation as seen in adipocytes and liver cells (Zahniser et al., 1984; Gammeltoft et al., 1984; Van Schravendijk et al., 1984).

In summary, although there is similarity in the binding characteristics of CNS and peripheral insulin receptors, brain receptors are present in lower numbers and appear to be regulated differently at the neural cell surface.

b.) Insulin Receptor Structure

As mentioned above, a major distinguishing feature of insulin receptors in nervous tissue is their lower apparent molecular weight (particularly in the α-subunit) due to a difference in the extent of protein glycosylation. The human brain insulin receptor is an exception, however, since Roth et al. (1986) have shown its subunit molecular weight is nearly identical to that of peripheral insulin receptors. It was of interest therefore to study the structure of the brain insulin receptor during embryonic development in an effort to understand the tissue specific differences in insulin receptor subunit molecular weight.

Figure 2 shows an autoradiogram of an SDS-PAGE of fetal and adult brain and adult rat liver receptors cross-linked with ^{125}I-insulin. As development proceeds from 16 days of fetal life to adulthood, the brain α-subunit travels faster, indicating a decrease in apparent molecular weight from 130 kDa at 16 days of fetal life to 120 kDa in the adult. In addition, the apparent molecular weight of the brain α-subunit in 16 day fetal brain is closer to that of adult liver (130 kDa vs 138 kDa respectively)

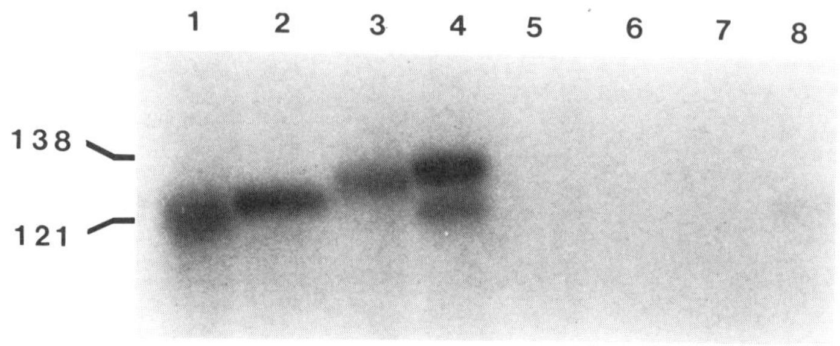

Figure 2. Autoradiogram of SDS-PAGE Under Reducing Conditions of Brain and Liver Receptors Cross-Linked With ^{125}I-Insulin Using DSS. Lanes 1,5: adult brain membranes; lanes 2,6: 20 day fetal brain membranes; lanes 3,7: 16 day fetal brain; lanes 4,8: adult rat liver. Lanes 5-8 correspond to non-specific binding controls in which cross-linking was carried out in the presence of 5 μM of porcine insulin.

To answer the question of whether this developmental decrease in the α-subunit molecular weight is due to differences in receptor glycosylation or protein molecular weight, affinity-labeled receptors were treated with endo F, endo H, and neuraminidase, then analyzed on SDS-PAGE. Figure 3 shows the effect of these enzymes on the apparent molecular weight of labeled α-subunits from fetal and adult brain and liver receptors. As development proceeds, the brain α-subunit loses sialic acid while the sialic acid content of the α-subunits of fetal and adult liver receptors remains constant. Overall, these data suggest the major differences between fetal and adult brain and between the adult brain and liver α-subunits are their content and composition of protein-linked oligosaccharide. Moreover, the data in Figure 3 suggest that there are no significant differences in the protein molecular weights of the fetal and adult brain α-subunits as compared to the α-chain of liver receptors.

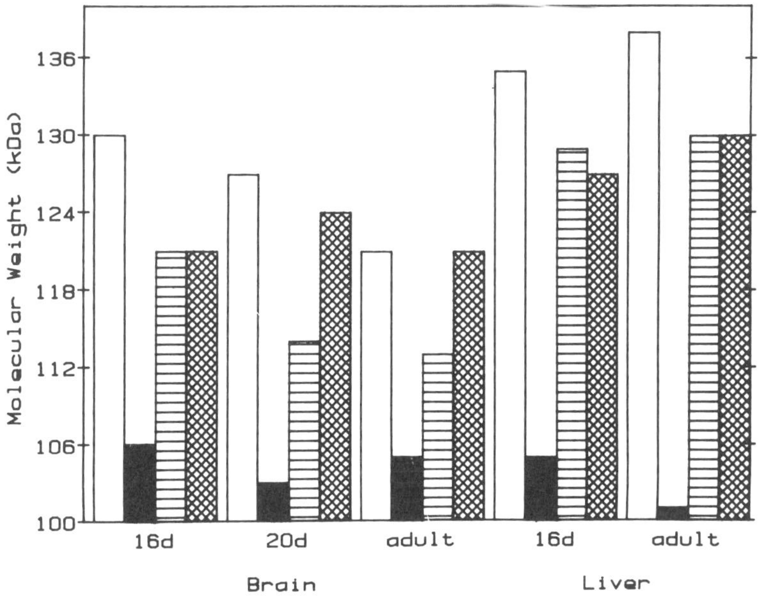

Figure 3. Comparison of Apparent Molecular Weights of Fetal and Adult Brain and Liver Insulin Receptor α-Subunits Following Deglycosylation. Molecular weight values were calculated from the relative mobility of ^{125}I-insulin cross-linked receptors run on SDS-PAGE under reducing conditions. Open bars, control; solid bars, endo F treated; horizontal bars, endo H treated; hatched bars, neuraminidase treated.

Table 1. Lectin Affinity Chromatography of Phosphorylated Receptors

Age	^{32}P in β-subunit (cpm) NAG-eluate	WGA flow through	% Retention
16d fetal	2023	612	76.7
20d fetal	1173	1674	41.2
Birth	728	2844	25.6
2d postnatal	879	3658	19.7
14d "	586	3864	15.1

Specific ^{32}P counts are shown (total counts in the insulin receptor β-subunit minus the non-specific background counts). Percent retention is calculated by dividing the total counts in the NAG-eluate by the sum of the eluate plus immunoprecipitated counts in the flow-through.

Further support for a decrease in receptor-linked sialic acid during brain development is shown by the experiment summarized in Table 1. Here the retention of autophosphorylated receptors on a wheat germ agglutinin (WGA) column was determined as a function of development. The results indicate that less autophosphorylated insulin receptor is retained by WGA as development proceeds, while recovery of the receptor in the flow-through by immunoprecipitation increases during development. In summary then, the adult brain and liver insulin receptor α-subunits differ in their content of sialic acid while the fetal brain represents an intermediate form of the α-subunit with regard to sialic acid content.

Loss of protein-linked sialic acid may be a general feature of neural development. Neural cell adhesion molecules, such as N-CAM, undergo extensive desialylation during development (Edelman, 1985). A similar phenomenon is seen throughout development in the whole brain (Margolis et al., 1976) and at the surface of the growth cones of neuroblasts (Pfenniger and Rees, 1976). In addition, sialidases, specific for neural glycoproteins, are active in fetal and early neonatal brain (Dawson, 1978; Yohe and Rosenburg, 1977; Meier et al., 1984). It has been suggested that these neural sialidases might influence synaptogenesis by affecting cell-cell interaction with the removal of highly negatively charged sialic acid residues from membrane glycoproteins (Yohe and Rosenburg, 1977). Alternatively, the temporal expression of lectin binding glycoproteins may be involved in the expression and recognition of cell surface receptors during brain development (Gombos et al., 1978).

c.) Functional Properties.

The preceding section on the structure of the brain insulin receptor raises the obvious question: "Is there a functional significance to the observed developmental changes in receptor molecular weight?". We have seen previously (Figure 2) that there are marked changes in the amount of insulin binding in the developing brain, which is most likely due to a fluctuation in receptor protein rather than a change in affinity for insulin (Table 2). Also, in Table 2 insulin-stimulated autophosphorylation changes in parallel with insulin binding. This suggests that changes in receptor glycosylation per se do not affect insulin binding and autophosphorylation. This is in agreement with a study by Lowe et al. (1986), who demonstrated a correlation between insulin binding and insulin-stimulated tyrosine kinase activity in primary cultures of neurons and glia from fetal and newborn rats. Interestingly, a remarkably similar developmental change in insulin receptor tyrosine kinase activity has been reported by Petruzzelli et al. (1985). In that study, insulin-dependent tyrosine kinase activity in insulin receptors isolated from heads of Drosophila peaked during late embryogenesis.

Table 2. Binding Affinities and Insulin-Stimulated Autophosphorylation During Brain Development

Developmental Age	Maximum binding fmol/mg	Average K_D (nM)	Phosphorylation Arbitrary units
16 Day Fetal	61±25	1.2	2.1±1.0
20 Day Fetal	364±42	3.7	12.8±0.5
Birth	112±19	1.9	4.7±1.2
2 Day Postnatal	150±20	2.3	5.6±1.8
14 Day Postnatal	63±15	1.4	1.4±0.7

Binding data is from Figure 1. K_D was calculated from Scatchard analysis of the binding data using a 2 site model. The number shown is the average of the high and low affinity site values. The number of high affinity sites remained essentially constant (5-8%) during the developmental period measured. Arbitrary units represent counts obtained from the excised β-subunits minus counts from an area of gel with no phosphorylated bands (1 unit = 100 cpm).

With regard to classical insulin-stimulated processes in the developing brain, the situation is less clear. Gorus et al. (1984) failed to detect insulin stimulation of glucose transport in freshly dissociated or cultured cells from embryonic mouse cerebral cortex. Similarly, Devaskar and Karycki (1985) showed insulin had no effect on amino acid or glucose uptake in freshly dissociated cells from 1-2 week old rabbit brain. In contrast, Clark et al. (1984) have shown that insulin stimulates glucose uptake in primary cultures of newborn rat glia, but not in neuronal cell cultures of similar developmental age (Boyd et al., 1985). It is possible that the ratio of glial cells to neurons present in the embryonic brain is sufficiently low that insulin effects on glucose transport are undetectable. Until quantitative information is available concerning the number and specific cellular localization of insulin receptors in embryonic brain, it will not be possible to reconcile these differences. Finally, again using cultured neuronal cells, Raizada et al. (1980) have demonstrated insulin-sensitive thymidine and uridine uptake in fetal cells as well as insulin-dependent inhibition of norepinephrine uptake in cells from newborn rat brain (Boyd et al., 1985). This latter effect is particularly interesting since it suggests a unique neuromodulatory function for insulin in the CNS.

In summary, although the role of insulin in the developing nervous system is still emerging, these data suggest that a relationship may exist between the specific temporal pattern of insulin receptor expression and the changes in neural cell growth and differentiation. This is supported by recent studies of insulin's effect on fetal nervous tissue in vitro. Puro and Agardh (1984) have shown insulin-mediated regulation of neuronal maturation in cultured fetal cholinergic neurons. Similarly, insulin promotes neurite formation and survival of cultured sympathetic and sensory neurons from chicken embryos (Recio-Pinto et al., 1986). Finally, insulin and insulin-like growth factors are potent inducers of oligodendrocyte development in cultures established from 1 day old rats (McMorris et al., 1986).

In conclusion, the preceding studies suggest that insulin receptors with properties similar to insulin receptors of other tissues are present in embryonic brain and may therefore play a significant role in brain growth, differentiation, and metabolism. Further work is clearly required, however, to define the specific function(s) of insulin and insulin receptors in the embryonic brain.

REFERENCES

Barnes, D. and Sato, G., 1980, Cell, 22:649-655.

Birch, N.P., Christie, D.L., and Renwick, A.G.C., 1984, Biochem. J., 218:19-27.

Boyd, F.T. and Raizada, M.K., 1983, Am. J. Physiol., 245:C283-287.

Boyd, F.T., Clarke, D.W., Muther, T.F., and Raizada, M.K., 1985, J. Biol. Chem., 260:15880-15884.

Brennan, W.A. Jr., 1987, J. Biol. Chem., (submitted).

Carey, E.M., 1982, In: Biochemical Development of the Fetus and Neonate, C.T. Jones, ed., Elsevier, pp 297-298.

Clarke, D.W., Boyd, F.T., Kappy, M.S., and Raizada, M.K., 1984, J. Biol. Chem., 259:11672-11675.

Cohen, N.M. and Turner, R.C., 1972, Biol. Neonate, 21:107-111.

Dawson, G., 1978, In: Mammalian Glycoproteins, Glycolipids and Proteoglycans, M.I. Horowitz and W. Pigonan, eds., Academic Press, New York, pp 285-325.

Devaskar, S.U. and Holekamp, N., 1984, Biochem. Biophys. Res. Comm., 120:359-367.

Devaskar, S.U. and Karycki, L., 1985, Biochem. Biophys. Res. Comm., 133:670-679.

Edelman, G., 1985, Ann. Rev. Biochem., 54:135-169.

Eng, J. and Yalow, R.S., 1981, Proc. Natl. Acad. Sci. (USA), 78:4576-4578.

Gammeltoft, S., Kowalski, A., Fehlmann, M., and van Obberghen, E., 1984a, FEBS Letts., 172:87-90.

Gammeltoft, S., Stauan-Olsen, P., Ottesen, B., and Fahrenkrug, J., 1984b, Peptides, 5:937-944.

Gombos, G., Ghandour, M.S., Vincendon, G., Reeber, A., and Zanetta, J.P., 1978, In: Maturation of Neurotransmission, A. Vernadakis, E. Giacobini, and G. Filogamo, eds., Krager, Basel, pp 10-22.

Gorus, F.K., Hooghe-Peters, E.L., and Pipeleers, D.G., 1984, J. Cellular Physiol., 121:45-50.

Havrankova, J., Roth, J., and Brownstein, M., 1978, Nature (Lond.), 272:827-829.

Heidenreich, K.A., Zahniser, N.R., Berhanu, P., Brandenburg, D., and Olefsky, J.M., 1983, J. Biol. Chem., 258:8527-8530.

Heidenreich, K.A. and Brandeburg, D., 1986, Endocrinology, 118:1835-1842.

Hendricks, S.A., Roth, J., Rishi, S., and Becker, K.L., 1983, In: Brain Peptides, D.T. Krieger, M.J. Brownstein, and J.B. Martin, eds., John Wiley and Sons, pp 903-939.

Hendricks, S.A., Agardh, C.D., Taylor, S.J., and Roth, J., 1984, J. Neurochem., 43:1302-1309.

Kappy, M.S. and Raizada, M.K., 1982, Brain Res., 249:390-392.

Kappy, M.S., Sellinger, S., and Raizada, M.K., 1984, J. Neurochem., 42:198-203.

LeRoith, D., Shiloach, J., Roth, J., and Lesniak, M.A., 1980, Proc. Natl. Acad. Sci. (USA), 77:6184-6188.

LeRoith, D., Shiloach, J., Roth, J., and Lesniak, M.A., 1981, J. Biol. Chem., 256:6533-6536.

Lowe, W.L. and LeRoith, D., 1986, Biochem. Biophys. Res. Comm., 134:532-538.

Lowe, W.L., Boyd, F.T., Clarke, D.W., Raizada, M.K., Hart, C., and LeRoith, D., 1986, Endocrinology, 119:25-35.

Margolis, R.K., Preti, C., Lai, D., and Margolis, R.U., 1976, Brain Res., 112:363-369.

McMorris, F.A., Smith, T.M., Desalvo, S., and Furlanetto, R.W., 1986, Proc. Natl. Acad. Sci. (USA), 83:822-826.

Meier, E., Regan, C.M., Balazs, R., 1984, J. Neurochem., 43:1328-1335.

Petruzzelli, L., Herrera, R., Garcia-Arenas, R., and Rosen, O.M., 1985, J. Biol. Chem., 260:16072-16075.

Pfenniger, L.H. and Rees, R.P., 1976, In: Neuronal Recognition, S.H. Barondes, ed., Plenum Press, New York, pp 131-173.

Posner, B.I., Kelly, P.A., Shiu, R.P.C., and Friesen, H.G., 1974, Endocrinology, 95:521-531.

Puro, D.G., and Agardh, E., 1984, Science, 225:1170-1172.

Recio-Pinto, E., Rechler, M.M., and Ishii, D.N., 1986, J. Neurosci., 6:1211-1219.

Rees-Jones, R.W., Hendricks, S.A., Quarum, M., Roth, J., 1984, J. Biol. Chem., 259:3470-3474.

Roth, R.A., Morgan, D.O., Beaudoin, J., and Sara, V., 1986, J. Biol. Chem., 261:3753-3757.

Sara, V.R., Hall, K., Misaki, M., Fryklund, L., Christensen, N., and Wetterberg, L., 1983, J. Clin. Invest., 71:1084-1094.

Van Schravendijk, C.F.H., Hooghe-Peters, E.L., De Meyts, P., and Pipeleers, D.G., 1984, Biochem. J., 220:165-172.

Yip, C.C., Moule, M.L., and Yeung, C.W.T., 1980, Biochem. Biophys. Res. Comm., 96:1671-1678.

Yohe, H.C. and Rosenburg, A., 1977, J. Biol. Chem., 252:2412-2418.

Young, W.S., Kuhar, M.J., Roth, J., and Brownstein, M.J., 1980, Neuropeptides, 1:15-22.

Zahniser, N.R., Goens, M.B., Hanaway, P.J., and Vinyeh, J.V., 1984, J. Neurochem., 42:1353-1362.

INSULIN DOWNREGULATES ALPHA-2 ADRENERGIC RECEPTORS IN CULTURED GLIAL CELLS

Elaine M. Richards, Mohan K. Raizada and Colin Sumners

Department of Physiology
College of Medicine
University of Florida
Gainesville, FL 32610

ABSTRACT

Our previous studies have suggested that insulin can modulate central catecholaminergic systems. In the present study we have investigated this further by examining the actions of this peptide on the regulation of α_2-adrenergic receptors in glial cells. Using [^{3}H]-yohimbine as a ligand for α_2-adrenergic receptors, we have demonstrated that insulin is able to decrease [^{3}H]-yohimbine binding to glia in a time- and dose-dependent manner. Saturation experiments followed by Scatchard analyses revealed that this was due to a decreased number of α_2-adrenergic receptors. These results suggest that insulin, by modulating α_2-adrenergic receptor levels, is able to regulate the amount of NE present in the synaptic cleft.

INTRODUCTION

There is now substantial evidence suggesting that insulin is a neuromodulator in the brain. Insulin and insulin receptors have been demonstrated on both neurons[1,2] and astrocytic glial[3] cells in culture as well as in the intact brain.[4-6] Insulin can be released through depolarization[7] and causes changes in the firing rate of nigrostriatal dopaminergic[8] and hippocampal neurons.[9] Its primary interaction appears to be with the monoamines as it affects the dopamine system of the olfactory bulbs[10] and at high doses stimulates release of dopamine, norepinephrine (NE) and epinephrine from hypothalamic slices.[11]

Recent studies from our laboratories have shown that insulin inhibits total bioamine uptake into neuronal cultures.[2] It can inhibit 95% of specific NE uptake into neurons. The specific NE uptake inhibitor, maprotiline, inhibits high affinity insulin binding at concentrations used to inhibit NE uptake, suggesting that maprotiline and insulin may act at the same receptors.[12]

In this study we were interested in examining the effects of insulin on α_2-adrenergic binding to glial cells. We have recently studied a glial binding site for [^{3}H]-yohimbine which has the characteristics of an α_2-adrenergic receptor. As α_2-receptors and insulin can both influence the amount of amine present in the synaptic cleft, we were interested in determining whether insulin could affect α_2-receptors. We have shown that insulin, in a time- and dose-dependent fashion, decreases glial [^{3}H]-yohimbine binding. Saturation and Scatchard analyses of insulin treated cells show that this decrease is primarily due to a reduction in the number of α_2-adrenergic receptors.

MATERIALS

One-day-old Sprague-Dawley rats were obtained from our breeding colonies, originally obtained from Charles River Farms. DMEM, fetal bovine serum and amphotericin B (Fungizone) were purchased from Gibco, Grand Island, NY; 1× crystallized trypsin was from Cooper Biomedical, Malvern, PA; cytosine arabinoside, poly-L-lysine (M.W. 150,000), deoxyribonuclease I, yohimbine, clonidine, norepinephrine, epinephrine, corynanthine, naphazoline, and dopamine were purchased from Sigma Chemical Company, St. Louis, MO. Rauwolscine HCl was a gift from Carl Roth, Karlsruhe, FRG. Yohimbine-[^{3}H-methyl] (Sp. Act. 50 - 70 Ci/nmol) was obtained from New England Nuclear, Boston, MA. Crystalline porcine insulin was a gift from Lilly Research Laboratories, Indianapolis, IN. Ascorbate was from Fisher Scientific, Pittsburgh, PA.

METHODS

Preparation of glial cultures

Glial cultures were prepared by a previously described method.[3] Brains were dissected free from 1-day-old Sprague-Dawley rats and placed in an isotonic salt solution containing 100 U penicillin G potassium, 100 μg streptomycin, and 0.25 μg amphotericin B (Fungizone) per ml, pH 7.4. All blood vessels and pia mater were removed. The brains were chopped into approximately 2-mm pieces, suspended in 20 ml of 0.25% (wt/vol) trypsin in isotonic salt solution (pH 7.4) and placed in a shaking water bath for 6 minutes at 37°C to dissociate the cells. After this time, the dissociated cells were removed and mixed with 10 ml Dulbecco's Modified Eagle's Medium (DMEM) containing 10% fetal bovine serum (FBS). The remaining undissociated tissue chunks were mixed with 160 μg deoxyribonuclease I (DNase I) and were incubated at 37°C for a further 6 minutes. The cells were then suspended in DMEM containing 10% fetal bovine serum (FBS), centrifuged at 1000 *g* for 10 min and washed with 50 ml DMEM containing 10% FBS. Cells were plated in DMEM containing 10% FBS into 100-mm Falcon culture dishes precoated with poly-L-lysine at a density of 15.0 × 10^6 cells. The cells were incubated for 3 days at 37°C in a humidified incubator with 5% CO_2-95% air. After this time, the medium was replaced by DMEM containing 10% FBS. After a further 3 days, cells were passaged and reinoculated at a concentration of 1 × 10^6 cells/100-mm diameter culture dish. The cells were then allowed to grow and divide for a further 20 days prior to use. The passaging resulted in cultures consisting primarily of non-neuronal cells.[3]

Membrane preparation

Cells were scraped from the dishes with the aid of a rubber policeman, and placed on ice in a centrifuge tube. They were spun for 10 minutes at 4°C and 1000 *g* and the supernatant discarded. The pellet was resuspended in phosphate buffered saline and either used or frozen in liquid nitrogen until use, preliminary experiments having shown that there was no significant difference between binding in fresh and frozen cells.

On the day of the binding, the cells were thawed on ice and then resuspended in 20 volumes of ice-cold 50 mM Tris-HCl, pH 7.0, + 0.1% ascorbic acid (binding buffer). They were homogenized in a polytron (setting 2.5 for 30 sec), then centrifuged at 50,000 *g* for 10 minutes at 4°C. The supernatant was discarded, the pellet resuspended in 20 volumes of binding buffer and the centrifugation step repeated. Following this, the pellet was resuspended in 1 ml of binding buffer and the protein content of an aliquot determined by the method of Lowry,[13] using bovine serum albumin as the standard.

Binding methods

Binding was performed in glass tubes. Glial membranes (175 μg) were incubated with 50 mM Tris-HCl, pH 7.0, 0.1% ascorbic acid and 10 μM [^{3}H]-yohimbine in a final volume of 250 μl for 5 mins at 25°C. For non-specific binding determinations 100 μM cold yohimbine was included in the incubation medium. The reaction was stopped by addition of 3 ml ice-cold buffer and rapid filtration under reduced pressure through Whatman GF/B filters, followed by 2 further 3-ml rinses of the tube and filter. The filters were placed in 10 mls Liquiscint overnight and counted in a liquid scintillation counter with an efficiency of 37% for [^{3}H]. Specific binding is calculated by subtracting the binding in the presence of cold yohimbine from that in its absence. Each data point represents six total and six non-specific tubes and n equals the number of times each experiment was repeated.

Insulin treatment

Insulin was dissolved in a small volume of 0.1 N NaOH and diluted to the correct concentration in buffer. It was then sterilized by filtration and added to the medium of the cells. For the time curves 167 nM insulin was added to the cells, which were then scraped 24 h later. For 48-h or longer incubations the cells received insulin treatments every 24 h to maintain the insulin concentration. Control cells received sterile vehicle instead of insulin and a control and an insulin-treated group were always performed together at each time point as we have previously determined that each group of glial cells demonstrates slightly different levels of [^{3}H]-yohimbine binding.

For concentration curves we used 24-hr time points with 16.7, 167 and 1670 nM insulin.

Scatchard analysis was achieved by binding insulin-treated (1670 nM for 48 h) and control membranes with 1.0 to 20 nM [^{3}H]-yohimbine and then analyzing the saturation data by the method of Scatchard.

TABLE ONE

Specificity of Glial [^{3}H]-Yohimbine Binding

	IC_{50} (nM) (mean ± SEM)			
Antagonists				
Rauwolscine	13.5			(n = 1)
Yohimbine	22.89	±	0.63	(n = 8)
Prazosin	740			(n = 2)
Corynanthine	6700	±	3700	(n = 3)
Agonists				
Naphazoline	30.4	±	16	(n = 3)
Clonidine	280.5	±	35	(n = 2)
Epinephrine	3200	±	1400	(n = 3)
Norepinephrine	8800	±	1620	(n = 7)
Dopamine	6250	±	1250	(n = 4)
Other				
Insulin	No displacement at 167 nM insulin.			

IC_{50} values are for the displacement of 10 nM [^{3}H]-yohimbine.

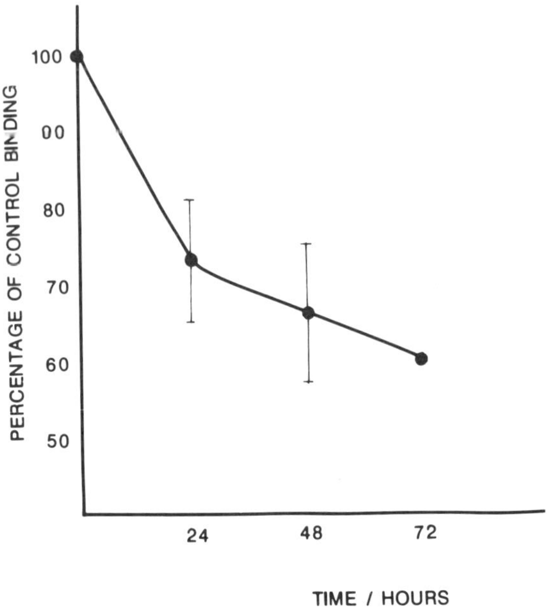

Figure 1. Time course for the decrease in [^{3}H]-yohimbine binding caused by insulin. 167 nM insulin was added to the cells and binding performed at the indicated times after treatment. Each point represents the mean ± SEM of 3 experiments in which 6 total and 6 non-specific binding tubes were used per data point, except the 72-h time point, which is of one experiment.

RESULTS

We have previously shown that membranes of glial cells bind [^{3}H]-yohimbine in a time-, protein concentration- and ligand concentration-dependent fashion. Binding at 25°C is between 70 and 80% specific and reaches equilibrium by 2.5 minutes and remains there for at least 20 min. The K_d is 21.42 ± 1.7 nM (n = 8) with a B_{max} of 1.95 ± 0.30 pmoles/mg protein (n = 8). The specificity of binding is shown in Table 1 and suggests a site with α_2-adrenergic characteristics.[14]

Insulin at 167 nM for 24, 48 or 72 hours causes a decrease in [^{3}H]-yohimbine binding. The decreases, expressed as a percentage of control, were 73 ± 8%, (n = 3), 66 ± 9% (n = 3) and 60 ± 8% (n = 1) at 24, 48 and 72 hours respectively (see Fig. 1). The dose dependency of the decrease is shown in Fig. 2. At 16.7 nM the binding was 88 ± 7% of control, at 167 nM 85 ± 3%, and at 1.67 μM 82 ± 5%. After 48 hours of treatment with 167 nM insulin, the binding was further decreased to 68 ± 7%.

Saturation experiments followed by Scatchard analyses revealed that insulin (1670 nM for 48 hrs) caused a 52% decrease in the maximal number of [^{3}H]-yohimbine binding sites compared with control cells. In addition, insulin treatment is associated with a slight decrease in the K_d of the binding site (summarized in Table 2). The decrease in binding is not caused by insulin competing for [^{3}H]-yohimbine binding, because even at the highest dose of insulin used there was no displacement of [^{3}H]-yohimbine binding when insulin was added to the binding buffer (Table 1).

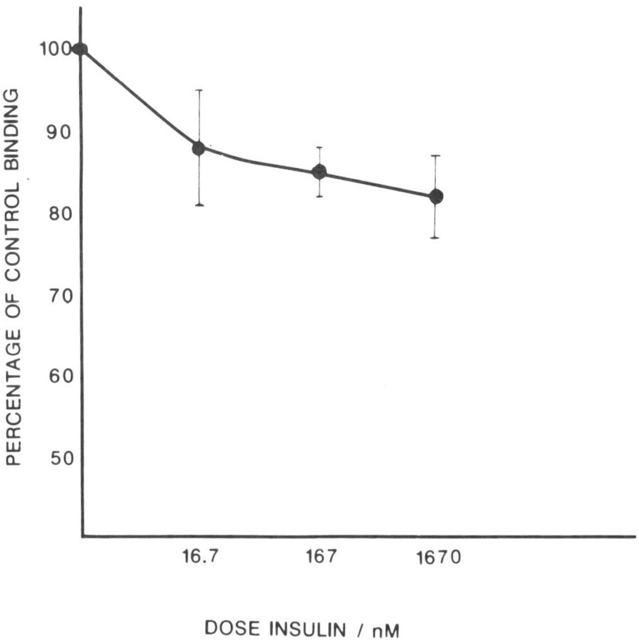

Figure 2. Dose response curve for the decrease in [^{3}H]-yohimbine binding with insulin. Each point represents the mean ± SEM of 6 total and 6 non-specific binding tubes at each point.

DISCUSSION

As mentioned in the introduction, insulin has many interactions with monoamines. One such interaction, that of inhibition of NE uptake, would tend to increase the amount of NE present in synapses. As a population of α_2-adrenergic receptors regulates the amount of NE in the cleft by affecting synthesis and release, it might be expected that insulin and α_2-adrenergic receptors would act in opposition in the control of this function. For example, insulin would increase NE in the cleft, which would feed back to increase α_2-adrenoceptors, which would, in turn, tend to return NE levels to normal. The present results do not support this hypothesis, as insulin downregulated α_2-adrenergic receptors. Several possible explanations of this phenomenon exist. Firstly, insulin may increase synaptic levels of NE not only by decreasing uptake but also by decreasing the level of "inhibitory" autoreceptors, suggesting that insulin is subserving an important physiological

TABLE TWO

Effects of insulin on the number and affinity of [^{3}H]-yohimbine binding sites in glial cultures

	K_d (nM)	B_{max} (pmoles/mg protein)
Control	21.3	2.83
Insulin (1670 nM for 48 hours)	15.1	1.35

Data represent mean values from two independent experiments in which a control and an insulin treated group were assayed concurrently.

pathway which has redundant systems. In other words, it seems that insulin can increase the amount of NE in the synaptic cleft by two mechanisms, inhibition of uptake and increased release via decreased α_2-adrenergic binding. This suggests that the neuromodulatory role of insulin in NE control is very important physiologically. Secondly, insulin may act at a post-α_2-adrenergic receptor site to increase the efficacy of α_2-adrenergic stimulation which, whilst maintaining homeostasis, would tend to decrease α_2-receptor binding. Thirdly, the α_2-adrenergic receptor we are examining is on glia, and may not have the same function as that of the neuronal α_2-adrenergic receptor.

The importance of these results, however, is that they again support the notion that insulin is a neuromodulator of the central monoaminergic system, and thus possesses an important physiological function.

ACKNOWLEDGEMENTS

We wish to thank Sue Rueth and Jacquie Perez for expert technical assistance. This work was supported by grants from NIH to C.S. and M.K.R. Mohan K. Raizada is an Established Investigator of the American Heart Association.

REFERENCES

1. F. T. Boyd, Jr., and M. K. Raizada, Effects of insulin and tunicamycin on neuronal insulin receptors in culture, Am. J. Physiol., 245:C283-C287 (1983).
2. F. T. Boyd, Jr., D. W. Clarke, T. F. Muther, and M. K. Raizada, Insulin receptors and modulation of norepinephrine uptake by insulin in neuronal cells in culture, J. Biol. Chem., 260:15880-15884 (1985).
3. D. W. Clarke, F. T. Boyd, Jr., M. S. Kappy, and M. K. Raizada, Insulin binds to specific receptors and stimulates 2-deoxy-D-glucose uptake in cultured glial cells from rat brain, J. Biol. Chem., 259:11672-11675 (1984).
4. J. Havrankova, D. Schmechel, J. Roth, and M. J. Brownstein, Identification of insulin in rat brain, Proc. Natl. Acad. Sci. U.S.A., 75:5737-5741 (1978).
5. J. Havrankova, J. Roth, and M. J. Brownstein, Insulin receptors are widely distributed in the central nervous system of the rat, Nature (London), 272:827-829 (1978).
6. J. Havrankova, J. Roth, and M. J. Brownstein, Insulin receptors in brain, in: "Advances in Metabolic Disorders," Vol. 10, "CNS Regulation of Carbohydrate Metabolism," A. J. Szabo, ed., Academic Press, New York (1983) pp. 259-268.
7. D. W. Clarke, F T Boyd, and M. K. Raizada, Insulin is released from neuronal cultures from the rat brain, J. Neurochem., 47:831-836 (1986).
8. C. F. Saller and L. A. Chiodo, Glucose suppresses basal firing and haloperidol-induced increases in the firing rate of central dopaminergic neurons, Science, 210:1269-1271 (1980).
9. R. A. Palovcik, M. I. Phillips, M. S. Kappy, and M. K. Raizada, Insulin inhibits pyramidal neurons in hippocampal slices, Brain Research, 309:187-191 (1984).
10. M. Barbaccia, D. Chuang, and E. Costa, Is insulin a neuromodulator? Adv. Biochem. Psychopharmacol., 33:511-518 (1982).
11. A. Sauter, M. Goldstein, J. Engel, and K. Ueta, Effect of insulin on central catecholamines, Brain Research, 260:330-333 (1983).
12. F. T. Boyd, Jr., D. W. Clarke, and M. K. Raizada, Insulin inhibits specific norepinephrine uptake in neuronal cultures from rat brain, Brain Research, 398:1-5 (1986).
13. O. H. Lowry, N. J. Rosebrough, A. L. Farr, and R. J. Randall, Protein measurement with folin-phenol reagent, J. Biol. Chem., 193:265-275 (1951).
14. E. M. Richards, M. K. Raizada, M. I. Phillips, and C. Sumners, Neuronal and glial cells in culture contain α_2-adrenergic receptors, in preparation.

SOMATOMEDINS (INSULIN-LIKE GROWTH FACTORS) AND THE NERVOUS SYSTEM

Yutaka Oomura and Carlos R. Plata-Salamán

Department of Physiology
Faculty of Medicine
Kyushu University 60
Fukuoka 812, Japan

INTRODUCTION

Somatomedin is a general term which refers to plasma factors that have both growth-promoting (stimulate sulfate incorporation into chondroitin sulfate of cartilage and increase thymidine incorporation into DNA in various tissues) and insulin-like effects (in adipose tissue and diaphragm, not neutralized by anti-insulin serum)[1,2]. "Somato" relates to somatotropin (growth hormone, GH) and also to the soma which is the target and "medin" to indicate it mediates the action of GH.

MOLECULAR FORMS OF SOMATOMEDINS

Many preparations have been designated as somatomedins. Somatomedin-A stimulated sulfate incorporation into glucosaminoglycans (sulfation factor activity) in chick cartilage[3-5]. Somatomedin-B stimulated DNA synthesis in glial cells[6]. Somatomedin-C had sulfation factor activity in rat cartilage[7]. Multiplication-stimulating activity had mitogenic activity in several cell types [8]. As radioimmunoassay for insulin was developed, it became apparent that human serum contained more insulin-like activity (ILA) than could be attributed to its content of immunoreactive insulin. The portion of ILA that was not inhibited by insulin antibodies was designated "atypical insulin", and "nonsuppressible insulin-like activity" (NSILA)[9,10], which yielded two active peptides, NSILA I and II[11,12]. One portion of

NSILA was later shown to consist of insulin-like growth factors I and II (IGF-I and -II)[11,12]. Another ILA was found to be similar to IGF-II[13]. All of these substances were isolated from human plasma except for multiplication-stimulating activity, which was derived from the rat liver cell line, BRL 3A. Somatomedin-A appears to be identical to IGF-I, with the possible exception of a glutamine deamidation at position 40[14]. Sequence analysis of somatomedin-C indicates that it is identical to IGF-I[15], and the term somatomedin-C/IGF-I (Sm-C/IGF-I) is now used to designate this peptide. Purification and analysis of one of the multiplication-stimulating activity fractions has revealed 93% homology with human IGF-II[16], so this peptide is now considered to be rat IGF-II[17]. Somatomedin-B is not included among the somatomedins, since its mitogenic activity is due to contamination by epidermal growth factor[18].

Thus, the substances now considered to be members of the somatomedin group as determined by purification, sequencing and immunological characterization and receptor reactivity are limited to Sm-C/IGF-I or IGF-I and IGF-II. However, there may be other peptides which have not yet been characterized. For example, a "big IGF-II" has been reported in human spinal fluid and serum[19]. This, and isolation of the somatomedins from plasma, and the study of cDNAs[20,21] make it evident that there are more somatomedins that need further study.

IGF-I is a basic peptide with a MW of 7649; it contains 70 amino acids in a single chain with three disulphide bridges, is highly growth hormone dependent and has potent growth-promoting activity[22-24]. IGF-II is a slightly acidic, single chain peptide with a MW of 7471; it contains 67 amino acids, appears to be less growth hormone dependent, and has less growth-promoting activity than IGF-I[25,26]. Both IGF-I and -II have high structural homology with human proinsulin; they consist of A, B, C and D domains. Parts of the sequences within the A and B domains are homologous to the A and B chains of insulin, with their interchain disulfide bridges. This sequence homology is 43% for IGF-I and 41% for IGF-II. No sequence homology exists between the C domains of IGF-I and -II (12 and 8 amino acids, respectively) and the C peptide region (35 amino acids) of human proinsulin[27-30]. In addition, the carboxyl-terminal extensions (D domains) of 8 and 6 amino acid residues are, respectively, typical structural features of IGF-I and -II which are not shared with proinsulin[27-29]. IGF-I has a 130-residue precursor, whereas the IGF-II has a 180-residue precursor[30a]. The sequence homology between IGF-I and -II is 62%. Three-dimensional models for IGF-I and -II indicate identical three dimensional conformation of the parts corresponding to the A and B chains of insulin, but the total amino acid content of the connecting peptides is less than that of the C-peptide in proinsulin[31]. The sequence and structural similarities between IGF-I and -II and proinsulin led to the suggestion that these molecules diverged from a common hormonal ancestor during evolution[32,33].

SITES OF PRODUCTION

Production of IGF-I and IGF-II by Adult and Fetal Tissues and Cultured Cells. General Description

The liver is a major source of IGF-I and -II[8,34-38]. Fibroblasts are also source of IGFs[39,40]. Extracts of liver contain only small amounts of IGFs or somatomedin-like activity. These peptides are therefore either not stored, or are stored in some biologically inactive form. Following growth hormone administration, there is a delay of several hours before plasma somatomedin concentrations begin to rise, suggesting that the somatomedins are synthetized and secreted de novo[34,37,41]. Other tissues (kidney, lung, testes, submaxillary gland, pancreas, heart and nervous system) and body fluids are also known to produce or contain somatomedins[30,42-49]. On the other hand, the main source of circulating IGF-II in adults is unknown. In incubated liver explants, IGF-I immunoreactivity increased exponentially and in parallel with liver growth from the 11th until the 16th day of gestation [26,46]. Immunoreactivity was also detected in media from the 17th day of gestation in intestine, heart, brain, lung and kidney[26,46].
Cultured human fibroblasts and smooth muscle cells, have been shown to synthesize or secrete somatomedin-like peptides[26,39,50-52]. It has been shown that the anterior and neurointermediate lobes of the rat pituitary gland, hypothalamus, cerebral cortex and cerebellum maintained in culture, release both IGF and its binding protein[53], which suggests local synthesis of both. Brain tissue binding proteins for IGFs appear to be different from those produced by the liver (see below). The physiological significance of the multiplicity of somatomedin production sites is unknown. These peptides may act locally to stimulate growth (replication and differentiation) without being released into the blood. This is the autocrine/paracrine hypothesis of somatomedin action[30] (Fig. 1); somatomedins can exert their biologic activity on their cells of origin or on cells near their sites of synthesis. In the central nervous system (CNS), paracrine and autocrine action may be predominant in the embryo/fetal life (growth), whereas the

endocrine and/or neuroregulatory (neurotransmitter and/or modulator) action may be expressed during adult life.

Production of IGF-I and -II by the Nervous System. Specific Description

IGF-I in the nervous system. There have been several failures in efforts to detect immunoreactive IGF-I in the CNS[54,55]. However, an additional human fetal brain form of somatomedin has been proposed[56]. This

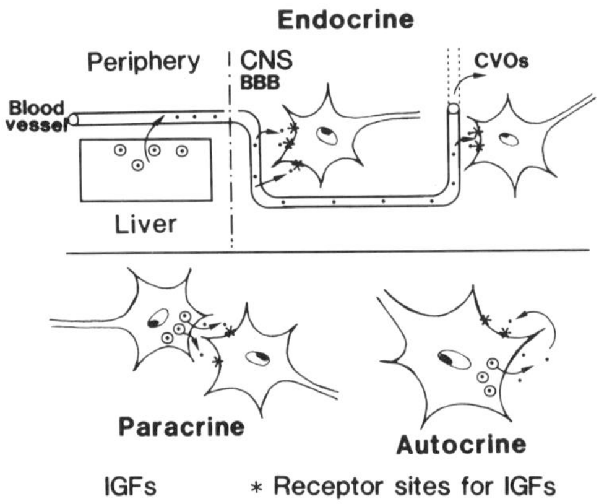

Fig. 1. Schematic representation of IGF action by endocrine, paracrine and autocrine mechanisms.

was suggested by evidence showing low or undetectable levels of immunoreactive IGF-I or IGF-II in human fetal serum[56] despite fetal tissue display of somatomedin receptors[57], and somatomedin growth-promoting activity on fetal cells in vitro[58]. A radioligand receptor assay was developed utilizing human fetal brain plasma membrane receptor as the matrix and IGF-I as the ligand[56]. This method revealed elevated levels of somatomedins (not attributed to either immunoreactive IGF-I or -II) in the fetal circulation (four-fold higher than in adults). These values decreased during maturation, and a transition from production of fetal to adult forms of somatomedins at about the time of birth was proposed[56]. In healthy newborns, a significant correlation was found between serum fetal brain somatomedin values and birth weight and length[56]. These results suggest the existence of embryonic/fetal somatomedin in humans that may regulate brain fetal and early brain postnatal growth. This embryonic/fetal somatomedin is related to a variant form of IGF-I identified in human fetal brain tissue. Structural analysis revealed that this variant of IGF-I has a truncated NH_2-terminal region compared to IGF-I isolated from serum[59]. The same variant of IGF-I has been identified in adult human brain[60]. This truncated variant IGF-I probably arises from post-translational modification of the prohormone form of IGF-I, and since it has so far been isolated from fetal and adult brain only[59,60], it might be specific to processing within the CNS.

In fact, in brains of fetal rats, a major mRNA (1.7 Kb) was identified that hybridized with the human IGF-I cDNA and four other mRNAs were found that hybridized with mouse IGF-I cDNA[61], whereas no IGF-I mRNAs were detected in adult rat brain[61]. It was further shown that IGF-I is synthesized in 17-day-gestation brain explant of fetal mouse[46], and extractable brain IGF-I concentration was the same in normal and hypophysectomized male rats[49]. This supports the notion of local synthesis of GH independent IGF-I.

<u>IGF-II in the nervous system</u>. IGF-II has been isolated from human fetal brain[59]. Human brain IGF-II-like immunoreactivity was present in two to five distinct size classes. The smallest component (7.5 Kda) was identical to the purified IGF-II from human serum[54,60]. The highest amounts of IGF-II-like immunoreactivity occur in the anterior pituitary where the 13 Kda species releases significant amounts of 7.5 Kda material[54]. Further, IGF-II and high MW forms have been extracted from synaptosomal preparations, implying granular storage of at least part of the IGF-II[54]. The dorsomedial hypothalamus and supraoptic nucleus were rich in IGF-II, and intermediate levels were found in the lateral and anterior hypothalamus and the paraventricular nucleus[54,55]. If there is a precursor-product relation, the predominance of higher MW forms in the hypothalamus would indicate that this region is a site for biosynthesis, but the conversion process is unknown. The amounts of IGF-II extracted from the liver and from the anterior pituitary are in the same range[54], so the pituitary may also serve as a site of synthesis and/or storage of IGF-II. In a clinical case of megaloencephaly, IGF-II levels in the frontal cortex of a 3-month-old child

were 10 times higher than those for adults, but the IGF-II level in plasma of this patient was in the lower normal range[54]. Thus seems to be no direct correlation between the levels of serum, and of brain IGF-II. In conclusion, the larger forms of brain IGF-II are synthesized locally[53,54]. The major form of the larger IGF-II in serum and brain has a MW of 9-10 Kda. Its concentration in serum is less than one-tenth of the total IGF-II determined by radioimmunoassay[62]. In contrast, about half of the IGF-II in CSF has a MW of 10 Kda[19]. The variants of IGF-II are evidence of the existence of more than one gene for IGF-II (product of an allelic or second gene)[62].

The gene coding for IGF-II is expressed in the brain of rats[63]. IGF-II mRNA has been detected in neonatal rat[63] and adult human brain[64]. The expression of IGF-II mRNA in the brain is consistent with the results of immunoassays of extracts of various regions of adult human brain including the anterior pituitary[54]. Multiple IGF-II mRNAs (4.7, 3.9, 2.2, 1.75 and 1.2 Kb) were observed in fetal rat brain[61]. The abundance of IGF-II mRNAs in rat fetal tissues compared to adult tissues lends verification that IGF-II is predominantly a fetal somatomedin. In one study, the brain was the only adult rat tissue in which 4.7 and 3.9 Kb IGF-II mRNAs were consistently detected[61]. In another study, six IGF-II mRNAs (6, 4, 3.8, 2.2, 1.7 and 1.2 Kb) were identified in the rat neonatal brainstem, cerebral cortex and hypothalamus[65]. In the brainstem, IGF-II mRNA was expressed at higher levels in the fetus than after birth, but the higher levels persisted into adulthood in the cerebral cortex and the hypothalamus[65]. The significance of these region-specific differences in the development related expression of IGF-II mRNAs remains to be determined. The different forms of IGF-II mRNAs may reflect differences in the processing of a single primary RNA transcript, or derivation from different IGF-II genes. Interestingly, although there is significantly more IGF-II mRNA in the liver than in the cerebral cortex and hypothalamus at the 16th day of gestation[65], it is as abundant in the cerebral cortex and more abundant in the hypothalamus than in the liver of 75-day old adult rats[65]. The persistence of IGF-II mRNA in the adult rat brain suggests several roles of IGF-II in the adult CNS. Acid extraction has shown IGF-I and -II to be widely distributed, not only throughout the nervous system of the cat (pituitary gland, hypothalamus, cerebral cortex)[44], but also in the sympathetic ganglia, vagus nerve and sciatic nerves. Electrical stimulation of the brachial and sciatic nerves released IGF-I and -II into perfusates from extirpated cut limbs[44]. Decrease to the pre-stimulation level before termination of the stimulus suggests the release of a readily accessible stored pool of limited size.

IGF-I and IGF-II in CSF. Somatomedin activity in human CSF was first reported in 1975[66]. IGF-II levels in normal human CSF are about 1.3 to 6% of the serum levels[67], whereas the levels of IGF-I like peptides are extremely low[68]. Radioimmunoassay revealed about 150 ng/ml of IGF-I and about 800 ng/ml of IGF-II in human serum[19]. In the same study, the spinal fluid contained only IGF-II in significant amounts (31 ng/ml). After acidification of the human spinal fluid, two IGF-II like peptides were detected; one was similar to the IGF-II purified from serum and the other had a larger MW (serum, 123 ng/ml; spinal fluid, 22 ng/ml)[19]. This "big" IGF-II is biologically active[19] and differs from "classical" IGF-II by substitution of cys-gly-arg for ser33 and a carboxyl terminal extension (E domain) of 21 amino acid residues[62]. The "big" IGF-II may be a precursor of IGF-II. The evidence that levels of IGF-I and -II in the CSF are independent of serum concentrations and of GH is further supported by clinical reports that CSF contents of IGF-I and -II are no different in acromegaly than in GH deficiency[67,68,69]. It is possible that blood, brain and CSF IGF-II might interact to generate certain responses in the CNS.

IGF-I and IGF-II Binding Proteins

The IGF-I and -II appear in the circulation bound to carrier proteins in high MW-mass complexes. In rat serum, tracer somatomedins were shown to be associated with two protein fractions with MWs of 150,000 and 40,000-60,000, which have also been identified in human serum[70-75]. The major somatomedin-binding protein complex of 150,000 appears to be a hexamer composed of subunits of about 24,000 MW each[76]. In human serum, about 72% of the endogenous somatomedins are associated with the 150,000 MW fraction and 25% with the 50,000 MW fraction[77], with less than 1% being found in the MW range of the isolated somatomedins. Other IGF-binding proteins with MW 24,000-39,000[78] have been identified. Complexes of the anterior pituitary gave two distinct bands at 39,000 and 52,000 MWs, and those of the posterior pituitary, hypothalamus and cerebral cortex yielded similar, but not identical profiles[78]. Results of competitive binding studies suggest that the different forms of binding proteins have different affinities for IGF-I and -II[78]. Two binding proteins, one with a selective affinity for IGF-I (type-I) and the other with selective affinity for IGF-II (type-II), have been identified[79]. In gel filtration both types of binding proteins of adult human serum eluted with the >100,000 and the 40,000-70,000 MW material[79]. The type-II binding protein predominated in the 40,000-70,000 material as well as in the nervous tissue (hypothalamus and cerebral cortex)[78] and CSF of adult human subjects[79]. This may indicate the predominance of IGF-II in CSF. The primary form of the type-II binding protein in the CSF has a MW of 34,000[79,80]. Rat astroglia also secrete two species of binding proteins that specifically bind IGF-I and -II with different affinities[81].

The roles of IGF-I and -II binding proteins might include prolongation in half-life of IGF-I and -II[82], provision of a reservoir for the peptides[49], prevention of rapid fluctuations in IGF-I and -II concentrations[83,84] and attenuation of biological activity[26]. The total serum concentration of IGF-I plus -II is 1000 times that of insulin, but hypoglycemia is not produced (this may explains why somatomedins cannot replace insulin in diabetes mellitus). The process of in vivo IGF-I and -II release from their macromolecular complexes to interact with cell surface receptors is unknown. It has been suggested that, at neutral pH, serum proteolytic enzymes reduce the affinity of IGF-I and -II binding proteins for their ligands, and that heparin, or other polyanions prevent reassociation, allowing the free IGF to remain available to its target sites[21,85,86]. The liver is a major site of production of IGF-I and -II binding proteins[37,38,87], and releases IGF-I in the circulation together with its binding protein[37,38]. Rat and human 150,000 MW binding proteins are regulated by GH[70,71,88-90].

RECEPTORS FOR IGF-I AND IGF-II

Receptors for IGF-I and -II have been identified in many cell and tissue preparations including pituitary and neural tissues[91,92]. Evidence of IGF receptors in the nervous system is rapidly expanding and many similarities exist between receptors in peripheral tissues and those in the nervous system (as for insulin). Knowledge of characteristics of IGF receptors in peripheral tissues thus provides a basis for understanding the potential mechanisms and biological effects activated in the nervous system.

Receptors in Peripheral Target Tissues

Molecular structure. Two distinct receptor types have been identified by affinity cross-linking experiments, biosynthetic labeling and hydrodynamic measurements (Fig. 2).

Type-I IGF receptors with high affinity for IGF-I (IGF-I receptors), are heterotetramers[93-99] with a native MW of 350,000 comprised of two α- and two β-subunits of MW 130,000 and 92,000-98,000, respectively. The larger subunit appears to contain the peptide binding site, although weak affinity labeling is also seen on the small subunit. The β-subunit contains an intrinsic tyrosine kinase (see below). The subunits are linked by interchain disulfide bridges. Since, under nonreducing conditions, up to three labeled species of MWs ranging from 290,000 to 350,000 are detected, it has been postulated that the subunits stoichiometries of the native unreduced IGF-I receptor are: $\alpha_2\beta_2$ (MW 350,000), $\alpha_2\beta\beta_1$ (MW 320,000) and $\alpha_2(\beta_1)_2$ (MW 290,000). The β_1-subunit appears to be a proteolytic fragment of the β-subunit. One construct for IGF-I action is that after binding to the α-subunit, the signal is transmitted to the β-subunit, perhaps involving conformational changes (Fig. 2). The β-subunit then continues the flow of information into the cell (e.g., phosphorylation of cellular proteins by the tyrosine kinase).

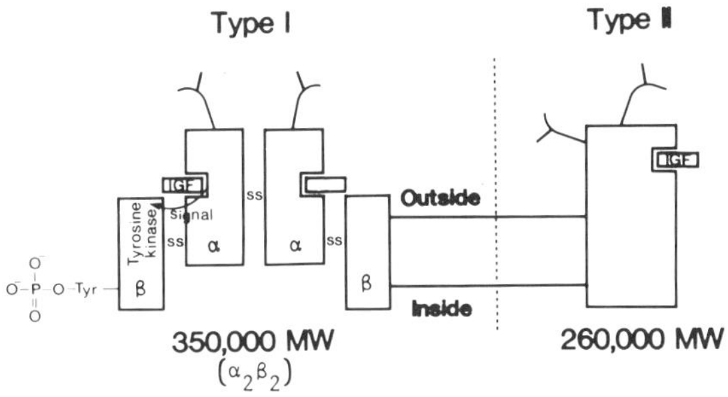

Fig. 2. Schematic representation of the current models of type-I (IGF-I) and type II (IGF-II) receptors.

Type-II IGF receptors which have high affinity for IGF-II (IGF-II receptors) consist of a single polypeptide chain of MW 258,000 to 268,000 that contains intrachain disulfide bonds[95,97]. This has been confirmed in studies on IGF-II receptors purified by affinity chromatography[100-102]. Both IGF-I and -II receptors are glycoproteins[27,94].

Many similarities between IGF-I receptors and insulin receptors are apparent in subunit structure and organization, peptide specificity, tyrosine autophosphorylation, biosynthesis, down-regulation and other characteristics[93,94,97,98,103,104]; although some differences have been reported by immunochemical techniques, showing nonidentical antigenic determinants[105-109]. However, it is not clear, whether the differences between insulin and IGF-I receptors reflect different primary structures or merely differences in glycosylation or some other post-translational modification. On the other hand, a subpopulation of atypical insulin receptors with moderate affinity for IGF-I and -II has been described[110]; as a "common" receptor for insulin-like peptides in which IGF-I and -II are equipotent and insulin is only slightly less so. These receptors have been proposed as type-III IGF receptors[110a].

Functional characteristics. The IGF-I receptor has a high affinity for IGF-I, a somewhat lower (but sometimes equal) affinity for IGF-II, and low affinity for insulin (0.1 to 1% of that for IGF-I). The IGF-II receptor has a high affinity for IGF-II, low to moderate affinity for IGF-I, and no affinity for insulin. In general, insulin and the IGF-I and -II express the same biological effects at appropriate concentrations[28,33,109]. It was proposed that acute metabolic effects of insulin and IGFs are mediated by insulin receptors, and that chronic growth effects (DNA synthesis and cell multiplication) induced by both peptides are mediated by the IGF receptors (Fig. 3). However, it is clear that there are many exceptions[104,111-113], and addition of maximally effective concentrations of both peptides is not additive. This suggests that pathways activated by both peptides converge either at or distal to the hormone-receptor interaction[109]. Because of the extensive cross-reactivity of IGF-I and -II with both IGF-I and -II receptors, it was postulated that either receptor could potentially mediate the biological responses of either peptide[109]. In all known cases, the heterologous IGF exhibits complete cross-reactivity with 10-100% the potency of the homologous IGF[114].

Receptor regulation. The number and affinity of IGF receptors are subjected to modulation by a variety of factors. As are other hormone receptors, IGF-I receptors are down-regulated (accounted by a decrease in receptor number rather than a change in binding affinity) by exposure of the cells to IGF-I[115], or insulin with a potency proportional to their ability to bind to the receptor[115,116].

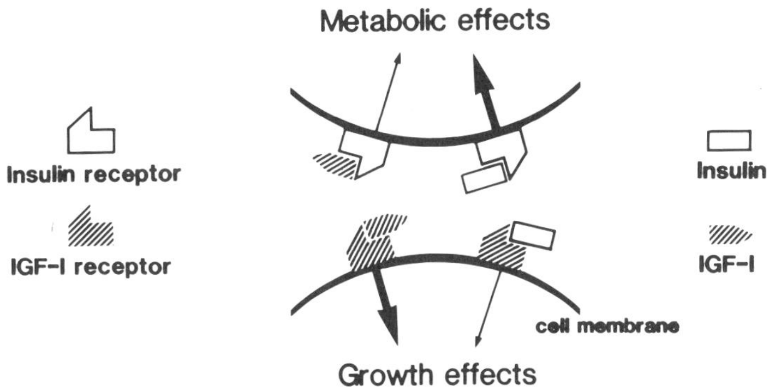

Fig. 3. Heterospecific receptor regulation between insulin and IGF.

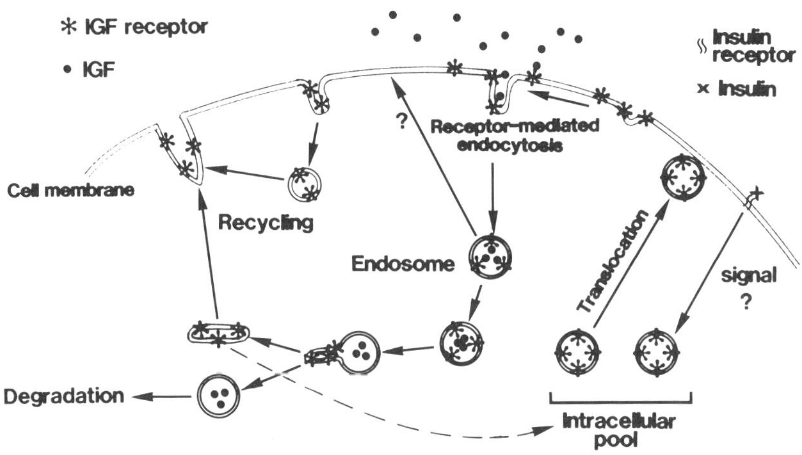

Fig. 4. Schematic representation of the proposed mechanism of the regulation of IGF receptor. Net receptor concentration on the cell surface represents active equilibrium between the rates of internalization and recycling, and the rates of receptor synthesis and degradation (not shown). Right side, insulin-induced translocation of type II IGF receptors from an intracellular pool to the cell surface.

Increased IGF-II binding to several cell types after incubation with insulin has been described[117,118]. Scatchard analysis indicated an insulin-induced redistribution or translocation (up-regulation) of IGF-II receptors from low-density microsomal (intracellular pool) to plasma membranes in rat adipocytes[117-119](Fig.4). By blocking receptor endocytosis with cyanide, it was calculated that 82% of the total estimated IGF-II receptors per cell in the basal state and 68% in insulin-treated cells reside intracellularly[119]. Internalized ligand-bound IGF-II receptors may segregate[119] and IGF-II receptors would be sequestered in one region of the endocytotic vesicles, and this region would then pinch off (Fig. 4) to produce a vesicle that is enriched in receptors. This vesicle recycles to the membrane where the receptors can bind more ligands[119]. The other vesicle, enriched in IGF-II, is directed to a degradation site(s)[121]. Alternatively, internalized IGF-II may remain associated with its receptor, which is replaced on the cell surface by unoccupied receptors from an intracellular pool. Some cell surface IGF-II receptors in insulin-treated cells may be rapidly internalized without ligand binding and rapidly recycle back to the plasma membrane[122](Fig. 4). The receptor-IGF-II complex is thus internalized and provides a mechanism for cellular uptake of IGFs. Both this and IGF receptors that are internalized without being bound can recycle to the membrane. The calcium ionophore A23187 has been shown to decrease the binding of IGF-II[118], and addition of calcium to microsomal membranes decreases IGF-I binding to these membranes by decreasing the affinity of high-affinity sites[123]. Calcium movements are thus implicated in the modulation of IGF receptor expression.

<u>Receptor phosphorylation</u> IGF-I receptors possess intrinsic tyrosine kinase activity[98,124-127]. Binding of IGF-I to the IGF-I receptor stimulates phosphorylation of one or more tyrosine residues on the β-subunit of the receptor[126,127](Fig. 2). The enzymatic and structural features of the IGF-I receptor-associated tyrosine kinase are remarkably similar to those of the insulin receptor kinase[99]. It has been proposed that tyrosine phosphorylation is important in transduction of the biological signal that follows binding of IGFs to their receptors[127]. The phosphorylation of intracellular substrates by a receptor tyrosine kinase may be an initial event in mediating the physiological effects of the IGF[128] including stimulation of cell growth. Although the IGF-II receptor does not have tyrosine kinase activity that is capable of autophosphorylation, the receptor is a substrate for a tyrosine protein kinase endogenous to the plasma membrane, and IGF-II renders the receptor a better substrate for this kinase[104,128].

Receptors in the Central Nervous System

Specific receptors for IGF-I and -II have been identified in brain membrane homogenates[91,92,92a], in primary cultures of rat anterior pituitary cells[129], in cultured human pituitary adenomas[130], in fetal murine neuronal cells[130a], and in human SH-SY5Y neuroblastoma cells[131]. The binding characteristics of IGF-I and -II receptors in rat anterior pituitary, hypothalamic, and other brain tissue are essentially the same[92], with IGF-II binding affinity three to five times that of IGF-I. The specific binding of [^{125}I]IGF-II, [^{125}I]IGF-I, and [^{125}I]insulin measured in 250,000 normal anterior pituitary cells[132] averaged 14.5, 2.6 and 0.6%, respectively. The presence of specific high affinity receptors for IGF-I and -II agree with the evidence that IGF-I and -II are involved in modulating brain (e.g., neuronal development, metabolism and neuroregulation) and pituitary functions. IGF-I receptors on the plasma membranes of adult rat and human brain display the typical heterotetrameric structure[132a]; α-subunits (MW, 115,000--slightly lower than in other tissues), which bind IGF-I and -II with almost equal affinity, and β-subunits (MW, 94,000--identical to that in other tissues) which contain tyrosine-kinase activity[132a,133] (Fig. 2). Moreover, the IGF-II receptor in brain is a monomer (MW, 250,000) like that in other tissues[132a]. Autoradiography shows IGF-I and -II binding in several brain areas including the olfactory bulb, cortex, hippocampus, amygdala, cerebellum and anterior pituitary[134,135]. However, within these regions each peptide binds in a different lamina, or cytoarchitecturally distinct region[134,135]. Density of IGF-I and -II binding in the choroid plexuses was high[134-136], suggesting that these may be sites for IGF-I and -II transport into the brain. In particular, specific binding of [^{125}I]IGF-I was localized in several rat brain regions associated with the neural regulation of food (olfactory bulb, paraventricular nucleus)[136] and fluid (subfornical organ, supraoptic and paraventricular nuclei)[136] intake. High specific binding of IGF-I was also present in the external palisade zone of the rat median eminence[137], where IGF-I may directly stimulate the release of somatostatin into the hypophyseal portal circulation[137]. Also, IGF-I receptors were identified on the oligodendrocytes[137a] and IGF-II receptors on astroblasts[138]. This might indicate an IGF-concentrating or distributing system and a mechanism for taking up IGF from CSF or plasma. Interestingly, IGF-I binding to membranes of rat olfactory bulb was reduced in genetically obese Zucker rats[139], and slight structural heterogeneity of IGF-I and insulin receptors in human brain may involve N-linked glycosylation[132a,140]; thus there is selective modification in the post-translational processing or proteolytic cleavage of IGF-I receptors in the brain[132a].

On the other hand, since the circumventricular organs (CVOs) mediate direct interaction between circulating peptide hormones and the CNS[141], CVO-binding sites may monitor concentrations and facilitate interaction of IGF-I and -II with the CNS by selectively taking up intact hormones from the blood and transporting them through brain interstitial fluid to CNS target sites behind the blood-brain barrier, and/or into the CSF through the blood-CSF barrier. Also, CVOs may contain potential target sites for IGF-I and -II action. The relative contributions of brain/CSF-derived and blood-borne IGF-I and -II may determine the dynamics of the CNS binding sites for IGF-I and -II. This could apply to other neuropeptides as well.

Receptor ontogeny Study of the ontogeny of IGF-I and -II receptors in human liver and brain revealed no change in IGF-II receptors of fetal liver membranes over a range of gestational ages, whereas IGF-I binding was barely detectable[57]. In the human fetus after 25 weeks of gestation and in the adult brain, IGF-I is three times as potent as IGF-II in inhibiting binding of labeled IGF-I, whereas the two peptides are equipotent against labeled IGF-II. In contrast, before 17 weeks of gestation, IGF-II is the most potent binding inhibitor of either labeled IGF-I or IGF-II[57]. Thus, IGF-II binding in the brain seems to be favored early in gestation, whereas high concentration, high affinity IGF-I receptors appear later[57]. Insulin was found to be 0.01 times as potent as IGF-I or -II in displacing $[^{125}I]$IGF-I, which agrees with the hypothesis that insulin reacts through IGF receptors. These differences between fetal and adult brain tissue led to the suggestion of a fetal form of somatomedin receptor[56,68].

Receptors in microvessels Specific receptors for IGF-I and -II have been shown in isolated brain capillaries[142]. In brain capillaries, 22% of the bound IGF-I and 43% of the bound IGF-II were internalized[142]. Several studies have characterized receptors for IGF-I and -II on cells from several micro- and macrovessels (endothelial cells, pericytes and smooth muscle cells)[142-147]. Micro- and macrovascular endothelial cells bind and process IGF-I by degradative and nondegradative pathways[147]. The predominance of nondegradative pathways for processing IGF-I, and the modulation of IGF-I receptors by physiological hormone concentrations suggests that endothelial cells may regulate the access of IGF-I to its target cells[147]. This specificity is further supported by the predominance of degradative pathways for IGF-II after internalization[146]. Thus, the brain microvessels are likely to play a major role in determining several nervous system functions that depend on IGF-I and -II: i) Since intact IGF-I and -II may be retained within endothelial cells[146], these cells may serve as a storage compartment for IGF-I and -II. ii) The receptor-mediated internalized IGF-I and -II may; a) Affect acute metabolic functions (IGF-mediated stimulation of glucose metabolism and thymidine incorporation into DNA in capillary endothelial cells have been shown)[145,146]; b) Mediate transport of blood-borne IGF-I and -II into underlying CNS target sites (transendothelial passage from blood to brain/CSF). Externalization of IGF at the brain capillary antiluminal membrane may normally occur in vivo as part of peptide transcytosis through the blood-brain barrier (receptor-mediated transcytosis system)[143,146-150]. The evidence implies that IGFs could be transferred in both directions between the brain-CSF and blood through the blood-brain barrier and across the CVOs. Brain levels of IGF-I and -II would be partly determined by such mechanisms. Of course, binding proteins for IGF-I and -II may alter the availability of these peptides to the CNS.

FUNCTIONAL SIGNIFICANCE OF IGF-I AND IGF-II IN THE NERVOUS SYSTEM

Interrelations of GH with IGF-I and IGF-II

Circulating levels of IGF-I in humans depend on GH secretion, being elevated during GH hypersecretion, and often almost undetectable during total GH deficiency. Levels of IGF-II may partially depend on GH.

Regulation of IGF-I by GH has been demonstrated in many systems[151-153]. In turn, IGF-I and -II have been found to inhibit basal and/or stimulated levels of GH in cultured rat and human pituitary tissue [92,130,154-157]. Insulin at high concentrations can mimic these effects[156]. Evidence shows that in rat[157,158], and human pituitary adenoma cells[159], IGF-I may modulate GH gene expression at the level of the somatotroph by inhibiting basal and GHRH-stimulated GH secretion and GH mRNA levels[157-159]. These effects may be due to direct inhibition of IGF-I on GH gene transcription, or by action at different post-transcriptional sites (by altering mRNA stability or suppressing GH translation). The inhibition was blocked by an IGF-I receptor antibody [159], indicating specificity of action, and may also involve inhibition in the rate of release[160]. Evidence in chronically cannulated conscious rats shows a highly significant association between secretory pulses of GH and IGF-I levels[161]. When injected intra-cerebroventricularly (ICV) into conscious rats, IGF-I has been found to markedly suppress the episodic bursts of pituitary GH secretion[162,163].

These results implicate IGF-I and -II in a negative feedback loop that inhibits GH secretion. This occurs at both the anterior pituitary level by decreasing the GH response to GHRH[154-157], and in the CNS by involving the inhibitory mechanism of hypothalamic somatostatin secretion[154]. Short- and ultra-short-loop inhibition of GH secretion might be mediated by IGFs generated locally in the pituitary or hypothalamus. In addition, increase in basal GH has been reported in anorexia nervosa[164]. Since anorexia nervosa decreases somatomedin activity[164], this may suppress the inhibitory effect of somatomedin on GH release and may raise the basal level of GH.

Direct CNS Effects of IGF-I and -II

As mentioned, IGF-I and -II can elicit the same biological effects as insulin[28,33,165,166]. The major difference is that, in general, insulin is more potent in affecting metabolic events, whereas the IGF-I and -II are more potent in growth-promoting activity. All purified IGFs have been shown to act as anabolic hormones *in vitro*[167,168] and *in vivo*[169-171]. On the basis of this evidence a role for somatomedins in fetal brain growth was suggested by studies showing that serum contained brain-growth-promoting activity that was related to sulphation factor activity[172]. Some possible CNS actions were described in the sections "Sites of Production" and "Receptors in the Central Nervous System". Additional evidence to support a role of IGF-I and -II in the CNS includes:

i) IGF-I and -II stimulated [^{3}H]thymidine incorporation into DNA of human glial cells[173], fetal rat brain cells[58,174], and human adrenergic neuroblastoma cells SH-SY5Y[131]; and stimulated ornithine decarboxylase activity in SH-SY5Y cells[131]. Neuronal and glial enzymes increase in the presence of IGF-I[174], suggesting influence on neuronal and glial precursor cell division (cell replication and differentiation). Telencephalic cells are more responsive than cells from hindbrain of the same fetal age[174]. The variant form of IGF-I previously described also stimulated DNA synthesis in fetal rat brain cells[60].

ii) Physiological concentrations of IGF-II enhanced neurite outgrowth in human neuroblastoma cells[175,176], chick embryo dorsal root ganglia[177], sympathetic cell cultures[178] and cortical neuronal cultures free of glial cells[179]. IGF-II supported the survival of several embryonic neurons[177-179]; and its half-maximal effective concentrations from study to study suggest dependence of the effects on neuronal tissue type. IGF-II also specifically increased the levels of α- and β-tubulin mRNAs in human neuroblastoma cells[176]. Capacity to increase tubulin transcripts correlates closely with enhancement of neurite formation[176]; increased tubulin concentration may promote microtubule formation associated with neurite outgrowth. The IGF-II modulation of neurite outgrowth expresses a different mechanism than that of nerve growth factor (NGF)[175,180]. In fact, physiological concentrations of IGF-II are permissive for NGF-directed neurite formation and can increase NGF-binding affinity in human neuroblastoma cells[180]; also, IGF-II potentiated the mitogenic effect of glia maturation factor at 0.001 times the concentration of insulin[137], and act synergistically with brain fibroblast growth factor[181]. These interactions are in sequential manner. Potentiation of activity of other mitogenic hormones may influence control of cell proliferation. This is consistent with the concept of competence and progression factors[182-184]; competence factors such as the platelet-derived growth factor[183] and fibroblast growth factor[181], which act in the G_0 phase, make the cells "competent" to begin DNA synthesis, and IGF-I and -II act in the subsequent G_1 phase as "progression" factors. On the other hand, increased IGF-I activity in regenerating sciatic nerves of adult rats (reaching peak values at two weeks) has been reported[185]. Reactive Schwann cells appear to be a major source of IGF-I synthesis[185]. It is possible that IGF-I exerts important growth supporting effects on regenerating peripheral nerves.

iii) ICV administration of a preparation enriched in IGFs suppressed food intake for 24 hr[162]. This reduction in food intake did not appear to be caused by illness or aversive effects[162]. It was reported that ICV administration of purified IGF-II (100 ng/rat) decreased food intake, whereas IGF-I had no effect[55]. IGF-II may contribute to regulation of food intake and body weight, but the action mechanism and interaction with other satiety signals are unknown. Cross-reactivity between insulin and IGFs might also participate in the regulation of food intake, since ICV insulin decreases food intake[186], but with potency lower than that of IGF-II[55,162].

PUTATIVE PARTICIPATION OF IGF-I AND IGF-II IN SOME SYNDROMES INVOLVING NERVOUS SYSTEM

It has been suggested that concentrations of IGF-I and -II change in mental retardation[187]. Serum IGF-I is deficient in patients with Down's syndrome[188,189]; it fails to rise during childhood and remains at a low concentration throughout life[188], whereas serum levels of IGF-II remain normal[189,190]. Since receptors for somatomedins have been found to be normal in fetuses with Down's syndrome[189], incomplete switching from production of the fetal form of somatomedin to IGF-I is suggested[189].

Concentrations of somatomedins[29,170] and intellectual quotients[172] are low in patients with Laron type dwarfism who are phenotypically hyposomatotropic. Significant growth retardation and delayed mental development of primary hypothyroid children are accompanied by low serum somatomedin concentration[29,191,192]. In patients with cerebral gigantism (Sotos syndrome) the serum somatomedin concentration has been variable[193-196]; however, levels of one or more of the somatomedins are high during the period of most excessive growth[195,196]. Direct participation of somatomedins in these three syndromes is not clear.

Increased serum and CSF levels of somatomedins have been found in patients with senile dementia disorders of the Alzheimer's type[197], and a defect of brain somatomedin receptors has been suggested. On the other hand, increased CSF somatomedin levels after subarachnoid haemorrhage have been reported in humans[198] and it was postulated that this could be a compensatory response to stimulate cerebral anabolism after injury[198].

Evidence indicates that IGF-I is a potent inducer of oligodendrocyte development[137a], and it promotes DNA synthesis and development of myelin-associated enzyme activity in fetal rat brain[174]. Since oligodendrocytes are critical in the synthesis and maintenance of myelinization in the CNS, a possible cause of hypomyelinization that results from early postnatal undernutrition in rats and humans is suggested to be IGF-I deficiency[137a].

In severe diabetes mellitus, circulating levels of IGF-I and -II are low[199,200], and inhibitors are very high[201,202]. This leads to very low levels of IGF activity, which may contribute to the higher incidence of congenital malformations among infants of diabetic mothers[202]. However, neurological effects of low somatomedin activity remain to be studied.

On the other hand, an involvement of IGF-I and -II in the automitogenic response for malignant transformation is suggested but unknown[203].

Acknowledgement. We thank Prof. A. Simpson, Showa University, for help with the manuscript.

REFERENCES

1. W. H. Daughaday, K. Hall, M. S. Raben, W. D. Salmon, J. L. Van den Brande, and J. J. Van Wyk, Somatomedin: A proposed designation for the "sulfation factor", Nature. 235:107 (1972).
2. R. H. Chochinov, and W. H. Daughaday, Current concepts of somatomedin and other biologically related growth factors, Diabetes. 25:994 (1976).
3. H. Sievertsson, L. Fryklund, K. Uthne, K. Hall, and B. Westermark, Isolation and chemistry of human somatomedins A and B, Adv. Metab. Disord. 8:47 (1975).
4. K. Hall, Human somatomedin: Determination, occurrences, biological activity and purification, Acta Endocrinol. 163:1 (1972).
5. J. J. Van Wyk, and L. E. Underwood, The somatomedins and their actions, Biochem. Actions Horm. 5:101 (1978).
6. K. Uthne, Human somatomedins. Purification and some studies on their biological actions, Acta Endocrinol. (Suppl.) 175:1 (1973).
7. J. J. Van Wyk, L. E. Underwood, R. L. Hintz, D. R. Clemmons, S. J. Voina, and R. P. Weaver, The somatomedins: A family of insulinlike hormones under growth hormone control, Recent Prog. Horm. Res. 30:259 (1974).
8. A. C. Moses, S. P. Nissley, P. A. Short, M. M. Rechler, and J. M. Podskalny, Purification and characterization of multiplication stimulating activity, Eur. J. Biochem. 103:387 (1980).
9. N. A. Samaan, W. J. Dempster, R. Fraser, M. W. Please, and D. Stillman, Further immunological studies on the form of circulating insulin, J. Endocrinol. 24:263 (1962).
10. E. R. Froesch, H. Bürgi, W. A. Müller, R. E. Humbel, A. Jacob, and A. Lambert, Antibody-suppressible and nonsuppressible insulin-like activity in human serum and their physiological significance. An insulin assay with adipose tissue of increased precision and specificity, J. Clin. Invest. 42:1816 (1963).
11. E. Rinderknecht, and R. E. Humbel, Amino-terminal sequences of two polypeptides from human serum with non-suppressible insulin-like and cell-growth-promoting activities: Evidence for structural homology with insulin B chain, Proc. Natl. Acad. Sci., U.S.A. 73:4379 (1976).
12. E. Rinderknecht, and R.E. Humbel, Polypeptides with nonsuppressible insulin-like and cell-growth promoting activities in human serum: Isolation, chemical characterization and some biological properties of forms I and II, Proc. Natl. Acad. Sci., U.S.A. 73:2365 (1976).
13. B. I. Posner, H. J. Guyda, M. T. Corvol, R. Rappaport, C. Harley, and S. Goldstein, Partial purification, characterization and assay of a slightly acidic insulin-like peptide (ILAs) from human plasma, J. Clin. Endocrinol. Metab. 47:1240 (1978).
14. G. Enberg, M. Carlquist, H. Jörnvall, and K. Hall, The characterization of somatomedin A, isolated by microcomputer - controlled chromatography, reveals an apparent identity to insulin-like growth factor I, Eur. J. Biochem. 143:117 (1984).
15. D. G. Klapper, M. E. Svoboda, and J. J. Van Wyk, Sequence analysis of somatomedin C: Confirmation of identity with insulin-like growth factor I, Endocrinology. 112:2215 (1983).
16. H. Marquardt, G. J. Todaro, L. E. Henderson, and S. Oroszlan, Purification and primary structure of a polypeptide with multiplication-simulating activity (MSA) from rat liver cell cultures: Homology with human insulin-like growth factor II (IGF-II), J. Biol. Chem. 256:6859 (1981).
17. A. C. Moses, S. P. Nissley, P. A. Short, M. M. Rechler, R. M. White, A. B. Knight, and O.Z. Higa, Increased levels of multiplication-stimulating activity, an insulin-like growth factor, in fetal rat serum, Proc. Natl. Acad. Sci., U.S.A. 77:3649 (1980).
18. C. H. Heldin, A. Wasteson, L. Fryklund, and B. Westermark, Somatomedin B: Mitogenic activity derived from contaminant epidermal growth factor, Science. 213:1122 (1981).

19. G. Haselbacher and R. Humbel, Evidence for two species of insulin-like growth factor II (IGF II and "big" IGF II) in human spinal fluid, Endocrinology 110:1822 (1982).
20. M. Jansen, F. M. A. Van Schaik, H. Van Tol, J. L. Van den Brande, and J. S. Sussenbach, Nucleotide sequences of cDNAs encoding precursors of human insulin-like growth factor II (IGF-II) and an IGF-II variant, FEBS Lett. 179:243 (1985).
21. J. L. Van den Brande, M. Jansen, C. M. Hoogerbrugge, P. de Pagter-Holthuizen, S. C. van Buul-Offers, F.M.A Van Schaik, and J. S. Sussenbach, Molecular aspects of the human somatomedins, Horm. Res. 24:131 (1986).
22. E. Rinderknecht, and R.E. Humbel, The amino acid sequence of insulin-like growth factor I and its structural homology with proinsulin, J. Biol. Chem. 253:2769 (1978).
23. J. Zapf, C. H. Schmid, and E. R. Froesch, Biological and immunological properties of insulin-like growth factors (IGF) I and II, Clin. Endocrinol. Metab. 13:3 (1984).
24. J. J. Van Wyk, The somatomedins: Biological actions and physiologic control mechanisms, in: "Human Proteins and Peptides," C. H. Li, ed., Academic Press, New York (1984).
25. E. Rinderknecht and R. E. Humbel, Primary structure of human insulin-like growth factor-II, FEBS Lett. 89:283 (1978).
26. L. E., Underwood, A. J. D'Ercole, D. R. Clemmons, and J. J. Van Wyk, Paracrine functions of somatomedins, Clin. Endocrinol. Metab. 15:59 (1986).
27. J. F. Perdue, Chemistry, structure, and function of insulin-like growth factors and their receptors: a review, Can. J. Biochem. Cell Biol. 62: 1237 (1984).
28. E. R. Froesch, and J. Zapf, Insulin-like growth factors and insulin: Comparative aspects, Diabetologia 28:485 (1985).
29. R. C. Baxter, The somatomedins: Insulin-like growth factors, Adv. Clin. Chem. 25:49 (1986).
30. D. R. Clemmons, and L. E. Underwood, Somatomedin-C/Insulin-like growth factor I in acromegaly, Clin. Endocrinol. Metab. 15: 629 (1986).
30a. G. I. Bell, J. P. Merryweather, R. Sanchez-Pescador, M. M. Stempien, L. Preistly, J. Scott, and L. B. Rall, Sequence of a cDNA clone encoding human preproinsulin-like growth factor II, Nature 310:775 (1984).
31. T. L. Blundell, S. Bedarkar, E. Rinderknecht, and R. E. Humbel, Insulin-like growth factor: A model for tertiary structure accounting for immunoreactivity and receptor binding, Proc. Natl. Acad. Sci., U.S.A. 75:180 (1978).
32. T. L. Blundell, and R. E. Humbel, Hormone families: Pancreatic hormones and homologous growth factors, Nature 287: 781 (1980).
33. J. Zapf, and E. R. Froesch, Insulin-like growth factors/somatomedins: Structure, secretion, biological actions and physiological role, Horm. Res. 24:121 (1986).
34. P. McConaghey, and C. B. Sledge, Production of "sulphation factor" by the perfused rat liver, Nature 225: 1249 (1970).
35. M. J. O. Francis, and D. J. Hill, Prolactin-stimulated production of somatomedin by rat liver, Nature 255:167 (1975).
36. M. Kogawa, K. Takano, K. Asakawa, N. Hizuka, T. Tsushima, and K. Shizume, Insulin stimulation of somatomedin A production in monolayer cultures of rat hepatocytes, Acta Endocrinol. 103:385 (1983).
37. J. C. Schwander, C. Hauri, J. Zapf, and E. R. Froesch, Synthesis and secretion of insulin-like growth factor and its binding protein by the perfused rat liver: Dependence on growth hormone status, Endocrinology. 113:297 (1983).
38. C. D. Scott, J. L. Martin, and R. C. Baxter, Production of insulin-like growth factor-I and its binding protein by adult rat hepatocytes in primary culture, Endocrinology 116:1094 (1985).
39. P. R. Atkinson, E. R. Weidman, B. Bhaumick, and R. M. Bala, Release of

somatomedin-like activity by cultured WI-38 human fibroblasts, Endocrinology. 106:2006 (1980).

40. D. R. Clemmons, Multiple hormones stimulate the production of somatomedin by cultured human fibroblasts, J. Clin. Endocrinol. Metab. 58:850 (1984).
41. L. S. Phillips, A. C. Herington, I. E. Karl, and W. H. Daughaday, Comparison of somatomedin activity in perfusates of normal and hypophysectomized rat livers with and without added growth hormone, Endocrinology. 98:606 (1976).
42. J. A. Romanus, A. Rabinovitch, and M. M. Rechler, Neonatal rat islet cell cultures synthesize insulin-like growth factor I, Diabetes 34:696 (1985).
43. K. Hall and M. Bozovic, Stimulation of ^{35}S incorporation into embryonic chick cartilage by extracts from rat muscle, Horm. Metab. Res. 1:235 (1969).
44. V. R. Sara, K. Uvnas-Moberg, B. Uvnas, K. Hall, L. Wetterberg, B. Posloncec, and M. Goiny, The distribution of somatomedins in the nervous system of the cat and their release following neural stimulation, Acta Physiol. Scand. 115:467 (1982).
45. K. Kawai, K. Takano, N. Hizuka, and K. Shizume, Properties and concentrations of somatomedin A in various rat tissues, Endocrinol. Jpn. 26:559 (1979).
46. A. J. D'Ercole, G. T. Applewhite, and L. E. Underwood, Evidence that somatomedin is synthesized by multiple tissues in the fetus, Dev. Biol. 75:315 (1980).
47. R. C. Baxter, Z. Zaltsman, and J. R. Turtle, Immunoreactive somatomedin-C/insulin-like growth factor-I and its binding protein in human milk, J. Clin. Endocrinol. Metab. 58:955 (1984).
48. R. C. Baxter, J. L. Martin, and D. J. Handelsman, Identification of human semen insulin-like growth factor-I/somatomedin-C immunoreactivity and binding protein, Acta Endocrinol. 106:420 (1984).
49. A. J. D'Ercole, A. D. Stiles, and L. E. Underwood, Tissue concentrations of somatomedin C: Further evidence for multiple sites of synthesis and paracrine or autocrine mechanisms of action, Proc. Natl. Acad. Sci., U.S.A. 81:935 (1984).
50. D. R. Clemmons, Variables controlling the secretion of a somatomedin-like peptide by cultured porcine smooth muscle cells, Circ. Res. 56:418 (1985).
51. D. R. Clemmons, and D. S. Shaw, Variables controlling somatomedin production by cultured human fibroblasts. J. Cell. Physiol. 115:137 (1983).
52. D. R. Clemmons and J. J. Van Wyk, Evidence for a functional role of endogenously produced somatomedin-like peptides in the regulation of DNA synthesis in cultured human fibroblasts and porcine smooth muscle cells, J. Clin. Invest. 75:1914 (1985).
53. M. Binoux, P. Hossenlopp, C. Lassarre, and N. Hardouin, Production of insulin-like growth factors and their carrier by rat pituitary gland and brain explants in culture, FEBS Lett. 124:178 (1981).
54. G. K. Haselbacher, M. E. Schwab, A. Pasi, and R. E. Humbel, Insulin-like growth factor II (IGF II) in human brain: Regional distribution of IGF II and of higher molecular mass forms, Proc. Natl. Acad. Sci., U.S.A. 82:2153 (1985).
55. T. J. Lauterio, L. Marson, W. H. Daughaday, and C. A. Baile, Intracerebroventricular injections of insulin-like growth factor II, but not insulin-like growth factor I, decrease food intake and body weight in rats, Soc. Neurosci. Abst. 12:795 (1986).
56. V.R. Sara, K. Hall, C. H. Rodeck, and L. Wetterberg, Human embryonic somatomedin, Proc. Natl. Acad. Sci., U.S.A. 78:3175 (1981).
57. V. R. Sara, K. Hall, M. Misaki, L. Fryklund, N. Christensen, and L. Wetterberg, Ontogenesis of somatomedin and insulin receptors in the human fetus, J. Clin. Invest. 71:1084 (1983).

58. G. Enberg, A. Tham, and V. R. Sara, The influence of purified somatomedins and insulin on foetal rat brain DNA synthesis in vitro, Acta Physiol. Scand. 125:305 (1985).
59. V. R. Sara, C. Carlsson-Skwirut, C. Andersson, E. Hall, B. Sjögren, A. Holmgren, and H. Jörnvall, Characterization of somatomedins from human fetal brain: Identification of a variant form of insulin-like growth factor I, Proc. Natl. Acad. Sci., U.S.A. 83:4904 (1986).
60. C. Carlsson-Skwirut, H. Jörnvall, A. Holmgren, C. Andersson, T. Bergman, G. Lundquist, B. Sjögren, and V.R. Sara, Isolation and characterization of variant IGF-1 as well as IGF-2 from adult human brain, FEBS Lett. 201:46 (1986).
61. P. K. Lund, B. M. Moats-Staats, M. A. Hynes, J. G. Simmons, M. Jansen, A. J. D'Ercole, and J. J. Van Wyk, Somatomedin-C/Insulin-like growth factor-I and insulin-like growth factor-II mRNAs in rat fetal and adult tissues, J. Biol. Chem. 261:14539 (1986).
62. P. P. Zumstein, C. Lüthi, and R. E. Humbel, Amino acid sequence of a variant pro-form of insulin-like growth factor II, Proc. Natl. Acad. Sci., U.S.A. 82:3169 (1985)
63. M. C. Soares, D. N. Ishii, and A. Efstratiadis, Developmental and tissue-specific expression of a family of transcripts related to rat insulin-like growth factor II mRNA, Nucleic Acids Res. 13:1119 (1985).
64. J. Scott, J. Cowell, M. E. Robertson, L. M. Priestley, R. Wadey, B. Hopkins, J. Pritchard, G. I. Bell, L. B. Rall, C. F. Graham, and T. J. Knott, Insulin-like growth factor-II gene expression in Wilms' tumour and embryonic tissues, Nature. 317:260 (1985).
65. A. L. Brown, D. E. Graham, S. P. Nissley, D. J. Hill, A. J. Strain, and M. M. Rechler, Developmental regulation of insulin-like growth factor II mRNA in different rat tissues, J. Biol. Chem. 261:13144 (1986).
66. G. R. Beaton, J. Sagel and L. A. Distiller, Somatomedin activity in cerebrospinal fluid, J. Clin. Endocrinol. Metab. 40:736 (1975).
67. M. Backstrom, K. Hall, and V. Sara, Somatomedin levels in cerebrospinal fluid from adults with pituitary disorders, Acta Endocrinol. 107:171 (1984).
68. K. Hall and V. R. Sara, Growth and somatomedins, Vit. Horm. 40:175 (1983).
69. K. Hall and V. R. Sara, Somatomedin levels in childhood adolescence and adult life, Clin. Endocrinol. J. Metabolism 13:91 (1984).
70. A. C. Moses, S. P. Nissley, K. L. Cohen, and M. M. Rechler, Specific binding of somatomedin-like polypeptide in rat serum depends on growth hormone, Nature 263:137 (1976).
71. R. L. Hintz, F. Liu, R. G. Rosenfeld, and S. F. Kemp, Plasma somatomedin-binding proteins in hypopituitarism: Changes during growth hormone therapy, J. Clin. Endocrinol. Metab. 53:100 (1981).
72. R. M. White, S. P. Nissley, A. C. Moses, M. M. Rechler, and R. E. Johnsonbaugh, The growth hormone dependence of a somatomedin-binding protein in human serum, J. Clin. Endocrinol. Metab. 53:49 (1981).
73. D. H. Morris, and D. S. Schalch, Structure of somatomedin-binding protein: Alkaline GH induced dissociation of an acid-stable, 60,000 molecular weight complex into smaller components, Endocrinology. 111:801 (1982).
74. D. A. Cohen and S. L. Blethen, Somatomedin binding proteins in GH-deficient children with normal plasma somatomedin levels, J. Clin. Endocrinol. Metab. 56:461 (1983).
75. S. L. S. Drop, D. J. Kortleve, and H. J. Guyda, Isolation of a somatomedin-binding protein from preterm amniotic fluid: Development of a radioimmunoassay, J. Clin. Endocrinol. Metab. 59:899 (1984).
76. J. R. Wilkins and J. D'Ercole, Affinity labeled plasma somatomedin-C/insulin-like growth factor I binding proteins: Evidence of growth hormone dependence and subunit structure, J. Clin. Invest. 75:1350 (1985).
77. W. H. Daughaday, A. P. Ward, A. C. Goldberg, B. Trivedi, and M.

Kapadia, Characterization of somatomedin binding in human serum by ultracentrifugation and gel filtration, J. Clin. Endocrinol. Metab. 55:916 (1982).

78. M. Binoux, P. Hossenlopp, S. Hardouin, D. Seurin, C. Lassarre, and M. Gourmelen, Somatomedin (Insulin-like growth factors) - binding proteins, Horm. Res. 24:141 (1986).

79. M. Binoux, S. Haradouin, C. Lassarre, and P. Hossenlopp, Evidence for production by the liver of two IGF binding proteins with similar molecular weights but different affinities for IGF I and IGF II. Their relations with serum and cerebrospinal fluid IGF binding proteins, J. Clin. Endocrinol. Metab. 55:600 (1982).

80. M. Binoux, C. Lassarre, and M. Gourmelen, Specific assay for insulin-like growth factor (IGF) II using the IGF binding proteins extracted from human cerebrospinal fluid, J. Clin. Endocrinol. Metab. 63:1151 (1986).

81. V. K. M. Han, D. F. Bell, J. M. Lauder, and A. J. D'Ercole, Characterization of somatomedin/insulin-like growth factor (Sm/IGF) binding proteins (BPs) in conditioned medium from rat astroglia by affinity labeling, Soc. Neurosci. Abst. 12:397 (1986).

82. K. L. Cohen and S. P. Nissley, The serum half-life of somatomedin activity: Evidence for growth hormone dependence, Acta Endocrinol. 83:243 (1976).

83. G. L. Smith, Somatomedin carrier protein, Mol. Cell. Endocrinol. 34:83 (1984).

84. R. L. Hintz, Plasma forms of somatomedin and the binding protein phenomenon, Clin. Endocrinol. Metab. 13:31 (1984).

85. D. R. Clemmons, L. E. Underwood, P. G. Chatelain and J. J. Van Wyk, Liberation of immunoreactive somatomedin-C from its binding proteins by proteolytic enzymes and heparin, J. Clin. Endocrinol. Metab. 56:384 (1983).

86. P. G. Chatelain, J. J. Van Wyk, K. C. Copeland, S. L. Blethen, and L. E. Underwood, Effect of in vitro action of serum proteases or exposure to acid on measurable immunoreactive somatomedin-C in serum, J. Clin. Endocrinol. Metab. 56:376 (1983).

87. E. M. Spencer, Synthesis by cultured hepatocytes of somatomedin and its binding protein, FEBS Lett. 99:157 (1979).

88. A. C. Moses, S. P. Nissley, J. Passamani and R. M. White, Further characterization of GH-dependent somatomedin-binding protein in rat serum and demonstration of somatomedin-binding protein produced by rat liver cells in culture, Endocrinology 104:536 (1979).

89. K. C. Copeland, L. E. Underwood, and J. J. Van Wyk, Induction of immunoreactive somatomedin C in human serum by growth hormone: Dose-response relationships and effect on chromatographic profiles, J. Clin. Endocrinol. Metab. 50:690 (1980).

90. M. Binoux, D. Seurin, C. Lassarre, and M. Gourmelen, Preferential measurement of insulin-like growth factor (IGF) I-related peptides in serum with the aid of IGF-binding proteins (IGF BPs) produced by rat liver in culture. Estimation of serum IGF BP levels, J. Clin. Endocrinol. Metab. 59:453 (1984).

91. V. R. Sara, K. Hall, H. Von Holtz, R. Humbel, B. Sjögren, and L. Wetterberg, Evidence for the presence of specific receptors for insulin-like growth factors I (IGF-I) and II (IGF-II) and insulin throughout the adult human brain, Neurosci. Lett. 34:39 (1982).

92. C. G. Goodyer, L. De Stephano, W. H. Lai, H. J. Guyda, and B. I. Posner, Characterization of insulin-like growth factor receptors in rat anterior pituitary, hypothalamus and brain, Endocrinology 114:1187 (1984).

92a. J. D. Grizzard, A. J. D'Ercole, J. R. Wilkins, B. M. Moats-Staats, and R. W. Williams, Affinity-labeled somatomedin-C receptors and binding proteins from the human fetus, J. Clin. Endocrinol. Metab. 58:535 (1984).

93. B. Bhaumick, R. M. Bala, and M. D. Hollenberg, Somatomedin receptor of human placenta: Solubilization, photolabeling, partial purification, and comparison with insulin receptor. Proc. Natl. Acad. Sci., U.S.A. 78:4278 (1981).
94. S. D. Chernausek, S. Jacobs, and J. J. Van Wyk, Structural similarities between human receptors for somatomedin C and insulin: Analysis by affinity labeling, Biochemistry 20:7345 (1981).
95. M. Kasuga, E. Van Obberghen, S. P. Nissley, and M. M. Rechler, Demonstration of two subtypes of insulin-like growth factor receptors by affinity cross-linking, J. Biol. Chem. 256:5305 (1981).
96. B. Bhaumick, G. D. Armstrong, M. D. Hollenberg, and R. M. Bala, Characterization of the human placental receptor for basic somatomedin, Can. J. Biochem. 60:923 (1982).
97. J. Massague, and M. P. Czech, The subunit structure of two distinct receptors for insulin-like growth factors I and II and their relationship to the insulin receptor, J. Biol. Chem. 257:5038 (1982).
98. D. O. Morgan, K. Jarnagin, and R. A. Roth, Purification and characterization of the receptor for insulin-like growth factor I, Biochemistry 25:5560 (1986).
99. K-T, Yu, M. A. Peters, and M.P. Czech, Similar control mechanisms regulate the insulin and type I insulin-like growth factor receptor kinases, J. Biol. Chem. 261:11341 (1986).
100. G. P. August, S. P. Nissley, M. Kasuga, L. Lee, L. Greenstein, and M. M. Rechler, Purification of an insulin-like growth factor II receptor from rat chondrosarcoma cell, J. Biol. Chem. 258:9033 (1983).
101. C. L. Oppenheimer, and M. P. Czech, Purification of the type II insulin-like growth factor receptor from rat placenta, J. Biol. Chem. 258:8539 (1983).
102. C. Thibault, J. K. Chan, J. F. Perdue, and W. H. Daughaday, Insulin-like growth factor receptors: Molecular radius and molecular weight determination using quantitative polyacrylamide gel electrophoresis, J. Biol. Chem. 259:3361 (1984).
103. M. P. Czech, C. L. Oppenheimer, and J. Massague, Interrelationships among receptor structures for insulin and peptide growth factors, Fed. Proc. 42:2598 (1983).
104. M. M. Rechler and S. P. Nissley, The nature and regulation of the receptors for insulin-like growth factors, Ann. Rev. Physiol. 47:425 (1985).
105. H. A. Jonas, R. C. Baxter, and L. C. Harrison, Structural differences between insulin and somatomedin-C/insulin-like growth factor-I receptors revealed by autoantibodies to the insulin receptor, Biochem. Biophys. Res. Commun. 109: 463 (1982).
106. M. Kasuga, N. Sasaki, C. R. Kahn, S. P. Nissley, and M. M. Rechler, Antireceptor antibodies as probes of insulinlike growth factor receptor structure, J. Clin. Invest. 72:1459 (1983).
107. F. C. Kull, S. Jacobs, Y. F. Su, M. E. Svoboda, J. J. Van Wyk, and P. Cuatrecasas, Monoclonal antibodies to receptors for insulin and somatomedin-C, J. Biol. Chem. 258:6561 (1983).
108. C. A. Stuart, R. Pietrzyk, A. K. Q. Siu, and R. W. Furlanetto, Size discrepancy between somatomedin-C and insulin receptors, J. Clin. Endocrinol. Metab. 58:1 (1984).
109. M. M. Rechler, and S. P. Nissley, Insulin-like growth factor (IGF)/somatomedin receptor subtypes: Structure, function, and relationships to insulin receptors and IGF carrier proteins, Horm. Res. 24:152 (1986).
110. H. A. Jones, J. D. Neuman, and L. C. Harrison, An atypical insulin receptor with high affinity for insulin-like growth factors copurified with placental insulin receptors, Proc. Natl. Acad. Sci., U.S.A. 83:4124 (1986).
110a. R. L. Hintz, A. V. Thorsson, G. Enberg, and K. Hall, IGF-II binding on human lymphoid cells: Demonstration of a common high affinity receptor

for insulin like peptides, Biochem. Biophys. Res. Commun. 118:774 (1984).

111. B. I. Posner, R. M. Gonzalez, and H. J. Guyda, Intracellular (golgi) receptors for insulinlike peptides in rat liver, Can. J. Biochem. 58:1075 (1980).

112. G. L. King, C. R. Kahn, M. M. Rechler, and S. P. Nissley, Direct demonstration of separate receptors for growth and metabolic activities of insulin and multiplication-stimulating activity (an insulinlike growth factor) using antibodies to the insulin receptor, J. Clin. Invest. 66:130 (1980).

113. M. M. Rechler, S. P. Nissley, G. L. King, A. C. Moses, E. E. Van Obberghen-Schilling, J. A. Romanus, A. B. Knight, P. A. Short, and R. M. White, Multiplication stimulating activity (MSA) from the BRL 3A rat liver cell line: Relation to human somatomedins and insulin, J. Supramol. Struc. Cell Biochem. 15:253 (1981).

114. S. J. Pilistine, A. C. Moses, and H. N. Munro, Insulin-like growth factor receptors in rat placental membranes, Endocrinology. 115:1060 (1984).

115. R. G. Rosenfeld, and L. A. Dollar, Characterization of the somatomedin-C/insulin-like growth factor 1 (SM-C/IGF-1) receptor on cultured human fibroblast monolayers: Regulation of receptor concentrations by SM-C/IGF-1 and insulin, J. Clin. Endocrinol. Metab. 55:434 (1982).

116. R. G. Rosenfeld, R. L. Hintz, and L. A. Dollar, Insulin-induced loss of insulin-like growth factor-I receptors on IM-9 lymphocytes, Diabetes. 31:375 (1982).

117. C. L. Oppenheimer, J. E. pessin, J. Massague, W. Gitomer, and M. P. Czech, Insulin action rapidly modulates the apparent affinity of the insulin-like growth factor II receptor, J. Biol. Chem. 258:4824 (1983).

118. N. Potau, J. Mossner, J. A. Williams, and I. D. Goldfine, Cholecystokinin and insulin regulate insulin-like growth factor II binding to pancreatic receptors; evidence of a role for intracellular calcium. Biochem. Biophys. Res. Commun. 119:359 (1984).

119. L. J. Wardzala, I. A. Simpson, M. M. Rechler, and S. W. Cushman, Potential mechanism of the stimulatory action of insulin on insulin-like growth factor II binding to the isolated rat adipose cell: Apparent redistribution of receptors recycling between a large intracellular pool and the plasma membrane, J. Biol. Chem. 259:8378 (1984).

120. Y. Oka, C. Mottola, C. L. Oppenheimer, and M. P. Czech, Insulin activates the appearance of insulin-like growth factor II receptors on the adipocyte cell surface, Proc. Natl. Acad. Sci., U.S.A. 81:4028 (1984).

121. Y. Oka, L. M. Rozek, and M. P. Czech, Direct demonstration of rapid insulin-like growth II receptor internalization and recycling in rat adipocytes, J. Biol. Chem. 260:9435 (1985).

122. Y. Oka and M. P. Czech, The type II insulin-like growth factor receptor is internalized and recycles in the absence of ligand, J. Biol. Chem. 261:9090 (1986).

123. R. C. Baxter and P. F. Williams, Reciprocal modulation of insulin and insulin-like growth factor-I receptor affinity by calcium. Biochem. Biophys. Res. Commun. 116:62 (1983).

124. S. Jacobs, F. C. Kull, H. S. Earp, M. E. Svoboda, J. J. Van Wyk, and P. Cuatrecasas, Somatomedin-C stimulates the phosphorylation of the β-subunit of its own receptor, J. Biol. Chem. 258:9581 (1983).

125. J. B. Rubin, M. A. Shia, and P. F. Pilch, Stimulation of tyrosine-specific phosphorylation in vitro by insulin-like growth factor I, Nature. 305:438 (1983).

126. Y. Zick, N. Sasaki, R. W. Rees-Jones, G. Grunberger, S. P. Nissley and M. M. Rechler, Insulin-like growth factor-I (IGF-I) stimulates tyrosine kinase activity in purified receptors from a rat liver cell line, Biochem. Biophys. Res. Commun. 119:6 (1984).

127. N. Sasaki, R. W. Rees-Jones, Y. Zick, S. P. Nissley, and M. M. Rechler, Characterization of insulin-like growth factor I-stimulated tyrosine kinase activity associated with the β-subunit of type I insulin-like growth factors receptors of rat liver cells, J. Biol. Chem. 260:9793 (1985).
128. S. Corvera, R. E. Whitehead, C. Mottola, and M. P. Czech, The insulin-like growth factor II receptor is phosphorylated by a tyrosine kinase in adipocyte plasma membranes, J. Biol. Chem. 261:7675 (1986).
129. R. G. Rosenfeld, G. Ceda, D. M. Wilson, L. A. Dollar, and A. R. Hoffman, Characterization of high affinity receptors for insulin-like growth factors I and II on rat anterior pituitary cells, Endocrinology. 114:1571 (1984).
130. G. P. Ceda, A. R. Hoffman, G. D. Silverberg, D. M. Wilson, and R. G. Rosenfeld, Regulation of growth hormone release from cultured human pituitary adenomas by somatomedins and insulin, J. Clin. Endocrinol. Metab. 60:1204 (1985).
130a. C. F. H. Van Schravendijk, E. L. Hooghe-Peters, J. L. Van den Brande, and D. G. Pipeleers, Receptors for insulin-like growth factors and insulin on murine fetal cortical brain cells, Biochem. Biophys. Res. Commun. 135:228 (1986).
131. M. E. K. Mattsson, G. Enberg, A.-I. Ruusala, K. Hall, and S. Pahlman, Mitogenic response of human SH-SY5Y neuroblastoma cells to insulin-like growth factor I and II is dependent on the stage of differentiation, J. Cell Biol. 102:1949 (1986).
132. R. G. Rosenfeld, G. Ceda, C. W. Cutler, L. A. Dollar, and A. R. Hoffman, Insulin and insulin-like growth factor (somatomedin) receptors on cloned rat pituitary tumor cells, Endocrinology. 117:2008 (1985).
132a. S. Gammeltoft, G. K. Haselbacher, R. E. Humbel, M. Fehlmann, and E. Van Obberghen, Two types of receptor for insulin-like growth factors in mammalian brain, EMBO J. 4:3407 (1985).
133. W. L. Lowe, Jr., and D. LeRoith, Tyrosine kinase activity of brain insulin and IGF-I receptors, Biochem. Biophys. Res. Commun. 134:532 (1986).
134. M. A. Leswiak, J. M. Hill, C. B. Pert, and J. Roth, Autoradiographic localization of ^{125}I-IGFI and ^{125}I-IGFII receptors in rat brain: Comparison with insulin receptors, Diabetes. 35, Suppl. 1:58A (1986).
135. L. G. Mendelsohn, G. A. Kerchner, J. A. Clemens, and M. C. Smith, Autoradiographic visualization of insulin-like growth factor-II receptors in rat brain, Fed. Proc. 45:325 (1986).
136. N. J. Bohannon, E. S. Corp, B. J. Wilcox, D. Porte, Jr., D. P. Figlewicz, and D. G. Baskin, Identification of specific binding sites for insulin-like growth factor-1 (IGF-1) in the rat brain by in vitro quantitative autoradiography, Appetite 7:243 (1986).
137. N. J. Bohannon, D. P. Figlewicz, E. S. Corp, B. J. Wilcox, D. Porte, Jr., and D. G. Baskin, Identification of binding sites for an insulin-like growth factor (IGF-I) in the median eminence of the rat brain by quantitative autoradiography, Endocrinology 119:943 (1986).
137a. F. A. McMorris, T. M. Smith, S. DeSalvo, and R. W. Furlanetto, Insulin-like growth factor I/somatomedin C: A potent inducer of oligodendrocyte development, Proc. Natl. Acad. Sci. USA 83:822 (1986).
138. R. Lim. J. F. Miller, D. J. Hicklin, A. C. Holm, and B. H. Ginsberg, Mitogenic activity of glia maturation factor, Exp. Cell Res. 159:335 (1985).
139. D. P. Figlewicz, D. G. Baskin, S. C. Woods, and D. Porte, Jr., Insulin and insulin-like growth factor-I (IGF-I) binding is decreased in the olfactory bulb (OB) but not the cerebral cortex of the obese Zucker fa/fa rat, Int. J. Obes. 9:A31 (1985).
140. K. A. Heidenreich, P. R. Gilmore, D. P. Figlewicz, and G. R. Freidenberg, The glycosylation of IGF-I receptors differs in human brain and placenta, Diabetes 35, Suppl.1:60A (1986).

141. M. Van Houten and B. I. Posner, Circumventricular organs: Receptors and mediators of direct peptide hormone action on brain, Adv. Metab. Disord. 10:269 (1983).
142. H. J. L. Frank, W. M. Pardridge, W. L. Morris, R. G. Rosenfeld, and T. B. Choi, Binding and internalization of insulin and insulin-like growth factors by isolated brain microvessels, Diabetes. 35:654 (1986).
143. R. S. Bar, and M. Boes, Distinct receptors for IGF-1, IGF-2, and insulin are present on bovine capillary endothelial cells and large vessel endothelial cells, Biochem. Biophys. Res. Commun. 124:203 (1984).
144. I. Jialal, M. Crettaz, H. L. Hachiya, C. R. Kahn, A. C. Moses, S. M. Buzney, and G. L. King, Characterization of the receptors for insulin and the insulin-like growth factors on micro- and macrovascular tissues, Endocrinology. 117:1222 (1985).
145. G. L. King, D. A. Goodman, S. Buzney, A. Moses, and C. R. Kahn, Receptors and growth-promoting effects of insulin and insulin-like growth factors on cells from bovine retinal capillaries and aorta, J. Clin. Invest. 75:1028 (1985).
146. R. S. Bar, M. Boes, and M. Yorek, Processing of insulin-like growth factors I and II by capillary and large vessel endothelial cells, Endocrinology. 118:1072 (1986).
147. N. K. Banskota, J.-L. Carpentier, and G. L. King, Processing and release of insulin and insulin-like growth factor I by macro- and microvascular endothelial cells, Endocrinology 119:1904 (1986).
148. W.M. Pardridge, J. Eisenberg, and J. Yang, Human blood-brain barrier insulin receptor, J. Neurochem. 44:1771 (1985).
149. K. D. Dernovsek, and R. S. Bar, Processing of cell bound insulin by capillary and macrovascular endothelial cells in culture, Am. J. Physiol. 248:E244 (1985).
150. G. L. King and S. M. Johnson, Receptor mediated transport of insulin across endothelial cells, Science. 227:1583 (1985).
151. D. R. Clemmons, L. E. Underwood, and J. J. Van Wyk, Hormonal control of immunoreactive somatomedin production by cultured human fibroblasts, J. Clin. Invest. 67:10 (1981).
152. M. Binoux, C. Lassarre, and N. Hardouin, Somatomedin production by rat liver in organ culture, Acta Endocrinol. 99:422 (1982).
153. C. D. Scott, J. L. Martin, and R. C. Baxter, Rat hepatocyte insulin-like growth factor-I and binding protein: Effect of growth hormone in vitro and in vivo, Endocrinology. 116:1102 (1985).
154. M. Berelowitz, M. Szabo, L. A. Frohman, S. Firestone, L. Chu, and R. L. Hintz, Somatomedin-C mediates growth hormone negative feedback by effects on both the hypothalamus and the pituitary, Science. 212:1279 (1981).
155. P. Brazeau, R. Guillemin, N. Ling, J. Van Wyk, and R. Humbel, Inhibition by somatomedin of growth hormone secretion stimulated by hypothalamic growth hormone releasing factor (somatocrinin, GRF) or the synthetic peptide hpGRF, C.R. Acad. Sci. [D] Paris. 295:651 (1982).
156. C. G. Goodyer, L. De Stephano, H. J. Guyda, and B. I. Posner, Effects of insulin-like growth factors on adult male rat pituitary function in tissue culture, Endocrinology. 115:1568 (1984).
157. S. Yamashita, and S. Melmed, Insulin-like growth factor I action on rat anterior pituitary cells: Suppression of growth hormone secretion and messenger ribonucleic acid levels, Endocrinology. 118:176 (1986).
158. S. Melmed, and S. Yamashita, Insulin-like growth factor-I action on hypothyroid rat pituitary cells: Suppression of triiodothyronine-induced growth hormone secretion and messenger ribonucleic acid levels, Endocrinology 118:1483 (1986).
159. S. Yamashita, M. Weiss, and S. Melmed, Insulin-like growth factor I regulates growth hormone secretion and messenger ribonucleic acid levels in human pituitary tumor cells, J. Clin. Endocrinol. Metab. 63:730 (1986).

160. M. S. Sheppard, and R. M. Bala, Insulin-like growth factor inhibition of growth hormone secretion, Can. J. Physiol. Pharmacol. 64:525 (1986).
161. R. C. Baxter, Z. Zaltsman, J. R. Oliver, and J. O. Willughby, Pulsatility of immunoreactive somatomedin-C in chronically cannulated rats, Endocrinology. 113:729 (1983).
162. G. S. Tannenbaum, H. J. Guyda, and B. I. Posner, Insulin-like growth factors: A role in growth hormone negative feedback and body weight regulation, Science. 220:77 (1983).
163. H. Abe, M. E. Molitch, J. J. Van Wyk, and L. E. Underwood, Human growth hormone and somatomedin C suppress the spontaneous release of growth hormone in unanesthetized rats, Endocrinology. 113:1319 (1983).
164. T. Tanaka, H. Maesaka, and S. Suwa, Changes in somatomedin activity in anorexia nervosa, Endocrinol. Japon. 32:891 (1985).
165. L. S. Phillips, and R. Vassilopoulou-Sellin, Somatomedins, N. Engl. J. Med. 302:371 (1980).
166. E. R. Froesch, C. Schmid, J. Schwander, and J. Zapf, Actions of insulin-like growth factors, Ann. Rev. Physiol. 47:443 (1985).
167. J. J. Van Wyk, L. E. Underwood, A. J. D'Ercole, D. R. Clemmons, W. J. Pledger, W. R. Wharton, and E. B. Leof, Role of somatomedins in cellular proliferation, in: "The biology of normal human growth," M. Ritzen, A. Aperia, K. Hall, A. Larsson, A. Zetterberg, and R. Zetterstrom, eds., Raven, New York (1981).
168. H. Rothstein, Regulation of the cell cycle by somatomedins, Int. Rev. Cytol. 78:127 (1982).
169. H. Rothstein, J. J. Van Wyk, J. H. Hayden S. R. Gordon, and A. Weinsieder, An in vivo study with somatomedin-C: Restoration of cycle traverse in G0/G1 blocked cells of hypophysectomized animals, Science. 208:410 (1980).
170. L. S. Phillips, and R. Vassilopoulou-Sellin, Somatomedins, N. Engl. J. Med. 302:438 (1980).
171. E. Schoenle, J. Zapf, and E. R. Froesch, Insulin-like growth factors I and II stimulate growth of hypophysectomized rats, Diabetologia. 23:199 (1982).
172. V. R. Sara, M. C. Stuart, R. Rutherford, S. Moore, and L. Lazarus, Brain growth-promoting activity in human serum: Relationship to growth hormone and somatomedin, J. Clin. Endocrinol. Metab. 47:1129 (1978).
173. L. Fryklund, K. Uthne, H. Sievertsson, and B. Westermark, Isolation and characterization of polypeptides from human plasma: Enhancing the growth of human normal cells in culture, Biochem. Biophys. Res. Commun. 61:950 (1974).
174. D. Lenoir and P. Honegger, Insulin-like growth factor I (IGF I) stimulates DNA synthesis in fetal rat brain cell cultures, Dev. Brain Res. 7:205 (1983).
175. E. Recio-Pinto and D. N. Ishii, Effects of insulin, insulin-like growth factor-II and nerve growth factor on neurite outgrowth in cultured human neuroblastoma cells, Brain Res. 302:323 (1984).
176. J. F. Mill, M. V. Chao, and D. N. Ishii Insulin, insulin-like growth factor II, and nerve growth factor effects on tubulin mRNA levels and neurite formation, Proc. Natl. Acad. Sci., U.S.A. 82:7126 (1985).
177. M. Bothwell, Insulin and somatomedin MSA promote nerve growth factor-independent neurite formation by cultured chick dorsal root ganglionic sensory neurons, J. Neurosci. Res. 8:225 (1982).
178. E. Recio-Pinto, M. M. Rechler, and D. N. Ishii, Effects of insulin, insulin-like growth factor-II, and nerve growth factor on neurite formation and survival in cultured sympathetic and sensory neurons, J. Neurosci. 6:1211 (1986).
179. Y. Aizenman, and J. de Vellis, Brain neuron development in a hormonally defined glial-free environment: Effects of transferrin, insulin, insulin-like growth factor-I and thyroid hormone, Soc. Neurosci. Abst. 12: 1104 (1986).

180. E. Recio-Pinto, F. F. Lang, and D. N. Ishii, Insulin and insulin-like growth factor II permit nerve growth factor binding and the neurite formation response in cultured human neuroblastoma cells, Proc. Natl. Acad. Sci., U.S.A. 81:2562 (1984).
181. S. D. Balk, A. Morisi, H. S. Gunther, M. F. Svoboda, J. J. Van Wyk, S. P. Nissley, and C. G. Scanes, Somatomedins (insulin-like growth factors), but not growth hormone, are mitogenic for chicken heart mesenchymal cells and act synergistically with epidermal growth factor and brain fibroblast growth factor, Life Sci. 35:335 (1984).
182. W. J. Pledger, C. D. Stiles, H. N. Antoniades, and C. D. Scher, An ordered sequence of events is required before BALB/C-3T3 cells become committed to DNA synthesis, Proc. Natl. Acad. Sci., U.S.A. 75:2834 (1978).
183. C. D. Stiles, G. T. Capone, and C. D. Scher, Dual control of cell growth by somatomedins and platelet-derived growth factor, Proc. Natl. Acad. Sci., U.S.A. 76:1279 (1979).
184. D. R. Clemmons, and J. J. Van Wyk, Somatomedin-C and platelet-derived growth factor stimulate human fibroblast replication, J. Cell. Physiol. 106:361 (1981).
185. H. A. Hansson, L. B. Dahlin, N. Danielsen, L. Fryklund, A. K. Nachemson, P. Polleryd, B. Rozell, A. Skottner, S. Stemme, and G. Lundborg, Evidence indicating trophic importance of IGF-I in regenerating peripheral nerves, Acta Physiol. Scand. 126:609 (1986).
186. C. R. Plata-Salamán, Y. Oomura, and N. Shimizu, Dependence of food intake on acute and chronic ventricular administration of insulin, Physiol. Behav. 37:717 (1986).
187. V. R. Sara, K. Hall, M. Rutter, L. Wetterberg, and A. Yuwiler, Hormonal regulation of brain growth: Implications for mental retardation, in: "Biological Psychiatry," C. Perris, G. Struwe and B. Jansson, eds., Elsevier, North Holland (1981).
188. V. R. Sara, K.-H. Gustavsson, G. Annerén, K. Hall, and L. Wetterberg, Somatomedins in Down's syndrome, Biol. Psychiatr. 18:803 (1983).
189. G. Annerén, V. R. Sara, K. Hall, and T. Tuvemo, Growth and somatomedin responses to growth hormone in Down's syndrome, Arch. Dis. Childhood. 61:48 (1986).
190. G. Annerén, G. Enberg, and V. R. Sara, The presence of normal levels of serum immunoreactive insulin-like growth factor 2(IGF-2) in patients with Down's syndrome, Ups. J. Med. Sci. 89:274 (1984).
191. B. Draznin, P. J. Burstein, U. E. Heinrich, C. J. Johnson, C. A. Emler, and D. S. Schalch, Insulin like growth factor and its carrier protein in hypopituitary and hypothyroid children and adults, Clin. Endocrinol. 12:137 (1980).
192. J. Marek, M. Schullerova, O. Schreiberova, and Z. Limanova, Effect of thyroid function on serum somatomedin activity, Acta Endocrinol. 96: 491 (1981).
193. B. Kjellman, Cerebral gigantism, Acta Paediatr. Scand. 54:603 (1965).
194. M. V. L. Du Caju, and J. L. Van den Brande, Plasma somatomedin levels in growth disturbances, Acta Paediatr. Scand. 62:96 (1973).
195. T. Sakano, T. Yoshimitsu, A. Tanabe, T. Tanaka, Y. Kobayashi, T. Usui, and K. Takano, Cerebral gigantism: A report of two cases with elevated serum somatomedin A levels and a review of the Japanese literature, Hirosh. J. Med. Sci. 26:311 (1977).
196. J. M. Wit, F. A. Beemer, P. G. Barth, J. W. E. Oorthuys, P. F. Dijkstra, J. L. Van den Brande, and N. J. Leschot, Cerebral gigantism (Sotos syndrome). Compiled data of 22 cases, Eur. J. Pediatr. 144:131 (1985).
197. V. R. Sara, K. Hall, K. Enzell, A. Gardner, R. Morawski, and L. Wetterberg, Somatomedins in aging and dementia disorders of the Alzheimer's type, Neurobiol. Aging. 3:117 (1982).
198. H. Von Holst, and V. Sara, Increased levels of somatomedins in human lumbar and central cerebrospinal fluid after subarachnoid haemorrhage, Acta Neurochirurgica. 78:157 (1985).

199. W. V. Tamborlane, R. L. Hintz, M. Bergman, M. Genel, P. Felig, and R. S. Sherwin, Insulin infusion pump treatment of diabetics influence of improved metabolic control on plasma somatomedin levels, N. Engl. J. Med. 305:303 (1981).

200. S. A. Amiel, R. S. Sherwin, R. L. Hintz, J. M. Gertner, C. M. Press, and W. V. Tamborlane, Effect of diabetes and its control on insulin-like growth factors in the young subject with type I diabetes, Diabetes. 33:1175 (1984).

201. L. S. Phillips, A. C. Fusco, and T. G. Unterman, Nutrition and somatomedin. XIV. Altered levels of somatomedins and somatomedin inhibitors in rats with streptozotocin-induced diabetes, Metabolism. 34:765 (1985).

202. T. W. Sadler, L. S. Phillips, W. Balkan, and S. Goldstein, Somatomedin inhibitors from diabetic rat serum alter growth and development of mouse embryos in culture, Diabetes 35:861 (1986).

203. A. S. Goustin, E. B. Leof, G. D. Shipley, and H. L. Moses, Growth factors and cancer, Cancer Res. 46:1015 (1986).

INSULIN-LIKE GROWTH FACTOR RECEPTORS IN THE BRAIN

Denis G. Baskin, Nancy J. Bohannon, and Dianne P. Figlewicz

Veterans Administration Medical Center
Seattle, WA 98108
and
Departments of Medicine, Biological Structure, and Psychology
University of Washington
Seattle, WA 98195

INTRODUCTION

A growing body of evidence now indicates that the central nervous system (CNS) is a target of peptides from the gut and pancreas. Insulin from the pancreatic islets, for example, enters the brain from the periphery and influences the physiology of the CNS (review by Baskin et al., 1987). The recent appreciation that insulin-like growth factors (IGF's), peptides with insulin-like structure and biological activity, are also present in the CNS has stimulated a great deal of current interest in brain IGF's and their possible functions in the CNS. The present article reviews the status of the IGF's as regulatory peptides in the CNS, and emphasizes recent developments concerning the anatomical location of receptors for IGF's in the brain.

The Insulin-like Growth Factors

Two principal types of IGF's are found in plasma: IGF-I and IGF-II (Zapf et al., 1984; Froesch and Zapf, 1985). Both have molecular weights of about 7500 and are also known as somatomedins. The main somatomedin of rat serum is identical to human IGF-I (somatomedin C), whereas the IGF-II homologue in rats (multiplication stimulating activity, or MSA) differs from human IGF-II by five amino acids. The IGF's are similar to proinsulin in three dimensional structure and share approximately 50% homology with the amino acid composition and sequence of the A and B chains of human insulin (Froesch and Zapf, 1985). The IGF's are secreted by liver cells, although evidence indicates that other tissues including brain may also synthesize them (Binoux et al., 1981,1985; Underwood and D'Ercole 1984).

IGF's in the Brain

Peptides with immunological properties of IGF-I and IGF-II have been detected in extracts of adult and fetal brain. Sara et al. (1982b) found somatomedins throughout the nervous system of the cat, with the highest concentrations in the hypothalamus and cerebral cortex. IGF-II immunoreactivity was detected in extracts of 24 grossly dissected regions of the human brain, with highest concentrations in cerebral cortex, cerebellum, forebrain, thalamus, and hippocampus, whereas IGF-I was almost undetectable (Hasselbacher et al., 1985). Immunoreactive IGF-I and IGF-II have been detected in human CSF, but the concentrations of IGF-II are much higher than those of IGF-I (Hasslebacher and Humbel, 1982; Widmer et al., 1984; Bäckstrom et al., 1984).

Origin of IGF's in the CNS

It is not known, however, if CNS IGF's are synthesized by neural tissue or derived from plasma. The uptake of plasma IGF's into the CNS by transport across the blood-brain barrier (BBB) is suggested by the presence of receptors for IGF-I and IGF-II in isolated brain capillaries (Frank et al., 1986). Data indicated that capillary internalization of IGF-II was higher than IGF-I, suggesting that brain capillaries may have a receptor mediated transport system for plasma IGF-II as has been proposed for insulin (Pardridge 1986). Fetal brain reportedly synthesizes somatomedins (D'Ercole et al., 1980; Binoux et al., 1985), and IGF secretion has been detected in cultures of rat pituitary and brain explants (Binoux et al., 1981). CNS synthesis of IGF's is supported by several recent studies indicating that IGF-like mRNA is present in nervous tissue (Perkins et al., 1986; Rall et al., 1986; Zangger et al., 1986).

IGF RECEPTORS IN THE BRAIN

Membrane Binding Studies

Binding sites with properties of receptors for insulin and the IGF's have been identified in membranes of adult rat and human brain, with highest binding generally found in limbic system regions. (Sara et al., 1982a; Goodyer et al., 1984; Gammeltoft et al., 1985). In the human brain, IGF-I receptors predominate (Gammeltoft et al., 1985). In the rat brain, it is not clear if receptors for IGF-I or IGF-II are in the majority. Goodyer et al. (1984) reported that IGF-II binding was higher than IGF-I binding to rat brain membranes, whereas Gammeltoft et al. (1985) concluded that IGF-II receptors are more abundant.

Characteristics of Brain IGF Receptors

Brain IGF receptors are classified into two principal types, as is true for IGF receptors of a variety of peripheral tissues including anterior pituitary gland (Rosenfeld et al., 1984, 1985). The Type 1 IGF receptor in the brain resembles the insulin receptor in the structure of its alpha and beta subunits. The alpha subunit of brain Type 1 IGF receptor has a lower molecular weight than that of the peripheral receptor (Gammeltoft et al., 1985), as a consequence of differences in N-linked glycosylation (Heidenreich et al., 1986). It has highest affinity for IGF-I, but also recognizes IGF-II and, at higher concentrations, binds insulin. The brain Type 2 IGF receptor, like its peripheral counterpart, is a monomer which has has highest affinity for IGF-II; it also recognizes IGF-I but does not bind insulin.

QUANTITATIVE AUTORADIOGRAPHIC DETECTION OF IGF RECEPTORS

One of the major unanswered questions about IGF's in the CNS is the identity of the cells that bear them. Anatomical information is lost in binding studies on membranes prepared from grossly dissected brain regions, and it is no longer possible to associate the receptors with cell types or microanatomical architecture such as nuclei, layers, or tracts. We have approached this problem with autoradiographic techniques that permit visualization of the location of receptors (Baskin and Dorsa, 1986; Dorsa and Baskin 1987).

Binding assay on brain slices

In this method, the brain is perfused with ice cold saline in situ, removed and frozen in Freon 22 (-45 C). The brain is sectioned with a cryostat and the frozen brain slices are thaw-mounted onto gelatin coated slides, then dried and stored at -90 C until use. The binding assays are done with the slide mounted brain slices, using appropriate concentrations of iodo[Thr^{59}]IGF-I. The binding is carried out for 18 hrs at 4 C in a 30 mM Hepes buffer, pH 7.6, with BSA and protease inhibitors (Bohannon et al., 1986b). In order to determine nonspecific binding, 1000-fold excess homologous unlabeled peptide is mixed with the labeled IGF-I. Specific binding of iodoIGF-I to brain or liver slices is typically 80-90% of the total binding. This basic protocol is modified as required to determine binding parameters and peptide specificity for the IGF-I binding sites in the intact brain slices. Afterwards, the sides are rinsed in 0 C buffer to remove unbound ligand, then dried and placed in contact with the emulsion of LKB Ultrofilm for 3-5 days.

Quantitation of IGF binding in situ

The developed autoradiographic images show the distribution of bound iodoIGF-I in the brain slices. Under standardized conditions, the optical density of the film can be quantitatively related to the radioactivity present in the brain slice. We use a computer digital image processing system to measure the optical density of small, anatomically defined regions of the autoradiographic film image (Baskin et al. 1986b; Baskin and Dorsa, 1986). Radioactive plastic sections that have been calibrated in terms of equivalent tissue radioactivity are coexposed with the labeled brain slices. The computer scans autoradiographic images produced by these radioactivity standards and establishes a curve relating optical density to DPM/sq. mm of tissue slice area. With this technique, now widely used for localizing and measuring receptors in situ, we have made progress in locating microanatomical brain regions which have high densities of receptors for IGF-I.

LOCATION OF IGF-I RECEPTORS IN BRAIN

Regions of high IGF-I receptor concentrations

Autoradiographic images of labeled brain slices reveal that specific binding sites for IGF-I are concentrated in discrete microanatomical regions. Figures 1-3 are photographs of the autoradiographic images produced on LKB Ultrofilm by brain slices labeled with iodoIGF-I. Measurements of iodoIGF-I binding by quantitative autoradiography have shown that the highest density of IGF-I receptors is in the choroid plexus and the olfactory bulbs (Bohannon et al., 1986a). In the olfactory bulbs, the binding is highest in the glomerular and nerve fiber layers; relatively high binding is also present in the accessory olfactory bulb (Fig. 1). High densities of IGF-I binding are also present in the pyriform cortex adjacent to the rhinal fissure. The concentration of synapses and pyramidal cells in these regions suggests that IGF-I may have a role in modulating synaptic transmission related to processing of olfactory stimuli. High binding in the choroid plexus (Figs. 2, 3) suggests that IGF-I may affect choroid plexus transport functions, perhaps influencing the composition of CSF. Interestingly, the choroid plexus also has a high density of insulin receptors (Baskin et al., 1986a). These autoradiographic binding observations are evidence that the choroid plexus may be a target organ of insulin and IGF-I. The median eminence also shows high binding for iodoIGF-I (Bohannon et al., 1986b).

Regions of moderate IGF-I binding

Visual examination of autoradiographic images of iodoIGF-I labeled brain slices show that moderate concentrations of IGF-I receptors are associated with other

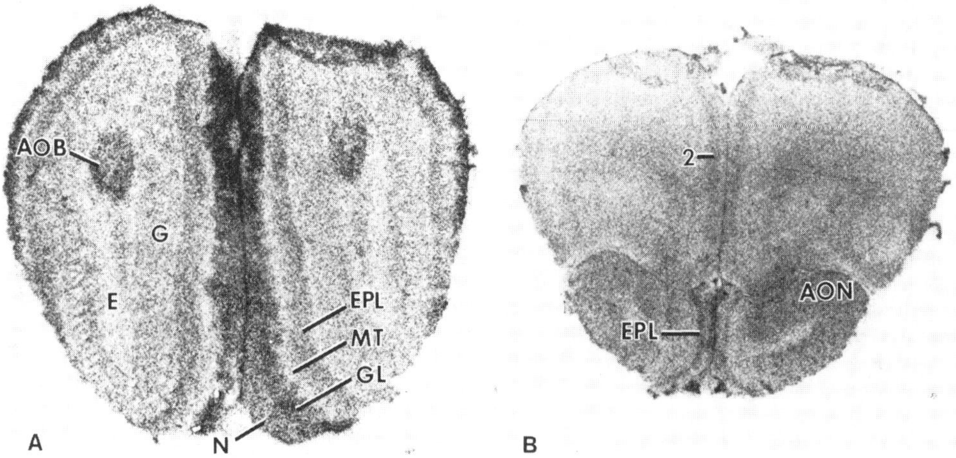

Fig. 1. Autoradiographic images of rat brain slices labeled with iodoIGF-I **A.** Olfactory bulbs. **B,** Level of anterior olfactory nucleus.

Abbreviations used in Figs 1-3:

AHi	amygdalohippocampal area	LD	laterodorsal thalamic nucleus
Am	amygdala complex	M	median eminence
AOB	accessory olfactory bulb	MG	medial geniculate body
AON	anterior olfactory nucleus	MT	middle tufted cell layer
AV	anteroventral thalamic nucleus	N	outer nerve fiber layer
ca1	CA1 region of hippocampus	P	pontine nucleus
ca2	CA2 region of hippocampus	PH	precommissural hippocampus
ca3	CA3 region of hippocampus	PO	primary olfactory cortex
CC	cingulate cortex	PT	posterior thalamus
CG	central grey	R	reticular thalamic nucleus
CP	choroid plexus	SC	superior colliculus
CPu	caudate-putamen	SFO	subfornical organ
D	dentate gyrus	v3	third ventricle
DG	dorsolateral geniculate	VL	ventrolateral thalamic nucleus
E	ependyma/subependyma layer	VM	ventromedial hypothalamus
EN	endopyriform nucleus	VMT	ventromedial thalamic nucleus
EPL	external plexiform layer	VT	ventroposterior thalamic nucleus
ER	entorhinal nucleus	Z	zona incerta
G	granule cell layer	1	layer I of cerebral cortex
GL	glomerular layer	2	layer II of cerebral cortex
GT	gelatinosus thalamic nucleus	6	layer VI of cerebral cortex

portions of the limbic system (Fig. 2). These include cerebral cortex, where the autoradiographic images are very dark in deep cortical layers (layer VI particularly), external plexiform layer of the olfactory bulb, nucleus accumbens, endopyriform nucleus, olfactory cortex, and amygdala. In the hypothalamus, there is moderate binding in the periventricular hypothalamus, ventromedial hypothalamus, supraoptic nucleus and suprachiasmatic nucleus. Moderate concentrations of IGF-I receptors are also located in the reticular thalamic nucleus, anteroventral thalamic nucleus, laterodorsal thalamic nucleus, ventromedial thalamic nucleus, ventroposterior thalamic nucleus, posterior thalamus, gelatinosus thalamic nucleus, ventral thalamic nucleus, posterior caudate-putamen, hippocampus (CA1, CA2, CA3, dentate gyrus, and precommissural hippocampus), and pontine area.

Regions of low IGF-I binding

Brain regions showing very low IGF-I binding include the inner glomerular layer of the olfactory bulb, anterior commissure, corpus callosum, globus pallidus, anterior medial thalamic nucleus, anterior caudate nucleus, and layers III and IV of the cerebral cortex. In the hypothalamus, lowest binding is in the arcuate nucleus.

Relationship to sensory pathways

Concentrations of iodoIGF-I binding sites are found in portions of the brain that are involved in integration of sensory processing (Figs. 2, 3). This includes the glomerular layer of the olfactory bulb, anterior olfactory nucleus, accessory olfactory nucleus, olfactory cortex, lateral geniculate, medial geniculate, superior colliculus, inferior colliculus, vestibular cochlear nucleus, and spinal trigeminal nucleus. IGF-I binding sites are also dense in many thalamic regions associated with sensory pathways. The function of IGF-I in these locations is unknown. IGF-I may possibly modulate synaptic transmission or influence synaptogenesis. The recent observation that IGF-I stimulates oligodendrocyte development in culture (McMorris et al., 1986) raises the possibility that IGF-I may play a role in establishing the glial architecture of sensory pathways.

Circumventricular organs

Circumventricular organs also show significant IGF-I receptor densities. The most conspicuous is the median eminence, which has the highest concentrations of iodoIGF-I binding sites to be found in the hypothalamus (Bohannon et al., 1986b). Our autoradiographic studies show that moderate concentrations of iodoIGF-I binding sites are also located in the subfornical organ, OVLT, and area postrema. We have not observed iodoIGF-I binding in the subcommissural organ. These observations suggest that IGF-I has important functions in the physiology of circumventricular organs.

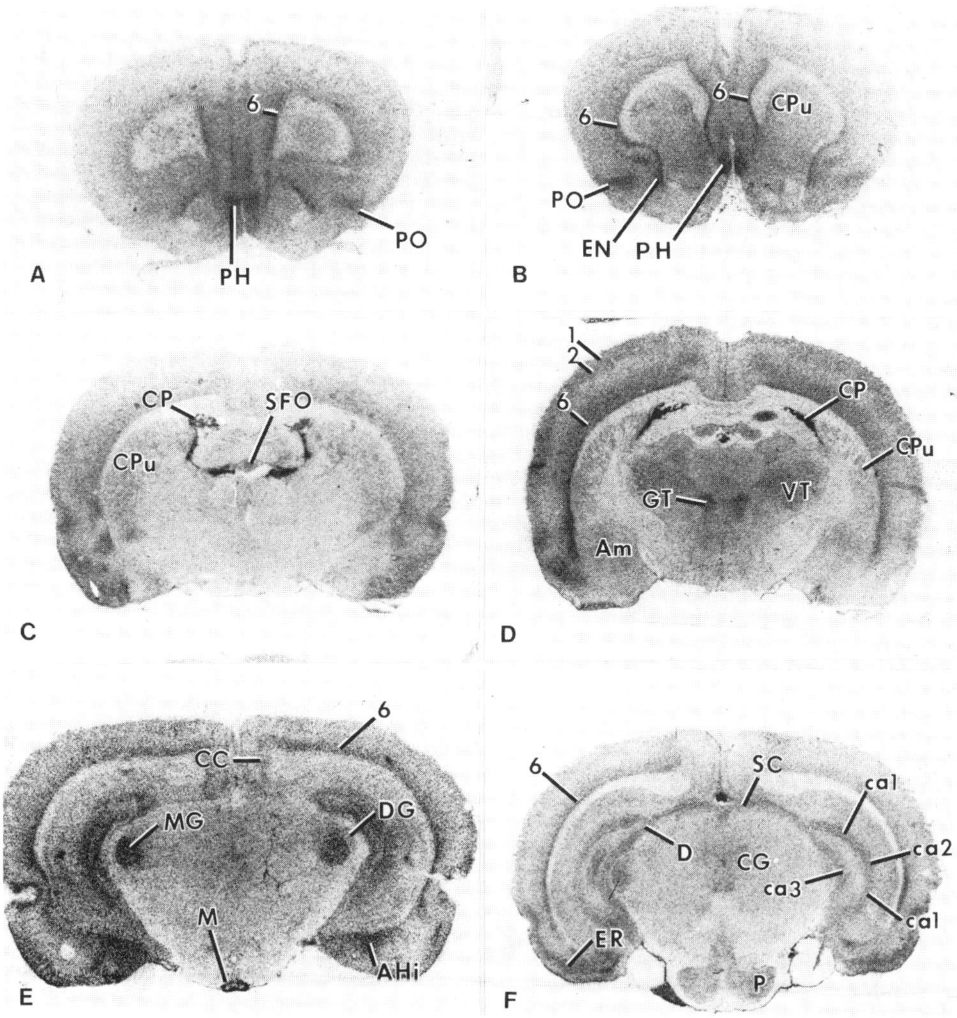

Fig. 2. Autoradiographic images of rat brain slices labeled with iodoIGF-I. **A**, level of frontal caudate-putamen. **B**, level of endopyriform nucleus. **C**, level of subfornical organ. **D**, level of anterior thalamus. **E**, level of median eminence. **F**, level of pontine nuclei. Abbreviations same as Fig. 1.

RELATIONSHIP OF RECEPTORS FOR IGF-I and INSULIN IN THE BRAIN

Although membrane binding data show that subdivisions of the limbic system have high densities of receptors for both insulin and IGF-I, quantitative autoradiographic techniques reveal that the locations of receptors for insulin and IGF-I are anatomically different. In the hypothalamus, for example, insulin binding sites are concentrated in the arcuate and dorsomedial nuclei (Corp et al., 1986),

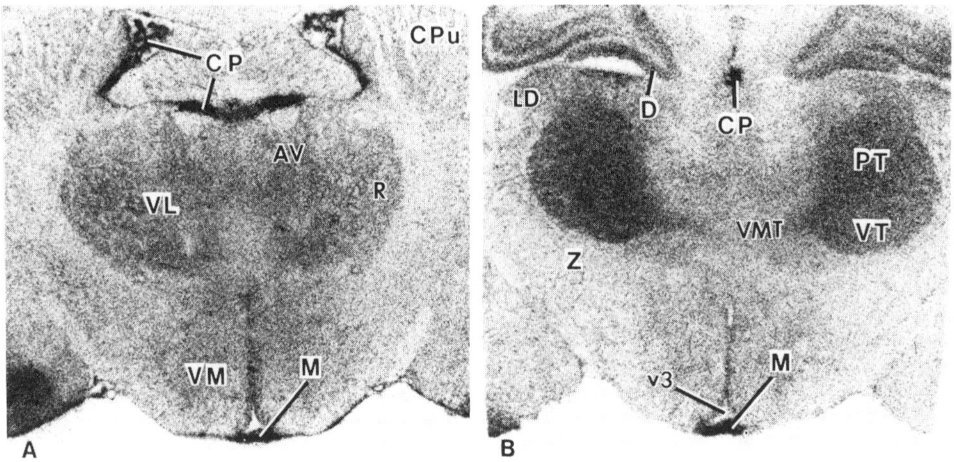

Fig. 3. IGF-I binding sites in the hypothalamus are concentrated in the median eminence (M), with moderate binding in the ventromedial hypothalamus (VM). **A,** intense binding in choroid plexus (CP) in lateral and dorsal third ventricle. **B,** dense binding in hippocampus ventricles. In both A and B, high levels of binding in regions of the thalamus are visible. Abbreviations same as Fig. 1.

whereas IGF-I binding sites are concentrated in the median eminence (Bohannon et al., 1986b). The arcuate nucleus contains relatively low concentrations of IGF-I receptors. In the olfactory lobes, insulin receptors are concentrated in the external plexiform layer (Baskin et al., 1986b), whereas IGF-I binding sites are densest in the the glomerular and nerve fiber layers (Bohannon et al., 1986a). Thus, insulin and IGF-I have distinctly separate sites of action in the brain. This argues for the conclusion that insulin and IGF-I also have different CNS functions.

CELLULAR LOCATION OF IGF RECEPTORS IN THE BRAIN

In vitro binding studies indicate that brain neurons, glia, and endothelial cells possess receptors for IGF's (Lenoir and Honegger 1983; Gammeltoft et al., 1985; Frank et al., 1986; McMorris et al., 1986). However, the identity of cells actually bearing IGF-I receptors in situ are not known, even in the anatomical regions that have been show to possess high receptor densities by quantitative autoradiographic techniques. Anatomical information is lost in binding studies with brain membrane homogenates; the resulting data represent an average of the receptor population of different neural cell types. Even the commonly used film apposition autoradiography techniques (e.g., LKB Ultrofilm) lack the resolution required to determine the precise cellular location of IGF-I receptors. Identification of the specific CNS cells which possess IGF-I receptors in situ is a major unsolved problem.

LOCATION OF IGF-II RECEPTORS IN THE BRAIN

We have recently initiated autoradiographic studies to localize neural pathways that may be regulated by IGF-II (Baskin and Bohannon, 1987). Slide mounted sections of olfactory bulbs and hypothalamus were incubated in iodoIGF-II (from Dr. Ron Rosenfeld) either alone or mixed with IGF-II (from Dr. R. Humbel), [Thr^{59}]IGF-I (Amgen), or IGF-II receptor (Type 2) antibodies (from Dr. Ron Rosenfeld). Binding was detected by LKB film autoradiography. Highest total binding for IGF-II appears to be present in the ventromedial nucleus and median eminence of the hypothalamus, and external plexiform layer of the olfactory bulbs. High binding is also present in the hippocampus. Binding is reduced equally by 1000-fold excess unlabeled IGF-II and by IGF-II receptor antibodies. IGF-II was more effective than [Thr^{59}] IGF-I in competing for iodoIGF-II binding sites. These preliminary results indicate that specific IGF-II receptors are concentrated in discrete regions of the brain, suggesting that IGF-II has an important role in the physiology or development of CNS pathways.

IGF-I RECEPTORS IN THE MEDIAN EMINENCE

We have recently shown that the iodoIGF-I binding site in the rat median eminence (Figs. 2, 3) is probably a Type 1 IGF receptor (Bohannon et al., 1987). Frozen brain sections were incubated in 0.1 nM iodo[Thr^{59}]IGF-I (Amersham) mixed with 0.01-500 nM unlabeled peptides: [Thr^{59}] IGF-I (Amgen), MSA (Collaborative Research), and porcine insulin (Lilly). Quantitative measurements of binding in the median eminence with computer image analysis showed that the rank of potency for competition was IGF-I>MSA>insulin. The data indicate that the ME has a single high affinity binding site (Kd c.a. 1-2 nM) for iodinated [Thr^{59}] IGF-I. Rat IGF-II receptor antibody (from Dr. Ron Rosenfeld) did not block iodo [Thr^{59}]IGF-I binding in the median eminence. Additional support for the hypothesis that the median eminence IGF I binding site is a Type 1 IGF receptor comes from recent data showing that the iodinated [Thr^{59}] analog of IGF-I that we used in our autoradiography studies exhibits very little cross reactivity with the Type 2 IGF receptor (Ewton et al., 1987). Thus, taken together, our quantitative autoradiographic data are consistent with the conclusion that the median eminence has a dense concentration of Type 1 receptors for IGF-I.

FUNCTIONS OF BRAIN IGF RECEPTORS

Growth Hormone Secretion

A little understood effect of IGF-I on the brain is its influence on hypothalamic mechanisms regulating secretion of growth hormone by the pituitary gland. Growth hormone secretion is regulated by somatostatin and growth hormone releasing factor (GRF), which are released into the hypophyseal portal circulation in the median eminence (Wehrenberg, 1986). Growth hormone stimulates IGF-I secretion by the liver (Clemmons and Van Wyk, 1984), and, in turn, IGF-I inhibits growth hormone secretion by a little understood negative feedback mechanism (Brazeau et al., 1982). Evidence points to IGF-I feedback on growth hormone secretion at the level of the anterior pituitary gland (Rosenfeld et al., 1984, 1985; Ceda et al., 1985) as well as hypothalamus, since IGF-I stimulates the release of somatostatin from hypothalamic slices in culture (Berelowicz et al., 1981a,b).

The site of action of this inhibition in the hypothalamus is not known, however. Presumably, IGF-I interacts with the brain at some location to influence the secretion of somatostatin and/or GRF. Studies in which growth hormone secretion was supressed by CSF infusions of IGF-I (Abe et al., 1983; Tannenbaum et al., 1983) suggest that plasma IGF-I may have to enter CSF to reach the effective feedback sites. Although there is evidence for IGF-I in CSF (Beaton et al., 1975; Hasselbacher and Humbel, 1982; Bäckstrom et al., 1984), it is not known if plasma IGF-I normally has access to CSF.

In the median eminence, receptors for IGF-I are concentrated mainly in the external zone (Bohannon et al., 1986b), where somatostatin and GRF neuron terminals release their peptides into hypophyseal portal blood. Since the median eminence has no vascular blood brain barrier, these terminals and their receptors are bathed in plasma. Thus, the median eminence is a logical candidate for a hypothalamic site for transducing plasma IGF-I concentrations into somatostatin release, thereby modulating growth hormone secretion. The IGF-I receptors in the median eminence appear to be strategically situated to mediate this negative feedback mechanism. Although the types of cells containing IGF-I receptors in the median eminence are unknown, it seems likely that many will be found associated with terminals of hypophysiotropic neuronal fibers.

Results of a study on median eminence IGF-I binding during a prolonged fast are consistent with this hypothesis. We found that in food restricted rats, in which basal plasma IGF-I levels were decreased by 67%, IGF-I receptors in the median eminence increased (Bmax) by 58% (Bohannon et al., 1987). This suggests that the median eminence becomes more sensitive to IGF-I when metabolic conditions produce lowered plasma IGF-I levels. Upregulation of median eminence IGF-I receptors may represent a mechanism for suppressing low growth hormone secretion during episodes of nutritional deprivation.

Development

Since the IGF's have well described growth promoting effects on non-neural cells, it is generally believed that IGF's also have similar functions in the CNS. The literature supports this view, although the data is fragmentary and much work remains to be done in this area. IGF-I stimulates DNA synthesis in serum-free cultures of fetal rat brain cells (Lenoir and Honegger, 1983), and induces oligodendrocyte development in vitro (McMorris et al., 1986). IGF receptors are present in the human fetal brain before the end of the first trimester (Sara et al., 1983). This suggests that IGF's are involved in early brain development, and may have an important role in the process of cellular proliferation and neuroblast formation in the CNS during that period.

Food Intake

IGF-I and IGF-II have also been implicated in central regulation of food intake. We have found that binding of IGF-I is decreased in membranes from olfactory bulbs of genetically obese Zucker rats, whereas other brain areas are not affected (Figlewicz et al., 1985). Mixtures of IGF's inhibit food intake when infused into brain CSF (Tannenbaum et al., 1983). A recent report suggests that intracerebroventricular IGF-II may be more potent than IGF-I in producing this effect (Lauterio et al., 1986). IGF effects on central food intake mechanisms are similar to those elicited by insulin infused into CSF (Woods and Porte, 1983). This raises the possibility that IGFs may interact with insulin receptors and vice versa in the central regulation of this behavior.

Interpretation of studies in which insulin and IGF's are infused into CSF have the caveats that the IGF's and insulin interact with each other's receptors, and that the concentrations of these peptides actually achieved in the environment of the receptors on neural cell membranes is unknown. The anatomical location of IGF receptors that participate in the satiety effects of CSF IGF's is unknown. IGF-I and IGF-II receptors in the olfactory bulb appear to be situated where afferent olfactory stimuli is processed and integrated. It is possible that food intake patterns are modified as a consequence of IGF action at these receptors.

CONCLUSIONS

Autoradiographic studies on IGF-I binding in the median eminence illustrate the power of quantitative autoradiography for characterizing IGF receptors in the CNS. IGF-I receptors are situated in extremely minute portions of brain microarchitecture, and this anatomical information is lost in the process of preparing membranes for binding analysis. Relatively low concentrations of IGF-I receptors have been reported in membrane preparations from the hypothalamus (e.g., Gammeltoft et al., 1985). The IGF-I receptors in the median eminence are included in hypothalamus membrane preparations, but because of its extremely small size relative to the hypothalamus the median eminence contributes a small fraction of the total IGF-I binding present in an entire hypothalamus. Quantitative autoradiography not only reveals that the median eminence has very high IGF-I binding capacity, but permits us to measure changes in binding and to characterize these sites as Type 1 IGF receptors with relatively few animals. Heroic efforts and many rats would be required to obtain enough median eminence tissue to duplicate these results with membranes. The approach has the added advantage that the binding is done with the IGF-I receptor in situ, in the context of the anatomical relationships in which it functions in vivo. This capability provides information that is not easily acquired with any other method, and gives new insights into possible functions of IGF's in the brain.

The presence of IGF's and their receptors in the CNS is now firmly documented but much remains to be learned about the origin and functions of IGF's in the brain. The brain, like other organs of the body, is undoubtedly subject to regulation by these peptides. Although preliminary studies suggest that IGF-like mRNA is present in brain, it is not yet certain whether the neural synthesis contributes in a major way to the IGF concentrations that can be extracted from brain tissue. It is perphaps natural to attempt to draw parallels between brain IGF and insulin systems, but this could be misleading in view of the largely separate locations of their receptors in the brain. Furthermore, although evidence for CNS secretion of IGF's is growing, the idea that brain cells synthesize a major proportion of insulin that is present in the brain is not well supported and remains conjectural (Baskin et al., 1987). The widespread distribution of IGF-I binding sites in regions associated with sensory pathways suggests an important role for this peptide in sensory physiology. Lack of data about the cellular location of receptors for the IGF's is perhaps one of the major gaps in our knowledge about IGF's as regulatory peptides in the CNS.

REFERENCES

Abe, H., Molitch, M., Van Wyk, J., and Underwood, L., 1983, Human growth hormone and somatomedin-C suppress the spontaneous release of growth hormone in unanesthetized rats, Endocrinology, 113:1319.

Bäckstrom, M., Hall, K., and Sara, V., 1984, Somatomedin levels in cerebrospinal fluid from adults with pituitary disorders, Acta. Endocrinol., 107:171.

Baskin, D., Brewitt, B., Davidson, D., Corp, E., Paquette, T., Figlewicz, D., Graham, M., Woods, S., and Dorsa, D., 1986a, Quantitative autoradiographic evidence for insulin receptors in the choroid plexus of the rat brain, Diabetes, 35:246-249.

Baskin, D., Davidson, D., Corp, E., Lewellen, T., and Graham, M., 1986b, An inexpensive microcomputer digital imaging system for densitometry: quantitative autoradiography of insulin receptors with ^{125}I and LKB Ultrofilm, J. Neurosci. Meth., 16:119.

Baskin, D., and Dorsa, D., 1986, Quantitative autoradiography and in vitro radioligand binding, in: "Functional Mapping in Biology and Medicine: Computer Assisted Autoradiography, Experimental Biology and Medicine, Vol. II", D. McEachron, ed, Karger, NY, pp. 204-234.

Baskin, D., Figlewicz, D., Woods, S., Porte, D., Jr., and Dorsa, D., 1987, Insulin in the brain, Ann. Rev. Physiol., 49:335.

Baskin, D., and Bohannon, N., 1987, Localization of binding sites for insulin-like growth factor-II (IGF-II) in rat brain by in vitro quantitative autoradiography, Endocrinology (Suppl.), 120 (in press).

Beaton, G., Sagel, J., and Distiller, L., 1975, Somatomedin activity in cerebrospinal fluid, J. Clin. Endocrinol. Metab., 40:736-737.

Binoux, M., Faivre-Bauman, A., Lassarre, C., Barret, A., and Tixier-Vidal, A., 1985, Triiodothyronine stimulates production of insulin-like growth factor (IGF) by fetal hypothalamus cells cultured in serum-free medium, Dev. Br. Res., 21:319.

Binoux, M., Hossenlopp, P., Lassarre, C., and Hardouin, N., 1981, Production of insulin-like growth factors and their carrier by rat pituitary gland and brain explants in culture, FEBS Lett., 124:178.

Berelowicz, M., Firestone, S., and Frohman, L., 1981a, Effects of growth hormone excess and deficiency on hypothalamic somatostatin content and release and on tissue somatostatin distribution, Endocrinology, 109:714.

Berelowicz, M., Szabo, M., Frohman, L., Firestone, S., Chu, L., and Hintz, R., 1981b, Somatomedin-C mediates growth hormone negative feedback by effects on both the hypothalamus and pituitary, Science, 212:1279.

Bohannon, N., Corp, E., Wilcox, B., Figlewicz, D., Dorsa, D., and Baskin, D., 1987, Insulin-like growth factor-I (IGF-I) binding in the median eminence of the rat is increased by food restriction, Endocrinology (Suppl.), 120 (in press).

Bohannon, N., Corp, E., Wilcox, B., Porte, Jr. D., Figlewicz, D., and Baskin, D., 1986a, Identification of specific binding sites for insulin-like growth factor-I (IGF-I) in the rat brain by in vitro quantitative autoradiography, Appetite, 7:243.

Bohannon, N., Figlewicz, D., Corp, E., Wilcox, B., Porte, Jr. D., and Baskin, D., 1986b, Identification of binding sites for an insulin-like growth factor (IGF-I) in the median eminence of the rat brain by quantitative autoradiography, Endocrinology, 119:943.

Brazeau, P., Guillemin, R., Ling, N., Van Wyk, J., and Humbel, R., 1982, Inhibition, by somatomedins of growth hormone secretion stimulated by hypothalamic growth hormone releasing factor (somatocrinin, GRF), or the synthetic peptide hGRP, C. R. Acad. Sci. (D) (Paris), 295-651.

Ceda, G., Hoffman, A., Silverberg, G., Wilson, D., and Rosenfeld, R., 1985, Regulation of growth hormone release from cultured human pituitary adenomas by somatomedins and insulin, J. Clin. Endocrinol. Metab., 60:1204.

Clemmons, D., and Van Wyk, J., 1984, Factors controlling blood concentrations of somatomedin C Clinics, in: "Endocrinology and Metabolism, Vol. 13, No. 1., Tissue Growth Factors," W.H. Daughaday, ed., Saunders, NY, pp. 113-144.

Corp, E., Woods, S., Porte, Jr., D., Figlewicz, D., and Baskin, D., 1986, Localization of ^{125}I-insulin binding sites in the rat hypothalamus by quantitative autoradiography, Neurosci. Lett., 70:17.

D'Ercole, A., Applewhite, G., and Underwood, L., 1980, Evidence that somatomedin is synthesized by multiple tissues in the fetus, Develop. Biol, 75:315.

Dorsa, D., and Baskin, D., 1987, Identification of neuropeptide receptors, in: "Advances in Neuromethods," A. Boulton, ed., Humana Press, Clifton, N.J. (in press).

Ewton, D., Falen, S., and Florini, J., 1987, The type II insulin-like growth-factor (IGF) receptor has low affinity for IGF-I analogs: Pleiotropic actions of IGFs on myoblasts are apparently mediated by the type I receptor. Endocrinology, 120:115.

Figlewicz, D., Baskin, D., Woods, S., and Porte, Jr., D., 1985, Insulin and insulin-like growth factor-I (IGF-I) binding is decreased in the olfactory bulb (OB) but not the cerebral cortex (C) of the obese Zucker (fa/fa) rat. Intl. J. Obesity, 9:233.

Frank, H., Pardridge, W., Morris, W., Rosenfeld, R., and Choi, T., 1986, Binding and internalization of insulin-like growth factors by isolated brain microvessels, Diabetes, 35:654.

Froesch, E., and Zapf, J., 1985, Insulin-like growth factors and insulin: comparative aspects, Diabetologia, 28:485.

Gammeltoft, S., Hasselbacher, G., Humbel, R. Fehlmann, M., and Van Obberghen, E., 1985, Two types of receptor for insulin-like growth factors in mammalian brain, EMBO J., 4:3407.

Goodyer, C., de Stephano, L., Lai, W., Guyda, H., and Posner, B., 1984, Characterization of insulin-like growth factor receptors in rat anterior pituitary, hypothalamus, and brain, Endocrinology, 114:1187.

Hasselbacher, G., and Humbel, R., 1982, Evidence for two species of insulin-like growth factor II (IGF-II and "big" IGF-II) in human spinal fluid, Endocrinology, 110:1822.

Hasselbacher, G., Schwab, M., Pasi, A., and Humbel, R., 1985, Insulin-like growth factor II (IGF II) in human brain: regional distribution of IGF II and of higher molecular mass forms, Proc. Natl. Acad. Sci. U.S.A., 82:2153.

Heidenreich, K., Freidenberg, G., Figlewicz, D., and Gilmore, P., 1986, Evidence for a subtype of insulin-like growth factor I receptor in brain, Reg. Peptides, 15:301-310.

Lenoir, D., and Honegger, P., 1983, Insulin-like growth factor I (IGF) stimulates DNA synthesis in fetal rat brain cell cultures. Devel Br. Res., 7:205.

Lauterio, T., Marson, L., Daughaday, W., and Baile, C., 1986, Intracerebroventricular injections of insulin-like growth factor II, but not insulin-like growth factor I, decrease food intake and body weight in rats. Soc. Neurosci. Abstr., 12:795.

McMorris, F., Smith, T., DeSalvo, S., and Furlanetto, R., 1986, Insulin-growth factor I/Somatomedin C: a potent inducer of oligodendrocyte development, Proc. Natl. Acad. Sci. U.S.A., 83:822.

Pardridge, W., 1986, Receptor-mediated peptide transport through the blood-brain barrier, Endocrine Rev., 7:314.

Perkins, S., Eberwine, J., Jansen, M., Hintz, R., Rosenfeld, R., Barchas, J., and Hoffman, A., 1986, Distribution of insulin-like growth factor II messenger RNA in human and rat tissues, Clin. Res., 34:63A.

Rall, L., Falloon, L., Styne D., and Bell, G., 1986, Insulin-like growth factor I and II mRNA are present in numerous tissues of the primate, Clin Res. 34:135A.

Rosenfeld, R., Ceda, G., Cutler, C., and Hoffman, A., 1985, Insulin and insulin-like growth factor (somatomedin) receptors on cloned rat pituitary tumor cells, Endocrinology, 117:2008.

Rosenfeld, R., Ceda, G., Wilson, D., Dollar, L., and Hoffman, A., 1985, Characterization of high affinity receptors for insulin and insulin-like growth factors I and II on rat anterior pituitary cells, Endocrinology, 114:1571.

Sara, V., Hall, K., von Holz, H., Humbel, R., Sjogren, B., and Wetterberg, L., 1982a, Evidence for the presence of specific receptors for insulin-like growth factors I (IGF-I) and 2 (IGF-2) and insulin throughout the adult human brain, Neurosci. Lett. 34:39.

Sara, V., Uvnas-Moberg, K., Uvnas, B., Hall, K., Wetterberg, L., Posloncec, B., and Goiny, M., 1982b, The distribution of somatomedins in the nervous system of the cat and their release following neural stimulation, Acta. Physiol. Scand., 115:467.

Sara, V., Hall, K., Misaki, M., Fryklund, L., Christensen, N., and Wetterberg, L., 1983, Ontogenesis of somatomedin and insulin receptors in the human fetus, J. Clin. Invest., 71:1084.

Tannenbaum, G., Guyda, H., and Posner, B., 1983, Insulin-like growth factors: a role in growth hormone negative feedback and body weight regulation via brain, Science, 220:77.

Underwood, L., and D'Ercole, A., 1984, Insulin and insulin-like growth factors/somatomedins in fetal and neonatal development, in: "Clinics in Endocrinology and Metabolism Vol. 13, No. 1. Tissue Growth Factors," W.H. Daughaday, ed., Saunders, NY, pp. 69-89.

Wehrenberg, W., 1986, The role of growth hormone-releasing factor and somatostatin on somatic growth in rats, Endocrinology, 118:489.

Widmer, U., Zapf, J., and Froesch, E., 1984, Insulin-like growth factors and their carrier proteins in cerebrospinal fluid of normals and acromegalics, Abstr. 7th. Int. Congr. Endocrinol., Amsterdam, (Excerpta Med.), p. 1413a.

Woods, S., and Porte, D., Jr., 1983, The role of insulin as a satiety factor in the central nervous system, in: "CNS Regulation of Carbohydrate Metabolism," A. Szabo, ed., Academic Press, New York, pp. 457-468.

Zapf, J., Schmid, Ch., and Froesch, E., 1984, Biological and immunological properties of insulin-like growth factors (IGF) I and II, in: "Clinics in Endocrinology and Metabolism, Vol. 13, No. 1, Tissue Growth Factors," W.H. Daughaday, ed., Saunders, NY, pp. 3-30.

Zangger, I., Eberwine, J., Barchas, J., Jansen, J., Rosenfeld, R., Hoffman, A., and Hintz, R., 1986, Tissue distribution of IGF-I mRNA, Clin. Res. 34:68A.

RECEPTORS FOR INSULIN AND INSULIN RELATED PEPTIDES IN THE CNS: STUDIES OF LOCALIZATION IN RAT BRAIN

J.M.Hill*, M.A.Lesniak**, M.Rojeshi**,
C.B.Pert* and J.Roth**

*Clinical Neuroscience Branch, NIMH
**Diabetes Branch, NIDDK
National institutes of Health, Bethesda, MD 20892

The central nervous system (CNS) has traditionally been excluded as an insulin target tissue because glucose metabolism in the CNS seems to be unaffected by insulin. We have found that insulin and specific receptors for insulin are present in rodent brain although their physiologic role is unknown. Recent work in rats has shown that receptors for IGF-I and IGF-II are also present in the CNS.

Insulin binding sites identified by binding of ^{125}-I-insulin to membrane preparations from several discrete areas of rat brain have been shown to be in highest concentration in the olfactory bulb and other components of the limbic system and hypothalamus, and are typical insulin receptors according to their physical properties and their competition with other insulin related peptides (Havrankova et al. 1978). These binding sites appear to be distributed amongst all of the cellular elements of the CNS. The brain insulin receptor of rat and other species demonstrates an α subunit that binds insulin and a β-subunit which contains an insulin stimulatable tyrosine specific protein kinase (Rees-Jones et al. 1984). Furthermore, within each species studied, brain insulin receptors are structually different in subtle ways from those in liver and probably most other peripheral tissues (Hendricks et al. 1984, Simon and LeRoith 1986, Lowe and LeRoith 1986) and is most likely due to alterations in the carbohydrate moieties of the subunit (Heidenreich 1985).

In contrast to many tissues, insulin receptors in brain tissue apparently do not upregulate or down regulate. In genetically obese (ob/ob) mice, an animal model of extreme hyperinsulinemia, insulin binding in brain is the same as thin littermates, whereas specific insulin receptors in liver are appropriately decreased in concentration (Havrankova et al. 1979). Conversely, in streptozotocin-induced diabetic rats, an example of hypoinsulinemia, brain receptors are again unmodified despite an appropriate increase in insulin receptors in liver. However, to address whether the blood-brain barrier might be protecting the adult CNS from exposure to peripheral insulin, another group (Devaskar et al. 1986) has studied the downregulating effect of varying states of systemic and intracranial hyperinsulinemia on fetal rabbit brain insulin receptors, since the blood brain barrier is not well developed in fetal life.

Alloxan-induced maternal diabetes produced mild fetal hyperinsulinemia and systemic administration of insulin to the fetus was used to produce moderate and severe hyperinsulinemia. All three states of peripheral hyperinsulinemia did not change brain insulin content or brain insulin receptor number or affinity. Intracranial administration of physiologic concentrations of insulin did not change receptor number, although a decrease in receptor number was observed when pharmacologic concentrations of insulin were achieved. In an earlier study (Havrankova et al. 1979), the 1 day old offspring of streptozotocin induced diabetic female rats had insulin levels lower than controls but insulin binding in whole brain was similar. The above studies demonstrate brain insulin receptors are unchanged in membrane preparations obtained from hyperinsulinemic and hypoinsulinemic animals, both adult and fetus, but do not exclude changes in insulin receptor binding in discrete areas of the brain.

Autoradiography of frozen rat brain tissue has shown that specific binding of ^{125}-I-labeled insulin is distributed throughout the brain in well defined neuroanatomic regions (Hill et al. 1986). Radioactivity bound in these regions was competed for when slices were incubated in the presence of both labeled insulin and nM concentration of unlabeled insulin (comparable to high circulating levels in vivo); binding disappeared when the unlabeled insulin was present in µM concentration (Fig 1). Non-specific binding was distributed throughout the tissue slice, whereas the specific binding was highly concentrated in well defined areas and accounted for 75-95% of total binding, indicating a high signal to noise ratio for the autoradiographic method.

^{125}-I-labeled insulin binds with high affinity to receptors for insulin and with lower affinity to receptors for the insulin-like growth factors (Rechler et al. 1980). Specific binding demonstrated by autoradiography in our study on slices of tissue from the olfactory bulb and cerebellum, which are areas dense in insulin receptors, was typical for an insulin receptor (Fig. 2): i.e. chicken insulin ≅ pork insulin > proinsulin > mixture of chemically modified A and B chains of insulin.

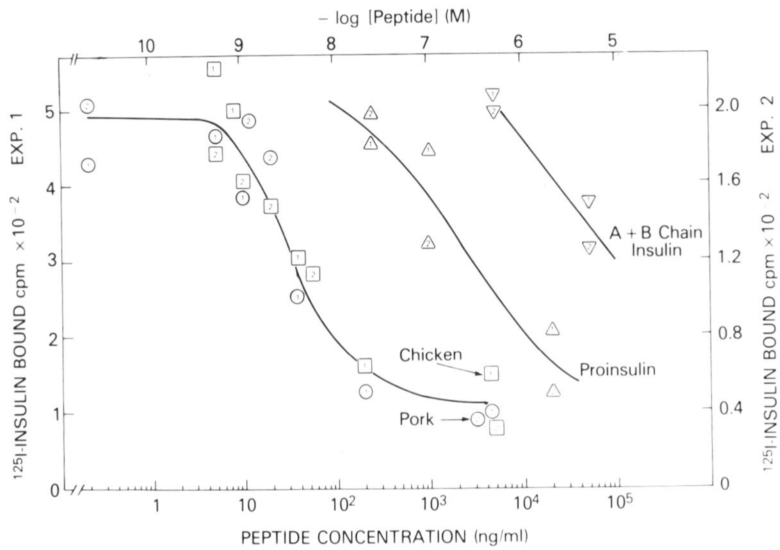

FIG. 1 Inhibition of ^{125}-I-insulin binding by unlabeled insulin and related peptides using olfactory bulbs. (For details see Hill et al. 1986).

These results are comparable to those obtained in insulin receptor binding assays of membranes from regions of the CNS obtained by dissection, including cerebellum and olfactory bulb (Havrankova et al. 1978) The specifity is distinct from the specificity of insulin-like growth factor-type receptors (Rechler et al. 1980). The effect of time and temperature on insulin binding was also determined in our study on olfactory bulb tissue slices; binding was directly related to temperature at earlier times and inversely related to temperature at steady state, which is also typical of an insulin receptor.

We also demonstrated that the specific binding of ^{125}-I-labeled insulin localized to discrete regions of the brain and could be correlated with underlying architecture. The patterns of distribution of binding is illustrated in Fig. 3. In general, the density of specific binding is proportional to both receptor concentration and affinity. Since insulin receptors throughout the brain are relatively homogeneous in affinity for ^{125}-I-insulin (Havrankova et al. 1978) we have tentatively concluded that the distribution of binding in different areas of the rat brain is related to differences in receptor concentration. The highest level of binding occurred in the olfactory bulb but other olfactory areas and the limbic structures to which they are connected were also dense in insulin receptors. In addition to the olfactory limbic areas, which are important in food seeking behavior, receptors were also prominent in areas of brain related to motor function, particularly the cerebellum. However, every slice of brain tissue that we examined had areas of specific binding. When ^{125}-I-insulin was located on cortical or laminated structures the highest binding occurred in the superficial or plexiform layer which is the stratum receiving afferent input. Similarly, binding in the neocortex occurred in the intermediate layers which are also the layers in which most afferent fibers terminate (Fig. 4). Microscopic examination of emulsion coated slices of ^{125}-I-labeled tissue showed the binding sites were in the neuropil and on cell bodies of glial cells, neurons, and endothelial cells.

In addition, we noted that insulin binding on the choroid plexus was also prominent. While we did not define the specificity of this binding, others (Baskin et al. 1986) have demonstrated that this (^{125}-I-insulin) binding is typical of insulin receptors. Binding to other auxillary structures of the CNS including the meninges, nonendothelial structures of large blood vessels and to the pineal gland was present but not especially prominent.

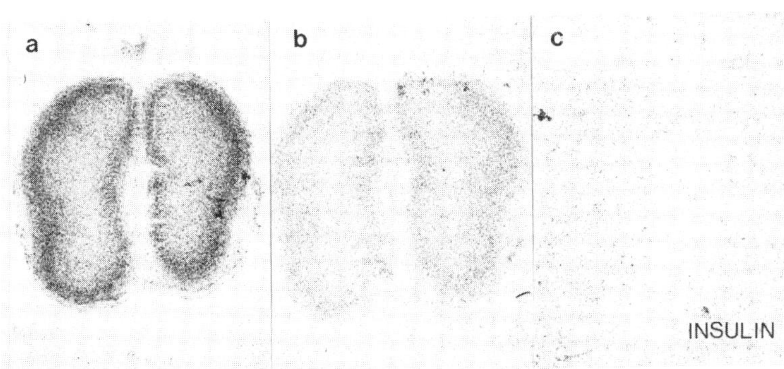

FIG. 2 Autoradiographs of 36 μm coronal sections of olfactory bulbs. a) Binding of ^{125}-I-insulin; b) competed for by a modest concentration (25 ng/ml); or c) an excess (5 μg/ml) of unlabeled insulin. (Hill et al. 1986)

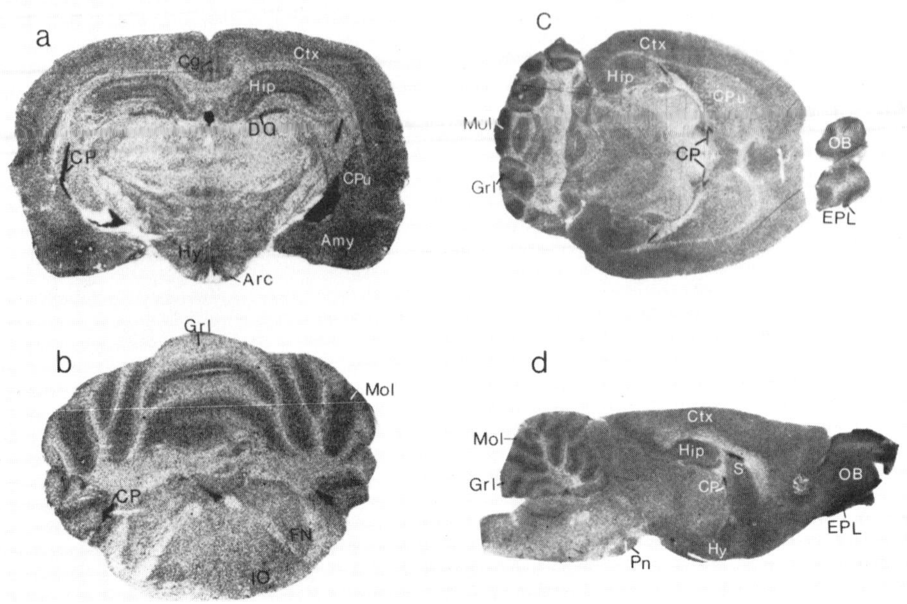

FIG. 3 Autoradiographs of coronal (a,b), horizontal (c), and sagittal (d) sections of rat brain incubated with ^{125}-I-insulin.
Abbreviations used: Amy, amygdala; Arc, arcuate nucleus; Cig, cingulate cortex; CP, choroid plexus; CPu, caudate putamen; DG, dentate gyrus; EPL, external plexiform layer; FN, facial nucleus; Grl, granule cell layer; Hip, hippocampus; Hy, hypothalamus; IO, inferior olive; Mol, molecular layer; OB, olfactory bulb; Pn, pontine nuclei; S, septum.

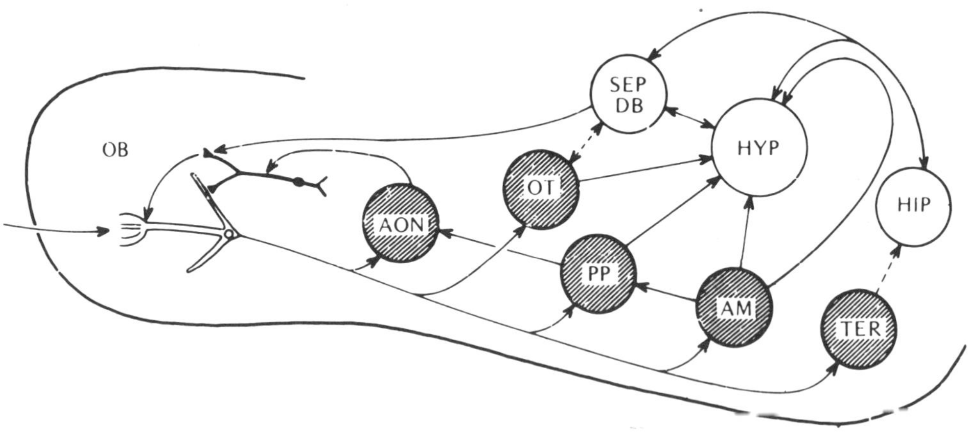

FIG. 4 Relationship between olfactory and limbic parts of the brain. Primary olfactory areas, which receive input from mitral cells of the olfactory bulb (OB), are shown as shaded circles: anterior olfactory nucleus (AON); olfactory tubercle (OT); prepyriform cortex (PP); amygdaloid complex (AM); and transitional entorhinal cortex (TER). Limbic structures are shown as open circles: septum and diagnonal band (SEP-DB); hypothalamus (HYP); and hippocampus (HIP). Note multiplicity of interconnections, including centrifugal pathways to granule cells of the olfactory bulb. (Reprinted with permission of Shepherd, 1979).

Table 1

RELATIVE DENSITY OF BINDING OF LABELED INSULIN, IGF-I, and IGF-II, TO SELECT BRAIN REGIONS

BINDING REGIONS	RECEPTORS		
	INSULIN	IGF-I	IGF-II
OLFACTORY BULB	++++	++++	++
HYPOTHALAMUS	++	+++	++
CEREBELLUM	++	++	++
MEDIAN EMINENCE	*	++++	++++
CHOROID PLEXUS	++++	++++	++++

Computer Densitometry Scoring ++++ High; +++ Moderately high; ++ Moderate; * present, but density not determined. Note: Table shows only a few of several regions studied.

We have also used autoradiography to study the binding of ^{125}-IGF-I (human) and ^{125}-I-IGF-II (rat) to receptors in rat brain and compared the binding patterns of the IGFs to those of insulin (Lesniak et al. 1986). Like insulin, the IGF receptors are widely distributed throughout the brain and are especially dense in regions similar to those of insulin i.e. choroid plexus, olfactory bulb, limbic regions, and cerebellum. In each area, the binding of each of the three peptides conforms to well defined cytoarchitectonic boundaries. Hc ever, each of the three peptides binds to a distinctive region within ea h area. Thus, except for the choroid plexus, it appears that the receptors for the three peptides are binding to nearby but distinctly different groups of cells.

Competition studies were performed in those regions of rat brain which exhibited high density of binding for the IGFs. The binding of IGF-I appears to be to a typical type I-IGF receptor; unlabeled IGF-I competes for labeled IGF-I more strongly than IGF-II or than insulin. However, there is an increase in the binding of labeled IGF-I in the presence of low concentrations of unlabeled IGF-II or insulin. Although this phenomenon is highly reproducible it is not understood. Degradation of labeled IGF-I was tested for by rebinding to rat brain membranes and was low. Since there was also an increase in binding of labeled IGF-I in the presence of unlabeled insulin,the known binding proteins for the IGFs are not likely to be the cause since insulin, unlike the IGFs, does not bind to these binding proteins (Rechler et al. 1980).

The binding of labeled IGF-II is competed for by unlabeled IGF-II but in an atypical manner. How closely the rat brain IGF-II receptor resembles the typical type II IGF receptor is therefore not entirely clear. Using a polyclonal anti IGF-II receptor antibody (a generous gift of S. P. Nissley and W. Keiss) we were able to show that the patterns of binding of both the labeled IGF-II and the antireceptor antibody were nearly identical (Hill et al. in press) Thus the brain receptor appears to be a type II IGF receptor despite the unusual results outlined in the competitive studies.

The autoradiographic studies described above demonstrate that receptors for insulin and IGFs are widely distributed in the CNS (see Table 1) with every slice having areas of specific binding. The distribution of receptors conforms to cytoarchitectonic boundaries, i.e. well defined anatomic regions of the brain. In regions that are rich in all three receptors, the binding sites are complementary more than overlapping. On the other hand, the choroid plexus but not circumventricular organs exhibits high density of binding for all three peptides.

The function of insulin and insulin-like growth factors in brain is not known. The wide distribution of these factors on discrete regions throughout the brain is typical for the binding patterns described previously for many neuroactive peptides. Other peptides with specific functions outside the brain have been localized in neural tissue including cholecystokinin (Beinfeld et al. 1981), vasoactive intestinal peptide (Said and Rosenberg 1976) and transferrin (Connor and Fine 1984). These peptides are postulated to function at specific sites in brain to modulate neuronal activity, distinct from their function in classic target tissues. Insulin and the insulin-like growth factors may also have a role in the CNS as neuromodulators.

REFERENCES

Baskin, D.G., Brewitt, B., Davidson, D., Corp, E., Paquette, T., Figlewicz, D., Lewellen, T., Graham, M., Woods, S., Dorsa, D., 1986, Quantitative autoradiographic evidence for insulin receptors in the choroid plexus of the rat brain, Diabetes 35:246A.

Beinfeld, M.C., Meyer, D.K., Eskay, R.L., Jensen, R.T., Brownstein, M.J. 1981, The distribution of cholecystokinin immunoreactivity in the control nervous system of the rat as determined by radioimmunoassay, Brain Res. 212:51-57.

Connor, J.R., and Fine, R.E., 1984, Localization of a transferrin-like protein in the adult rat CNS, Soc. Neurosci. 10:154A.

Devaskar, S.V., Karycki, L., Devaskar, V.P., 1986, Varying brain insulin concentrations differentially regulate the fetal brain insulin receptor, Biochem. Biophys. Res. Comm. 136:208-219.

Havrankova, J., and Roth, J., 1978, Insulin receptors are widely distributed in the central nervous system of the rat, Nature 272:827-829.

Havrankova, J., Roth, J., Brownstein, M.J., 1979, Concentration of insulin and of insulin receptors in brain are independent of peripheral insulin levels, J. Clin. Invest. 64:636-642.

Heidenreich, K.A., 1985, The Mr difference between insulin receptors in brain and peripheral tissues is due to variation in carbohydrate content, Diabetes [Suppl] 34:56A.

Hendricks, S.A., Agardh, C-D., Taylor, S.I., Roth, J., 1984, Unique features of the insulin receptor in rat brain, J. Neurochem 43:1302-1307.

Hill, J.M., Lesniak, M.A., Kiess, W., Nissley, S.P., 1987, Radioimmunohistochemical localization of IGF-II receptors in rat brain, Peptides (in press).

Hill, J.M., Lesniak, M.A., Pert, C.B., Roth, J., 1986, Autoradiographic localization of insulin receptors in rat brain:prominence in olfactory and limbic areas, Neuroscience 17:1127-1138.

Lesniak, M.A., Hill, J.M., Roth, J., Pert, C.B., 1986, Autoradiographic localization of ^{125}-I-IGF-I and ^{125}-I-IGF-II receptors in rat brain: comparison with insulin receptors, Diabetes 35:58A.

Lowe, W.L. Jr. and LeRoith, D., 1986, Insulin receptors from guinea pig liver and brain: structural and functional studies, Endocrinology 118:1669-1677.

Rechler, M.M., Zapf, J., Nissley, S.P., Froesch, E.R., Moses, A.C. et al., 1980, Interactions of insulin-like growth factors I and II and multiplication stimulating activity with receptors and serum carrier proteins, Endocrinology 107:1451-1459.

Rees-Jones, R.W., Hendricks, S.A., Quarum, M., Roth, J., 1984, The insulin receptor of rat brain is coupled to tyrosine kinase activity, J. Biol. Chem. 259:3470-3478.

Said, S.I. and Rosenberg, R.N., 1976, Vasoactive intestinal polypeptide: abundant immunoreactivity in neural cell lines and normal nervous tissue, Science 192:907-908.

Shepherd, G.M., 1979, Olfactory cortex, in: "The Synaptic Organization of the Brain", Oxford University Press, N.Y.

Simon, J. and LeRoith, D., 1986, Insulin receptors of chicken liver and brain. Characterization of α and β subunits properties, Eur. J. Biochem. 158:125-132.

VISUALIZATION OF IGF-2 RECEPTORS IN RAT BRAIN

Laurane G. Mendelsohn

Central Nervous System Research
Lilly Research Laboratories
Indianapolis, IN 46285

The notion that trophic factors are present in the brain and serve to maintain neurons, promote target tissue innervation, and stimulate synaptogenesis has been a well-accepted theory for some time. The transport of trophic factors to neuronal endings has been a favorite explanation for the axonal flow of materials in neurons which was first discovered by Weiss in 1948. More recently, reports of trophic effects of NGF on lesioned CNS neurons and evidence suggesting that insulin and the somatomedins are present in the CNS encouraged us to explore the localization of their receptors. In the experiments described here, we used iodinated human insulin-like growth factor-2 and autoradiography to visualize the receptors for this peptide in rat brain.

Human IGF-2 (hIGF-2) was prepared through recombinant DNA technology. The cloned material was expressed as a fused gene product with the tryp LE_1 operon in *E. coli*. After purification, the amino acid sequence, disulfide bond formation, and secondary structure were confirmed by amino acid analyses, N-terminal amino acid sequencing, and fast atom bombardment of fragments prepared by pepsin digestion. Biological activity and potency were evaluated using a competitive serum protein binding assay and evaluation of the potency to stimulate amino acid transport in human fibroblasts. In that assay, hIGF-2 had an ED_{50} of 2-3 ng/ml and was roughly equipotent with human IGF-1. Human insulin was approximately 10-fold less potent than either of the somatomedins in this assay.

Brains were removed from freshly decapitated rats and rapidly frozen in liquid 4% carboxymethyl cellulose by immersion in isopentane cooled with an acetone dry-ice bath. Serial sections of these frozen rat brains were thaw-mounted onto slides and stored under vacuum at 4°C overnight. The dehydrated sections were either stained with thionine or incubated with ^{125}I-IGF-2 (10 pM) for 16 hrs at 4°C. The specificity of IGF-2 binding was assessed by incubating adjacent sections with labeled IGF-2 in the presence of human insulin (80 nM) or hIGF-2 (80 nM). The assays were terminated by three brief washes in ice-cold buffer. After drying, the slices were exposed to X-ray film for 4-7 days at 4°C.

Autoradiographs of IGF-2 receptors showed that these sites were present in many brain regions but were also discretely localized. The most striking observation was the presence of receptors in hippocampal CA_1-CA_4 regions and the dentate gyrus (Fig. 1A). Labeling in the CA_3 and CA_4 areas was consistently heavier than in the CA_1 and CA_2 regions and was present over neuronal elements. Other labeled areas included the entorhinal cortex, which projects to the hippocampus, and the deep layers of the cortex. Incubation in the presence of

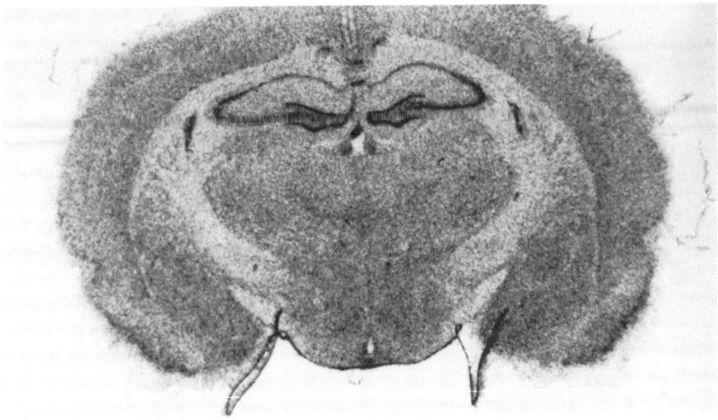

Figure 1A. Autoradiograph of dorsal hippocampus of rat brain labeled with ^{125}I-hIGF-2.

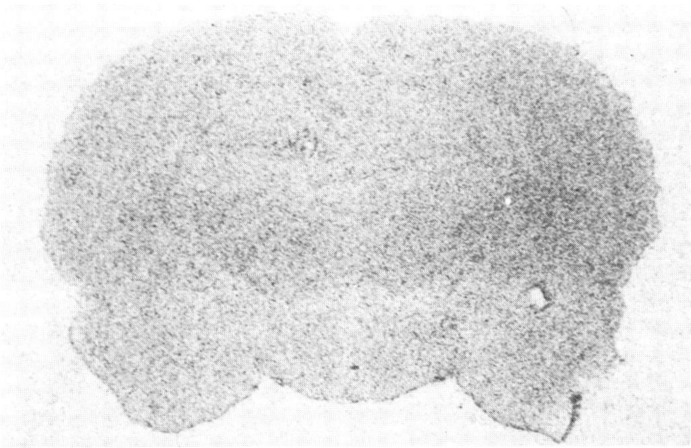

Figure 1B. Autoradiograph of dorsal hippocampus of rat brain in the presence of excess unlabeled hIGF-2.

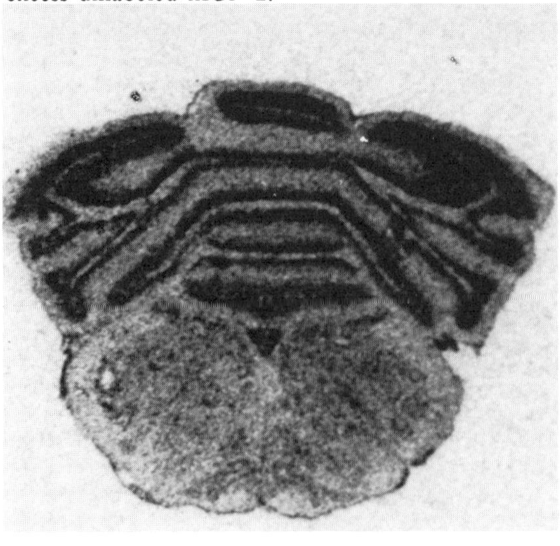

Figure 2A. Autoradiograph of cerebellum of rat brain labeled with ^{125}I-hIGF-2.

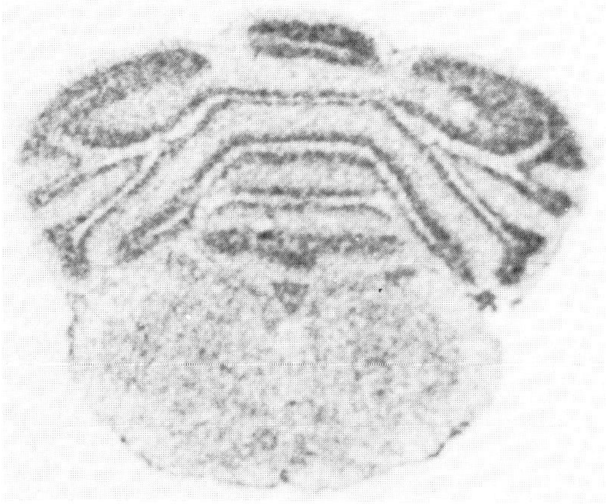

Figure 2B. Autoradiograph of cerebellum of rat brain in the presence of excess h-insulin.

excess insulin produced a slight decrease in the amount of ^{125}I-IGF-2 bound (not shown). In contrast, the presence of excess IGF-2 produced a dramatic decrease in specifically bound ^{125}I-IGF-2 (Fig. 1B).

Another area heavily labeled by IGF-2 is the granule cell layer of the cerebellum (Fig. 2A). As before, insulin slightly displaced ^{125}I-IGF-2, while unlabeled IGF-2 produced a dramatic reduction of binding to these layers (Figs. 2B and 2C). Other areas to which ^{125}I-IGF-2 bound included the granule cell layer of the olfactory bulb and the piriform cortex. The anterior pituitary was neavily labeled (not shown). In some preparations, labeling of the thalamus and subiculum was observed. The pineal gland was densely labeled; and in the brain stem, the central gray, interpeduncular nucleus, and the red nucleus were more heavily labeled than other areas (Fig. 3).

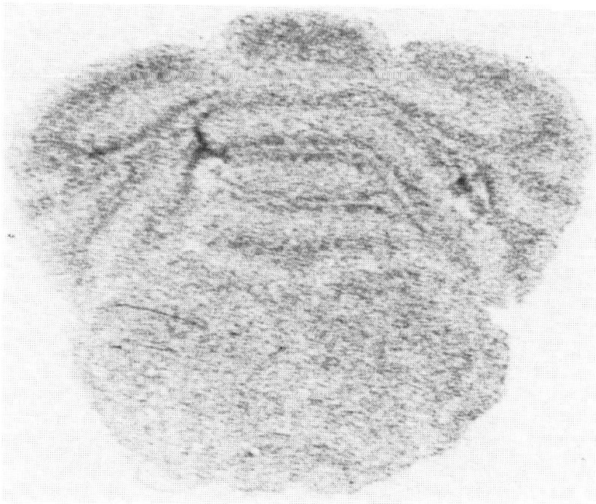

Figure 2C. Autoradiograph of cerebellum of rat brain in the presence of excess h-IGF-2.

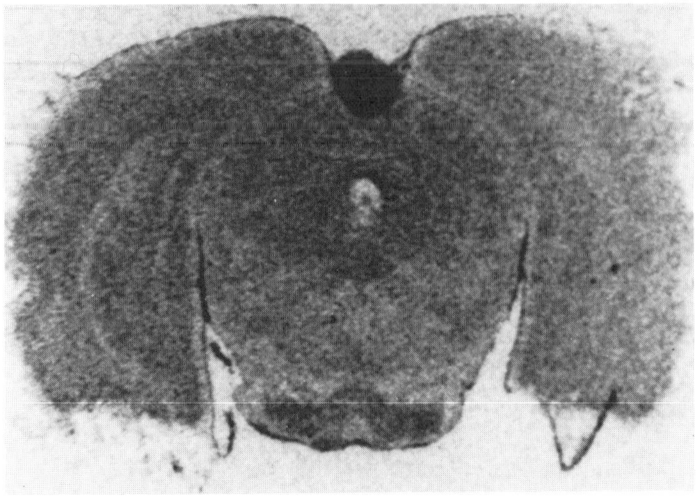

Figure 3. Autoradiograph of section through pineal gland of rat brain. Labeling by ^{125}I-IGF-2 is heaviest in the pineal and central gray.

In other studies, we investigated the localization of the cerebellar receptors more closely. Dr. Bernardino Ghetti, Indiana University School of Medicine, Indianapolis, Indiana, provided us with mutant mice which have well-characterized neuronal cell deficiencies (Figs. 4A, 4B, and 4C). One mutant, the PCD (Purkinje Cell Deficient), loses its Purkinje cells during development. Another, the Weaver mutant, suffers a selective loss of granule cells of the cerebellum. Each trait is recessively inherited.

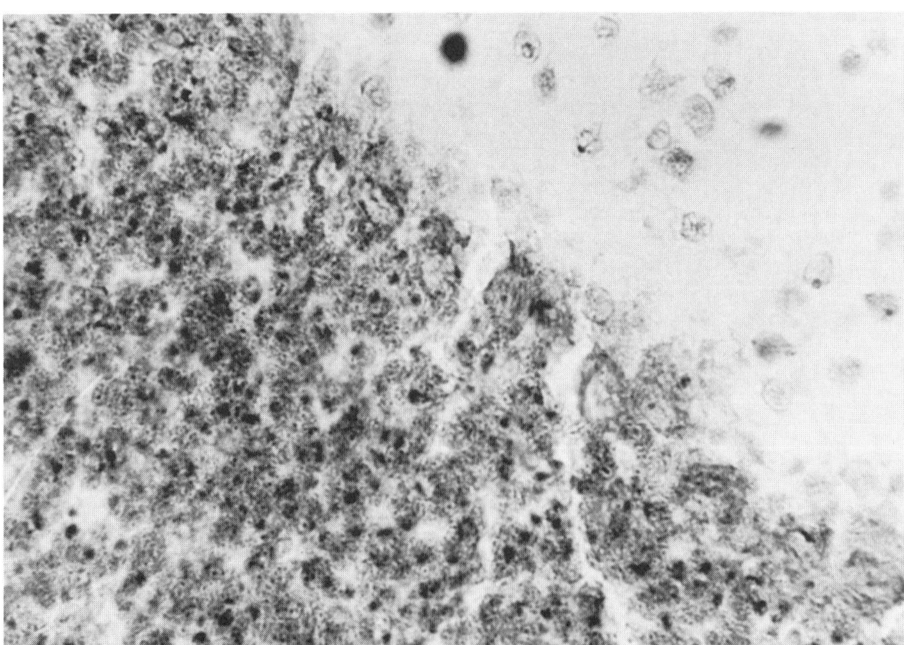

Figure 4A. Micrographs from thionine-stained cerebella of normal mice.

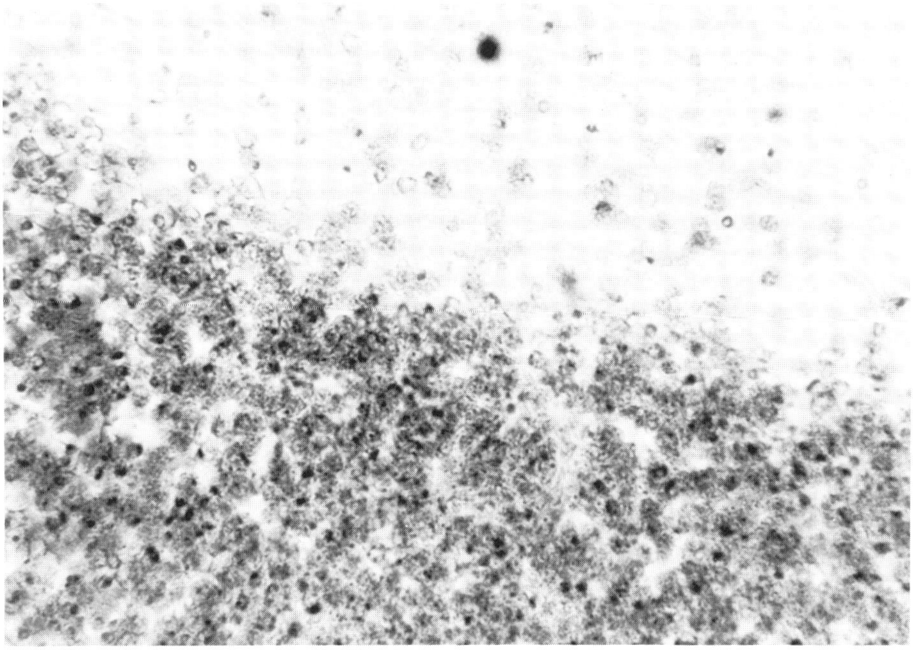

Figure 4B. Micrographs from thionine-stained cerebella of Purkinje Cell Deficient (PCD) mice. The large Purkinje cells are missing in PCD cerebella.

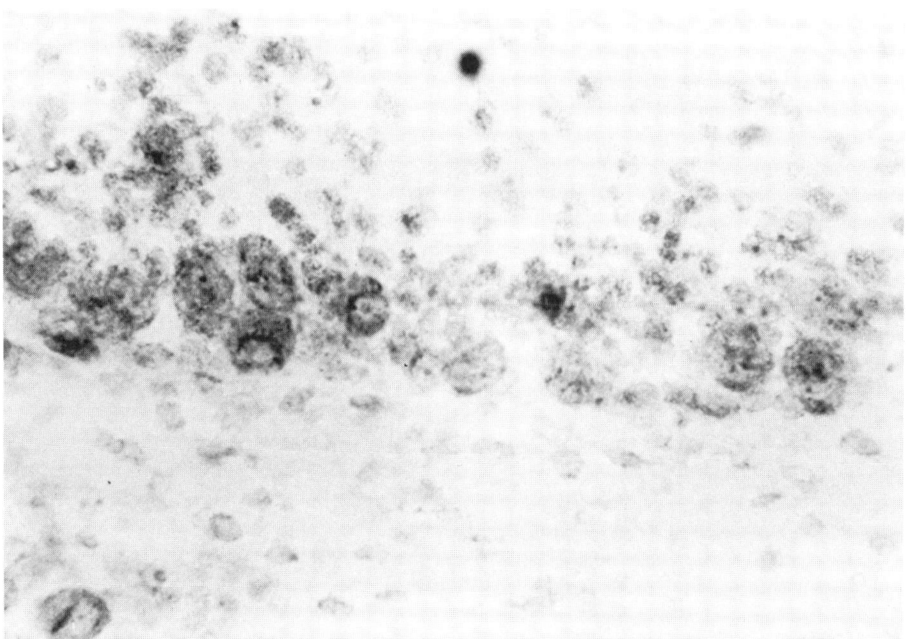

Figure 4C. Micrographs from thionine-stained cerebella of Weaver mice. Granule cells are absent in Weaver cerebella.

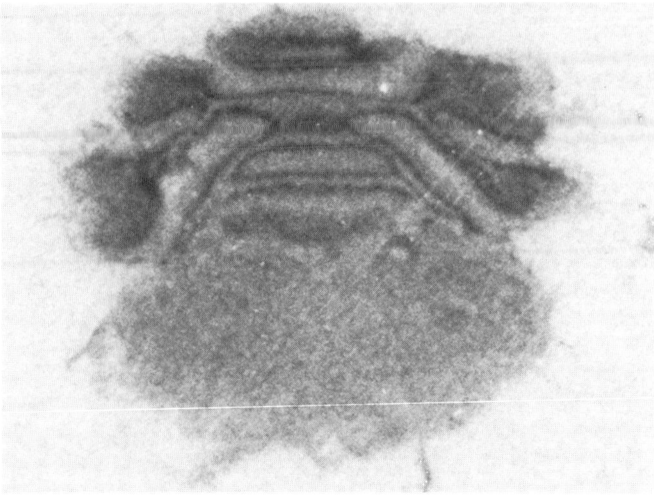

Figure 5A. Autoradiograph of IGF-2 binding sites in cerebellum of a normal mouse.

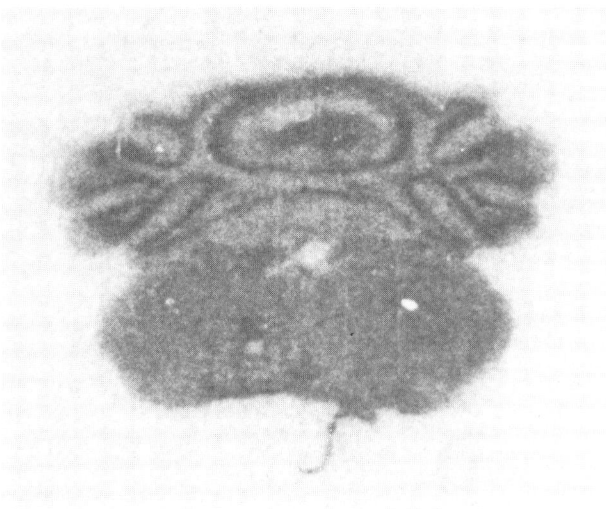

Figure 5B. Autoradiograph of IGF-2 binding sites in cerebellum of a PCD mouse.

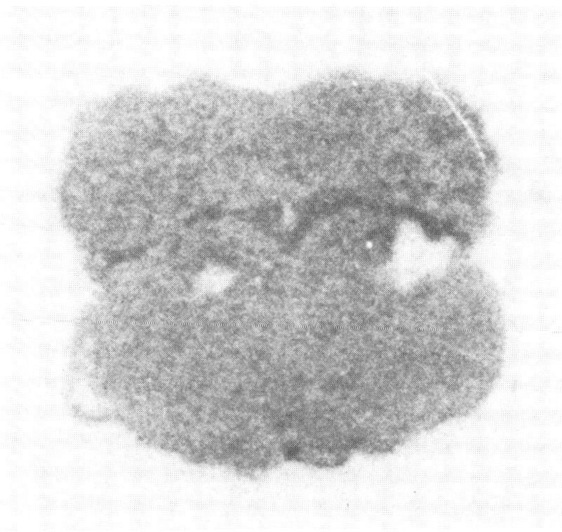

Figure 5C. Autoradiograph of IGF-2 binding sites in cerebellum of a Weaver mouse.

Cerebellar slices from these mutant mice and control normal litter mates were incubated with labeled IGF-2. Adjacent sections were stained with thionine to identify the densely labeled nuclei observed on the autoradiographs. Autoradiographs show that binding of labeled IGF-2 to granule cell layers from normal control litter mates and PCD mice was similar (Figs. 5A and 5B). Autoradiographs of affected Weaver mice show severe atrophy of the cerebellum and severely reduced binding of IGF-2 (Fig. 5C) reflecting the loss of receptors and the missing cells. Thus in the cerebellum, the evidence suggests that the IGF-2 receptor is present on granule cells.

In conclusion, we have used autoradiography to visualize IGF-2 receptors in rat brain. Receptors are present in the deep layers of the cortex, the piriform and entorhinal cortex, the CA_{1-4} regions of the hippocampus, and the dentate gyrus. Other areas labeled included the pineal gland, anterior pituitary, and the granule cell layer of the olfactory bulbs.

In the cerebellum of rats and mice, granule cells were densely labeled by IGF-2 and these receptors were absent in mutants deficient in granule cells.

The presence of IGF-2 in brain is provocative to say the least. Although it has many growth-related anabolic-like activities, its normal function is poorly understood. Its unique distribution and high affinity for brain receptors suggest that it may be a neurotransmitter or a neuronotrophic substance.

INSULIN-LIKE GROWTH FACTORS AND THEIR RECEPTORS IN THE PITUITARY AND HYPOTHALAMUS

Ron G. Rosenfeld and Andrew R. Hoffman

Departments of Pediatrics and Medicine
Stanford University Medical Center
Stanford, California

SOMATOMEDINS: BACKGROUND

The somatomedins, or insulin-like growth factors (IGFs), constitute a family of peptide hormones which are growth hormone dependent, possess insulin-like activity, and have mitogenic activity in a wide variety of cell lines[1]. Two human somatomedins have been purified and sequenced: IGF-I has a molecular weight of 7649, and consists of 70 amino acids, while IGF-II has a molecular weight of 7471, with 67 amino acids[2,3]. A rat equivalent of IGF-II, termed multiplication stimulating activity (MSA), has also been purified and sequenced; it differs from human IGF-II in four of the 67 amino acid positions[4]. The sequences of cDNAs encoding for human prepro-IGF-I and -II have been elucidated, and the respective 130 and 180 amino acid precursors predicted[5,6]. IGF-II has been mapped to the short arm of chromosome 11, tightly linked to both the insulin gene and the c-Ha-ras1 proto-oncogene[7]. IGF-I maps to chromosome 12, which is evolutionarily related to chromosome 11, and carries the gene for the c-Ki-ras2 proto-oncogene[8].

These striking homologies suggest evolutionary conservation of a common critical peptide skeleton, and raise important questions concerning the precise role of each peptide and how cells specifically mediate each peptide's biological activities. As their structural homology would suggest, IGF-I and -II have weak insulin-like metabolic effects, while insulin shares the mitogenic and growth-promoting actions of the IGFs. While competitive binding and affinity cross-linking studies have indicated the existence of specific receptors for each peptide, it has been difficult to discriminate among the functional roles of each receptor because of: 1) overlapping affinities of insulin and IGFs for each other's receptors; 2) use of incompletely purified IGF preparations in both binding and biological studies; and 3) possible heterogeneity in binding properties of these receptors in different tissues and species[9].

The interrelationship of the insulin and IGF receptors has been clarified by efforts to purify and structurally characterize these membrane proteins[9-11]. On the basis of affinity cross-linking studies, followed by SDS-PAGE, both the insulin and IGF-I receptors have been found to be heterotetramers, composed of two 135,000 dalton α-subunits and two 90,000 dalton β-subunits linked by interchain disulfide bonds. Both subunits are glycosylated and are exposed on the external surface of the cell. Interestingly, the α-subunit of both the insulin and IGF-I receptors in the brain has a lower apparent molecular weight than the α-subunit of peripheral tissue, presumably due to differences in the N-terminal glycosylation of the proteins[12]. The α-subunit contains the binding site for insulin or IGF-I; the β-subunit contains a transmembrane domain, an ATP-binding site and a probable site for tyrosine auto-phosphorylation[13]. These findings are consistent with the observation that insulin and IGF-I can induce the phosphorylation of a tyrosine residue on the β-subunit of their own receptors, as well as on exogenous protein substrates. Cloned cDNAs encoding for the entire 1370-1382 amino acid sequence of the human insulin receptor precursor[14] and the 1367 amino acid sequence of the human IGF-I receptor precursor[15] have been identified, and found to have significant sequence homologies to the EGF receptor and to the src family of tyrosine-specific protein kinases. Nevertheless, the role(s) of receptor (or other substrate) phosphorylation in the biological actions of both insulin and IGF-I remains unestablished.

Studies performed with IGF-II have indicated the existence of a structurally and immunologically distinct receptor (type II)[9-11]. Following cross-linking and SDS-PAGE, this receptor migrates with an apparent Mr of 220,000 in the unreduced state and 250,000 following reduction, suggesting that it is a single-chain polypeptide with internal disulfide bridges. Binding of [^{125}I]IGF-II to this receptor is preferentially inhibited by IGF-II > IGF-I, with no affinity for insulin, which actually appears to activate the appearance of additional type II receptors on the cell surface[16]. Although phosphorylation of the type II receptor in intact cells has been observed, and can be stimulated by the addition of IGF-II, this action could be mediated through the IGF-I receptor[17]. At this time, there is still no definitive evidence for the type II receptor having intrinsic tyrosine kinase activity.

SOMATOMEDIN RECEPTORS IN THE PITUITARY AND HYPOTHALAMUS

By analogy with the CRF-ACTH-cortisol axis and the TRH-TSH-thyroxine axis, it is reasonable to hypothesize that the IGFs may be capable of regulating GH secretion by a negative feedback mechanism at the pituitary and/or hypothalamic level (see below). Accordingly, confirmation of the presence of specific receptors for the IGFs (and insulin) in the pituitary and hypothalamus has been eagerly sought. To date, three distinct pituitary models have been employed: 1) rat anterior pituitary (either membrane preparations or monolayer cultures of freshly dispersed cells); 2) membrane preparations from human pituitary adenomas; and 3) cloned rat pituitary tumor cell lines.

Rat Anterior Pituitary

Employing crude membrane preparations of anterior pituitaries from normal adult, male Sprague Dawley rats, Goodyer et al[18] demonstrated specific receptors for IGF-I, IGF-II and insulin. Specific binding per 100 ug membrane protein averaged 3.6% for IGF-I, 16.1% for IGF-II, and 1.3% for insulin. When expressed as specific binding per unit protein weight, [^{125}I]IGF-II binding to pituitary membranes was four-fold greater than in hypothalamic membranes, and eight-fold greater than in brain membranes. Interestingly, displacement of both [^{125}I]IGF-I and [^{125}I]IGF-II binding was greater by unlabeled IGF-II than by IGF-I. Insulin, at concentrations as high as 2000 ng/ml, weakly displaced both radioligands.

Concurrently, Rosenfeld and coworkers[19] characterized high affinity receptors for both IGF-I and -II on primary monolayer cultures of dispersed anterior pituitary cells derived from adult, male Sprague-Dawley rats. Quantification of specific binding of iodinated ligands revealed a pattern similar to that reported by Goodyer et al[18]. Specific binding of [^{125}I]IGF-I, [^{125}I]IGF-II and [^{125}I]insulin to 100-150,000 cells averaged 0.8%, 9.5% and 0.1%, respectively. In contrast to the results reported by Goodyer et al[18], IGF-I was 5-fold more potent than IGF-II at displacing [^{125}I]IGF-I, and 1000-fold more potent than insulin (Figure 1). On the other hand, IGF-II was twice as potent as IGF-I in displacing [^{125}I]IGF-II, while insulin was totally nonreactive.

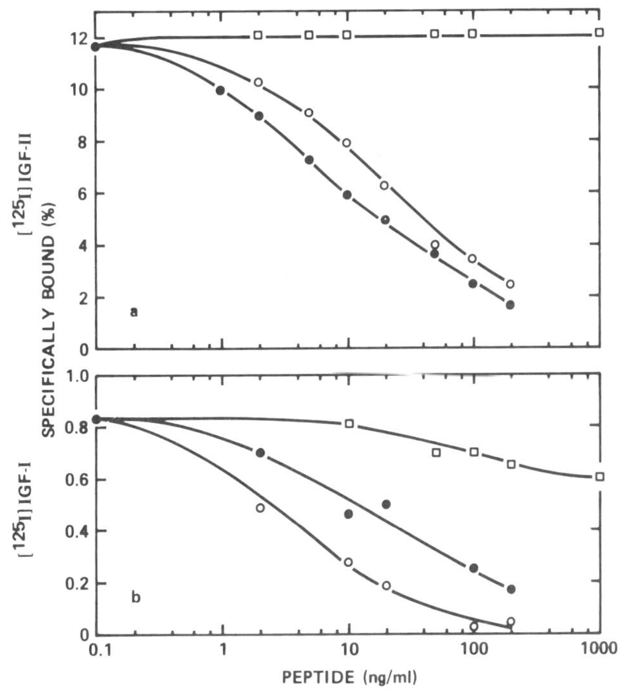

Figure 1. Competition for IGF-II (a) and IGF-I (b) binding to 130,000 rat anterior pituitary cells per well. ● IGF-II; o IGF-I; □ insulin.
From Reference 19, with permission of authors.

Scatchard analysis of [^{125}I]IGF-II binding to pituitary monolayers demonstrated a curvilinear plot (Figure 2). Using a two-component model, this plot could be resolved into a high affinity receptor with a Ka of 7.0 x $10^8 M^{-1}$ and 120,000 receptor sites/cell, and a low affinity receptor with a Ka of 1.1 x $10^8 M^{-1}$ and approximately 720,000 receptor sites/cell. As is characteristic of type II IGF-II receptors elsewhere, preincubation of pituitary cells with insulin, somatomedin, and rGH, as well as rGRF and rSRIF, did not alter specific binding of [^{125}I]IGF-II. On the other hand, preincubation of cells with insulin (1 and 100 ug/ml) or with somatomedin (200 ng/ml IGF-II plus 400 ng/ml IGF-I) resulted in a 30% reduction in the subsequent specific binding of [^{125}I]IGF-I.

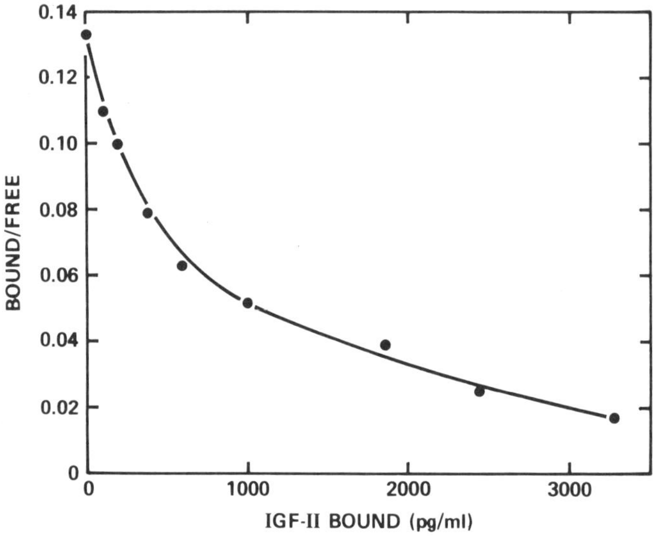

Figure 2. Scatchard plot of IGF-II binding to rat anterior pituitary cells. From Reference 19, with permission of authors.

In sum, these data demonstrate the presence of abundant specific high affinity receptors for IGF-II on rat anterior pituitary cells. These receptors appear qualitatively similar to classical type II receptors on adipocytes, fibroblasts and hepatocytes, all of which share the following characteristics: 1) a greater affinity for IGF-II than for IGF-I, 2) no affinity for insulin, and 3) an inability to be down-regulated after prolonged exposure to IGF-I, IGF-II, or insulin.

Human Pituitary Adenomas

In subsequent experiments, Ceda et al[20] performed competitive radioligand studies on membranes prepared from four GH-secreting human pituitary adenomas. Specific binding of insulin, IGF-I and IGF-II was demonstrable in all membranes tested, and ranged from 3.3-9.4% per 100 ug membrane protein for [^{125}I]insulin, from 2.5-9.7% for [^{125}I]IGF-I, and from 3.3-12.5% for [^{125}I]IGF-II. Thus, unlike the situation in rat anterior pituitary cells, specific binding of insulin and IGF-I was almost as high as for IGF-II. Competition studies were consistent with specific receptors for each radioligand. Fifty percent displacement of [^{125}I]insulin was observed at insulin concentrations of 20 ng/ml (3.7×10^{-9} M/L). Fifty percent displacement of [^{125}I]IGF-I occurred at 9 ng/ml of unlabeled IGF-I (1.2×10^{-9} M/L); insulin competed weakly for this receptor, with 40% displacement of [^{125}I]IGF-I at insulin concentrations of 100 ug/ml (1.9×10^{-5} M/L). When [^{125}I]IGF-II was employed as radioligand, insulin was totally noncompetitive, even at concentrations as high as 100 ug/ml (1.9×10^{-5} M/L), while 50% displacement was observed at IGF-II concentrations of approximately 30 ng/ml (4×10^{-9} M/L).

Cloned Rat Pituitary Tumor Cells

Because of the great difficulty of maintaining either human or rat adenohypophyseal cells in prolonged culture, we subsequently extended our investigations to cloned strains of rat pituitary tumor cells[21]. GH_3, GH_1 and GC cells constitute three distinct clonal lines, which have been successfully propagated for over 20 years, and which have retained the capacity to both synthesize and secrete GH. Several previous studies had demonstrated the presence of insulin receptors in these cell lines. As early as 1979, Hollander et al[22] reported specific insulin receptors in both GH_1 and GC cells. More recently, Corin et al[23] characterized insulin binding to GH_3 cells, while Turyn and co-workers[24] described insulin binding to GH_1 cells.

Table 1 compares specific binding of insulin, IGF-I and IGF-II to normal rat anterior pituitary cells and GH_1, GH_3 and GC cells. Specific binding of all three radioligands was readily demonstrable in each cell line, ranging from 8.9-11.6% per 250,000 cells for [^{125}I]insulin, 4.7-6.6% for [^{125}I]IGF-I, and 9.3-9.7% for [^{125}I]IGF-II. This pattern clearly contrasts with that observed in rat anterior pituitary cells, which preferentially bind IGF-II over IGF-I, and have limited insulin binding.

Competitive binding studies in each cell line demonstrated specific high-affinity receptors for each ligand (Figures 3 and 4). Scatchard analysis of [^{125}I]insulin binding to GH_3 cells (Figure 5) yielded a curvilinear plot, which could be resolved into a high affinity receptor with a Kd of 1.0×10^{-10} M/L, and a low affinity receptor with a Kd of 5.6×10^{-9} M/L. The number of high affinity insulin receptors per cell for GH_3, GC, and GH_1 cells were 9,700, 9,200, and 16,000, respectively. By contrast, the Scatchard plot of [^{125}I]IGF-I binding was generally linear (Figure 6: GC cells), with a Kd ranging from 1.2-1.6 x 10^{-9} M/L, and approximately 80,000 receptors per cell.

Table 1. Specific binding of [^{125}I]insulin, [^{125}I]IGF-I, and [^{125}I]IGF-II to rat pituitary cells.

Cells	Insulin	IGF-I	IGF-II
Normal rat pituitary	0.6±0.3 (3)	2.6±1.4 (3)	14.5±2.2 (6)
GC	9.5±3.1 (7)	6.6±1.7 (9)	9.7±1.2 (4)
GH_3	11.6±2.4 (5)	4.7±1.1 (5)	9.3±3.2 (5)
GH_1	8.9±1.7 (5)	5.4±1.4 (5)	9.6±1.9 (5)

[^{125}I]Insulin, [^{125}I]IGF-I, or [^{125}I]IGF-II was added to cell monolayers in HEPES buffer with 1% BSA (pH 6.5 for [^{125}I]IGF-II; pH8.0 for [^{125}I]Insulin and [^{125}I]IGF-I) at 15C for 3h in the absence or presence of an excess of unlabeled peptide (10 ug/ml unlabeled insulin for [^{125}I]insulin binding; partially purified somatomedin preparation containing 800 ng/ml IGF-I and 400 ng/ml IGF-II for [^{125}I]IGF-II binding). Nonspecific binding was subtracted from total binding for determination of specific binding. Data are expressed at the percent specific binding per 250,000 cells and represent the mean ± SEM of the number of separate experiments in parentheses.

Cross-linking of [^{125}I]insulin and [^{125}I]IGF-I to GH_3 cells demonstrated classical type I receptors, with apparent molecular weights greater than 300,000 in the unreduced state, and 125,000 following reduction of disulfide bonds with dithiothreitol (Figures 7 and 8). Affinity cross-linking of [^{125}I]IGF-II demonstrated binding to both type I and type II receptors.

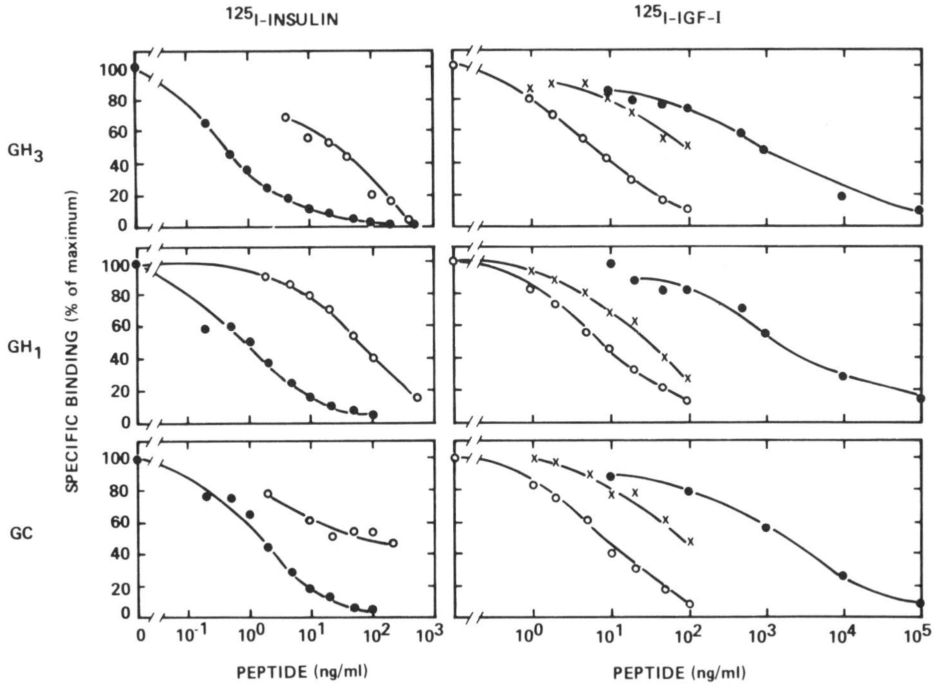

Figure 3. Competition for insulin (left) and IGF-I (right) binding to GH$_3$, GH$_1$, and GC cells. ● insulin; o IGF-I; x IGF-II. From Reference 21, with permission of authors.

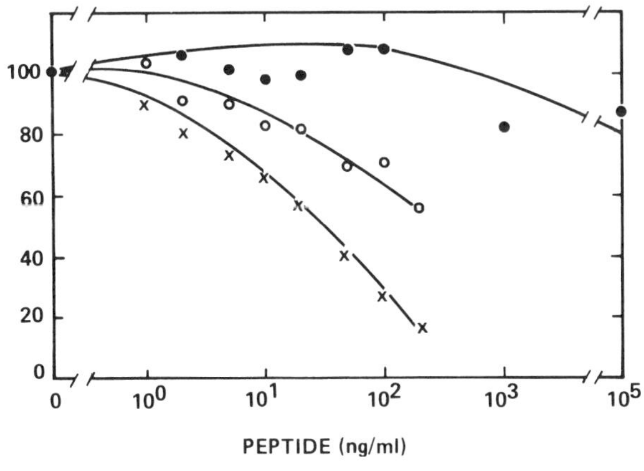

Figure 4. Competition for IGF-II binding to GH$_3$ cells. ● insulin; o IGF-I; x IGF-II. From Reference 21, with permission of authors.

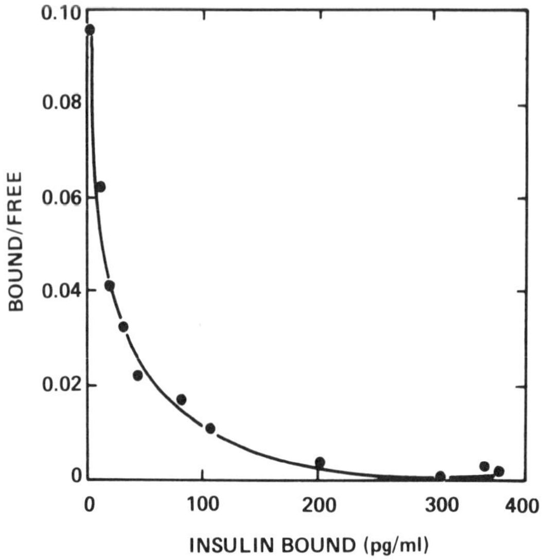

Figure 5. Scatchard plot of insulin binding to GH_3 cells. The high affinity receptor has a K_d of 1.0×10^{-10} M/L and 9,700 binding sites/cell. The low affinity receptor has a K_d of 5.6×10^{-9} M/L and 94,000 sites/cell. From Refernce 21, with permission of authors.

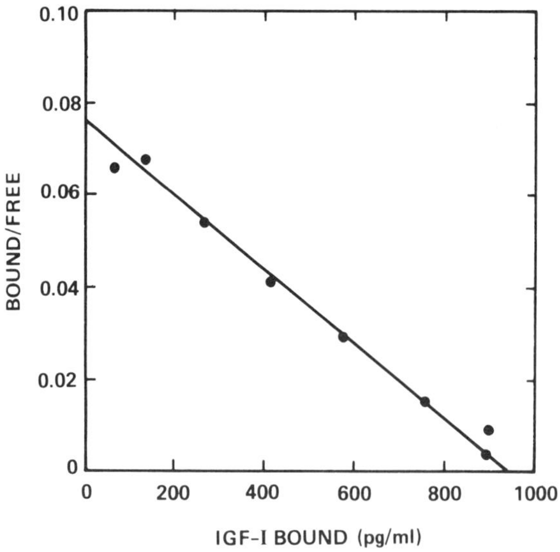

Figure 6. Scatchard plot of IGF-I binding to GC cells. The K_d is 1.6×10^{-9} M/L, with 63,000 binding sites/cells. From Reference 21, with permission of authors.

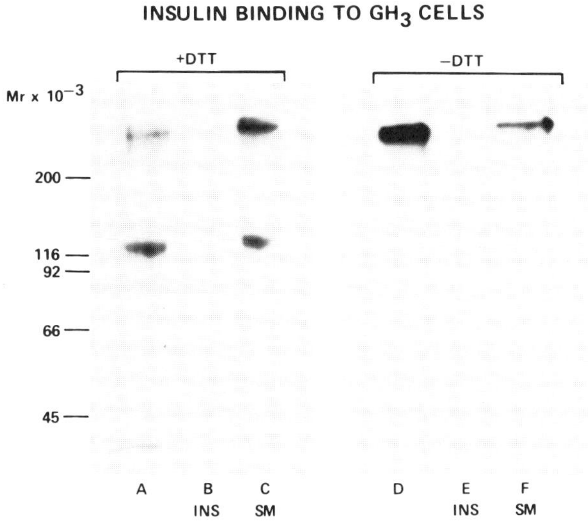

Figure 7. Autoradiogram of SDS gel, showing the specificity of insulin-receptor complexes cross-linked to GH_3 cells under reducing (lanes A-C) and nonreducing (lanes D-F) conditions. From Reference 21, with permission of authors.

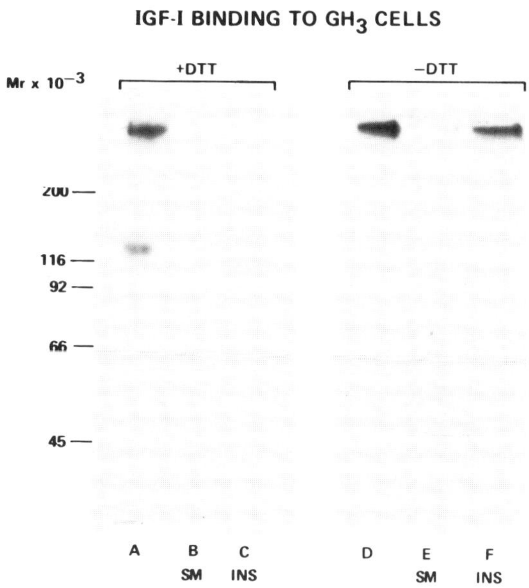

Figure 8. Autoradiogram of SDS gel, showing the specificity of IGF-I-receptor complexes cross-linked to GH_3 cells under reducing (lanes A-C) and nonreducing (lanes D-F) conditions. From Reference 21.

SOMATOMEDIN RECEPTORS IN THE HYPOTHALAMUS

In a study of insulin receptors in the rat central nervous system, Havrankova et al[25] reported that the anterior hypothalamus was relatively rich in insulin receptors, especially when compared with the pituitary. In subsequent studies in rat brain, Gammeltoft et al[12] demonstrated specific binding of insulin, IGF-I and IGF-II to hypothalamic membranes, although binding of all three radioligands was rather modest compared with other regions of the rat brain. Goodyer et al[18] also reported specific binding of all three ligands to rat hypothalamic membranes, with the highest specific binding found with [^{125}I]IGF-II (as was the case with rat anterior pituitary). Specific binding of IGF-I, IGF-II, and insulin to 200 ug of hypothalamic membrane protein averaged 3.0, 9.3, and 2.2%, respectively. In comparing these and similar studies, it is important to recall that such membrane preparations are derived from a heterogeneous collection of cells, and may vary in the relative contributions of neuronal vs. mesenchymal cells.

Studies of hypothalamic somatomedin receptors in other species have lagged behind studies in the rat. Sara et al[26] have reported specific binding of insulin, IGF-I and IGF-II to crude hypothalamic membrane preparations derived from human adult brain. Interestingly, these investigators also found relatively high specific binding of all three radioligands to human pituitary, similar to observations in human pituitary adenomas (see above)[20].

Recent studies by Bohannon et al[27] have provided data concerning microanatomical localization of IGF receptors in the rat brain. These experiments employ autoradiography of slide-mounted sections of frozen brain. Incubation of rat brain slices with [^{125}I]IGF-I resulted in a dense grain concentration in the region of the external palisade zone of the median eminence. This autoradiographic image was significantly reduced in the presence of excess unlabeled IGF-I. Such studies are consistent with a biological role for the somatomedins in hypothalamic development and/or regulation, and suggest that the IGFs may regulate GH secretion on both a hypothalamic and pituitary level. The obvious advantage of such a method is the ability to localize binding to small anatomical regions of the brain or hypothalamus. However, as is the case with crude membrane preparations, one is still dealing with heterogenous cell populations. More precise studies will require additional methodologies, such as cultures of hypothalamic neurons, immunofluorescence and in situ hybridization.

SOMATOMEDIN PRODUCTION IN BRAIN AND PITUITARY

In order for the somatomedins to interact with the hypothalamic-pituitary network, IGF must be present in the brain, in the CSF, in the pituitary gland or in the hypothalamic-hypophyseal portal circulation. The somatomedin peptides were originally purified from blood, and the potential sites of synthesis were unknown. Since GH receptors could be demonstrated in liver, and perifused livers respond to GH by producing peptides with somatomedin activity[28], it was initially suggested that the liver was a major source of somatomedin production. It was soon discovered, however, that numerous organs had the capacity to synthesize and secrete somatomedins. D'Ercole and colleagues[29] studied IGF-I production from a variety of fetal mouse organs in explant culture. Except for the liver, the brain was the most prolific producer of radioimmunoassayable somatomedin. Using similar organ culture techniques, Binoux et al[30] demonstrated that IGF and IGF carrier proteins were synthesized by young rat anterior and posterior pituitary, hypothalamus, cerebral cortex, and cerebellum. When cycloheximide was added to the culture medium, the incorporation of [^{3}H]leucine into secreted proteins was inhibited, and the concentration of IGF in the medium was also decreased. These studies suggested that the IGF was synthesized in situ by the cultured explants. IGF-I was also demonstrated in rat brain tissue extracts; unlike IGF-I in other organs, the concentration of brain IGF-I was not GH dependent[31]. Triiodothyronine, however, has been shown to increase IGF secretion from cultured fetal mouse hypothalamic cells[32].

Recently, it has been learned that human cerebrospinal fluid contains large quantities of IGF-II, but very little IGF-I[33,34]. Much of the IGF-II consisted of a "big" IGF-II[33], which has been identified as a precursor of a variant IGF-II[35]. This high molecular weight immunoreactive IGF was detectable in extracts derived from essentially every part of the human brain, except the pons[36]. The anterior pituitary gland was particularly rich in this large form of IGF-II. In addition, a variant, amino-terminally trucated form of IGF-I has been characterized in human fetal brain tissue[37].

Local synthesis of IGF-I and IGF-II in the central nervous system and the pituitary gland has now been elegantly confirmed by finding specific IGF mRNA in those organs. IGF-II mRNA has been detected in fetal rat brain[38-40]. While IGF-II mRNA levels decline dramatically after the neonatal period in liver and other organs, the mRNA is readily detectable in adult rat cerebral cortex and hypothalamus, strongly suggesting that IGF-II plays a regulatory role throughout development in the rat CNS[39,40]. ICF-I mRNA, on the other hand, could only be detected in rat brain during fetal life[40]. While the question of whether insulin is synthesized in brain has long been a matter of controversy[41], a recent report also describes the presence of insulin mRNA, as detected by in situ hybridization, in rat periventricular hypothalamic cells[42].

FEEDBACK REGULATION: SOMATOMEDIN INHIBITION OF GH RELEASE AND SYNTHESIS

Somatomedin may regulate GH synthesis and release by interacting at all three loci of the hypothalamic-somatotroph-somatomedin axis.

Central Nervous System

Only two studies have dealt directly with the hormonal role of somatomedins in the central nervous system. IGF-I stimulated the release of somatostatin from cultures of rat medial-basal hypothalamus in a concentration-dependent manner[43]. Furthermore, IGF-I substantially inhibited GHRH release from cultured rat hypothalamus[44]. Thus, IGF-I can decrease the release of pituitary GH both by inhibiting the secretion of the most potent GH releasing factor and by stimulating the release of a GH-release-inhibitory factor.

Anterior Pituitary Gland

The role of IGFs in the regulation of GH secretion has been studied in vivo and in vitro. When Tannenbaum et al[45] injected a preparation enriched in somatomedins into the ventricles of unanesthetized, freely moving rats, they noted a decrease in the number of GH secretory episodes. Employing a similar experimental design, Abe and colleagues[46] obtained comparable results, using a highly purified IGF-I preparation. Studying primary cultures of rat anterior pituitary cells, Berelowitz et al[43] showed that IGF-I inhibited basal and stimulated GH release after 24 hours of incubation. Brazeau et al[47] demonstrated that both IGF-I and IGF-II inhibited GHRH-stimulated GH release from cultured rat pituitary cells after 3-4 or 24 hours of incubation; IGF-I was more potent than IGF-II, and neither EGF nor FGF duplicated this action. The short-term (3-4 hour) inhibition of GH release by the somatomedins was also reported by Goodyer et al[48], who showed, additionally, that the effect could be maintained for up to 5 days in culture, and by Sheppard and Bala[49], who found a much smaller inhibition of GH synthesis and release.

Melmed and colleagues[50-56] have studied the regulation of Gh synthesis and release by somatomedins and insulin in rat pituitary cells. Using the pituitary tumor GH_3 cell line, they showed that prolonged (4-8 day) incubation with both insulin and IGF-I inhibited GH secretion[50]; moreover, insulin inhibited hydrocortisone[50] and triiodothyronine[51] stimulated GH release. Insulin was shown to suppress rat GH mRNA levels in untreated and hydrocortisone-exposed GH_3 cells[52] and to inhibit the transcription of the GH gene in these cells[53]. In a similar series of experiments, these investigators showed that insulin and IGF-I inhibited basal and GHRH-stimulated GH secretion and mRNA synthesis in cultures derived from normal rat anterior pituitary cells[54,55]. Using anterior pituitary cells derived from hypothyroid rats, they demonstrated that IGF-I also inhibited GH secretion and mRNA synthesis in triiodothyronine-stimulated cells[56].

Although these experiments demonstrated that the IGFs can mediate GH release, it had not been shown that the somatomedins could directly and rapidly inhibit pituitary GH release. Ceda et al[57] therefore perifused normal rat pituitary cells to study dynamic feedback regulation at the pituitary level. Cells were exposed to hourly 150 second pulses of GHRH, with or without added IGF or insulin. With this system, the cells responded in a consistent manner to repeated boluses of 1 nM GHRH. As depicted in Figure 9 and summarized in Table 2, IGF-I and IGF-II both inhibited GHRH-stimulated GH release in a dose-dependent manner, with IGF-I being somewhat more potent than IGF-II. Insulin was an extremely weak inhibitor of GHRH-elicited GH release, and only at extremely high concentrations, suggesting that its activity in normal rat cells might in fact be mediated via the IGF-I receptor.

The regulation of GH release from cultured human pituitary cells has also been investigated by Ceda et al[20,58]. They demonstrated that somatomedins inhibit basal and GHRH-stimulated GH release from normal human pituitary cells, as well as from cells derived from somatotroph adenomas. Insulin was also effective in suppressing GH release in both human systems. Goodyer and her colleagues[59] showed that both IGF-I and IGF-II inhibited GH release from cultured human fetal pituitaries, and a semi-purified IGF preparation inhibited GH release from adult pituitaries, but did not alter GH release from cultures of pituitary adenomas. Yamashita et al[60] confirmed the observations of Ceda and colleagues[20,58] in cultured human pituitary adenomas, and also showed that IGF-I specifically inhibited human GH mRNA levels in the tumor Cells.

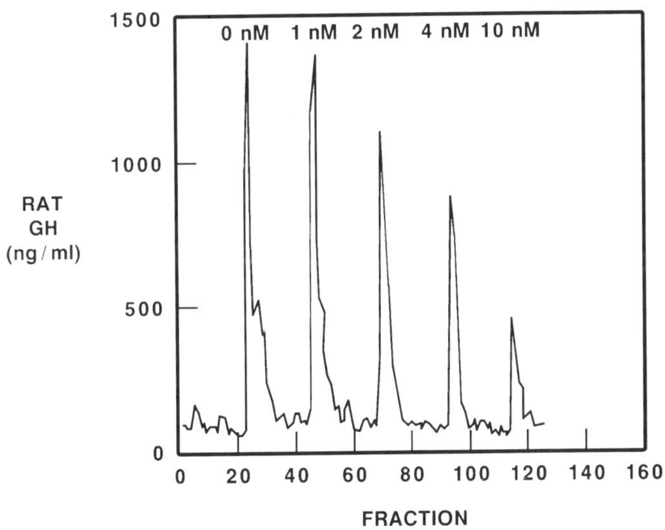

Figure 9. Effect of IGF-I on GHRH-stimulated GH release from perifused rat pituitary cells. After 4 hours equilibrium, perifused rat pituitary cells (25×10^6 cells) were exposed to hourly boluses of 1 ml of 1 nM GHRH plus the designated concentrations of IGF-I. Cells were perifused at a rate of 0.4 ml/min and samples collected every 2.5 minutes. From Reference 57, with permission of authors.

Table 2. Inhibition of GH release from perifused rat pituitary cells.

PEPTIDE	CONCENTRATION (nM)	GH RELEASED (area under the curve expressed as of % of control)
IGF-I	0	100
	1	93
	2	75
	4	60
	10	29
IGF-II	0	100
	5	89
	10	69
INSULIN	0	100
	1	94
	10	87
	100	89

Somatomedin Production: Direct Feedback by Somatomedin?

In addition to modulating GH secretion, the somatomedins could, also, potentially regulate IGF synthesis in peripheral tissues. Wilson and colleagues[61] have recently developed an animal model in which a rat IGF-II secreting cell line, 18,54-SF, is transplanted into nude rats, resulting in chronically elevated plasma IGF-II levels. As plasma IGF-II levels increased, both plasma IGF-I levels and liver IGF-I mRNA tended to decrease. Despite the elevated IGF-II concentrations, the GH response to GHRH was not blunted, suggesting that chronic increases in plasma IGF-II levels may not alter GH secretory dynamics. Investigations are currently in progress to explore the possibility that IGF-II can act through a non-hypothalamic-pituitary mechanism (perhaps via the liver or other peripheral tissues) to suppress IGF-I production.

CONCLUSIONS

Over the last five years, increasing evidence has been accumulated concerning the presence (and, possibly, the synthesis) of the somatomedin peptides IGF-I and -II in the brain, hypothalamus and pituitary. The existence of specific receptors for these growth factors in the hypothalamus and anterior pituitary is consistent with a role for the SMs in the regulation of CNS and pituitary growth and function. At the very least, there are sufficient data to hypothesize that the somatomedins may: 1) be important in fetal (and, possibly, postnatal) CNS growth and development; 2) be capable of functioning through autocrine, paracrine, as well as endocrine routes; 3) modulate GH synthesis and secretion at both a hypothalamic

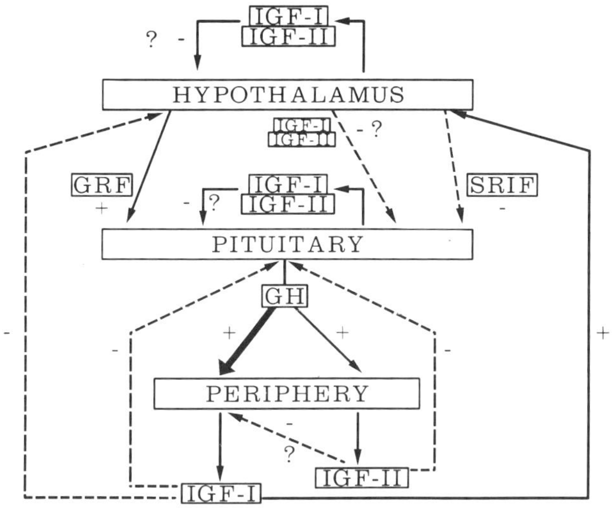

Figure 10. Schematic model of IGF feedback regulation of GH and somatomedin production. Questionmarks indicate still unproven levels of feedback control.

and pituitary level; and 4) regulate somatomedin production at a peripheral level, independent of GH. Figure 10 provides a theoretical model for the multiple levels of somatomedin regulation of both GH and IGF production. Although still speculative, this model provides for a feedback regulatory role of locally produced IGF-I and -II in both the hypothalamus and pituitary. The possibility of GH auto-feedback at the pituitary level must also be considered, although not depicted in this schematic model. Finally, as discussed above, preliminary data now suggest that peripheral production of IGF-I (and, perhaps, IGF-II) may be regulated by the somatomedins, themselves.

Supported by NIH Grants DK 28229, AG01312, and DK 36054. RGR is a recipient of a Research Career Development Award (DK 01275) from the NIH.

REFERENCES

1. J. Zapf, E. Rinderknecht, R. E. Humbel, and E. R. Froesch, Nonsuppressible insulin-like activity (NSILA) from human serum: Recent accomplishments and their physiologic implications, Metabolism 27:1803 (1978).
2. E. Rinderknecht and R. E. Humbel, The amino acid sequence of human insulin-like growth factor I and its structural homology with proinsulin, J. Biol. Chem. 253:2769 (1978).
3. E. Rinderknecht and R. E. Humbel, Primary structure of human insulin-like growth factor II, FEBS Lett. 89:283 (1978).
4. H. Marquardt, G. J. Todaro, L. E. Henderson, and S. Oroszlan, Purification and primary structure of a polypeptide with multiplication-stimulating activity from rat liver cell cultures, J. Biol. Chem 256:6859 (1981).

5. M. Jansen, F. M. A. Van Schaik, A. T. Ricker, B. Bullock, D. E. Woods, K. H. Gabbay, A. L., Nussbaum, J. S. Sussenbach, and J. L. Van den Brande, Sequence of cDNA encoding human insulin-like growth factor I precursor. Nature 306:609 (1983).
6. G. I. Bell, J. P. Merryweather, R. Sanchez-Pescador, N. M. Stempien, L. Preistly, J. Scott, and L. B. Rall, Sequence of a cDNA clone encoding human preproinsulin-like growth factor II, Nature 310:778 (1984).
7. J. E. Brissenden, A. Ullrich, and U. Francke, Human chromosomal mapping of genes for insulin-like grwoth factors I and II and epidermal growth factor, Nature 310:781 (1984).
8. J. V. Tricoli, L. B. Rall, J. Scott, G. I. Bell, and T. B. Shows, Localization of insulin-like growth factor genes to human chromosomes 11 and 12, Nature 310:784 (1984).
9. R. G. Rosenfeld and R. L. Hintz, Somatomedin receptors: Structure, function, and regulation, in: "The Receptors, Vol. III," P. M. Conn, ed., Academic Press, Inc., Orlando (1986).
10. J. Massague and M. P. Czech, The subunit structures of two distinct receptors for insulin-like grwoth factors I and II and their relationship to the insulin receptor, J. Biol. Chem. 257:5038 (1982).
11. M. Kasuga, E. Van Obberghen, S. P. Nissley, and M. M. Rechler, Demonstration of two subtypes of insulin-like growth factor receptors by affinity crosslinking, J. Biol. Chem. 256:5305 (1981).
12. S. Gammeltoft, G. K. Haselbacher, R. E. Humbel, M.Fehlmann, and E. Van Obberghen, Two types of receptors for insulin-like growth factors in mammalian brain, EMBO 4:3407 (1985).
13. S. Jacobs, F. C. Kull, Jr., H. S. Earp, M. E. Svobada, J. J. Van Wyk, and P. Cuatrecasas, Somatomedin-C stimulates the phosphorylation of the β-subunit of its own receptor, J. Biol. Chem. 258:9581 (1983).
14. A. Ullrich, J. R. Bell, E. Y. Chen, R. Herrera, L. M. Petruzzelli, T. J. Dull, A. Gray, L. Coussens, Y. C. Liao, M. Tsubokawa, A. Mason, P. H. Seeburg, C. Grunfeld, O. M. Rosen, and J. Ramachandran, Human insulin receptor and its relationship to the tyrosine kinase family of oncogenes, Nature 313:756 (1985).
15. A. Ullrich, A. Gray, A. W. Tam, T. Yand-Feng, M. Tsubokawa, C. Collins, W. Henzel, T. Le Bon, S. Kathuria, E. Chem, S. Jacobs, U. Francke, J. Ramachandran, and Y. Fujita-Yamaguchi, Insulin-like growth factor I receptor primary structure: comparison with insulin receptor suggests structural determinants that define functional specificity, EMBO 5:2503 (1986).
16. Y. Oka, C. Mottola, C. L. Oppenheimer, and M. P. Czech, Insulin activates the appearance of insulin-like growth factor II receptors on the adipocyte cell surface, Proc. Natl. Acad. Sci. U.S.A. 81:4028 (1984)
17. J. F. Haskell, S. P. Nissley, M. M. Rechler, N. Sasaki, L. Greenstein, and L. Lee, Evidence for the phosphorylation of the type II insulin-like growth factor receptor in cultured cells, Biochem. Biophys. Res. Commun. 130:793 (1985).
18. C. G. Goodyer, L. De Stephano, W. H. Lai, H. J. Guyda, and B. I. Posner, Characterization of insulin-like

growth factor receptors in rat anterior pituitary, hypothalamus, and brain, Endocrinology 114:1187 (1984).
19. R. G. Rosenfeld, G. Ceda, D. M. Wilson, L. A. Dollar, and A. R. Hoffman, Characterization of high affinity receptors for insulin-like growth factors I and II on rat anterior pituitary cells, Endocrinology 114:1571 (1984).
20. G. P. Ceda, A. Hoffman, G. Silverberg, D. M. Wilson, and R. G. Rosenfeld, Regulation of growth hormone release from cultured human pituitary adenomas by somatomedins and insulin, J. Clin. Endocrinol. Metab. 60:1204 (1985).
21. R. G. Rosenfeld, G. P. Ceda, C. W. Cutler, L. A. Dollar, and A. R. Hoffman, Insulin and insulin-like growth factor (somatomedin) receptors on cloned rat pituitary tumor lines, Endocrinology 117:2008 (1985).
22. P. Hollander, F. Stanley, and H. H. Samuels, Thyroid and glucocorticoid hormones induce insulin receptors and inhibit insulin degradation in cultured GH cells, 61st Annual Meeting of The Endocrine Society, Anaheim CA (abstract 497) (1979).
23. R. Corin, F. C. Bancroft, M. Sonenberg, and D. B. Donner, Binding and degradation of 125-I-labeled insulin by a clonal line of rat pituitary tumor cells, Biochem. Biophys. Acta 762:503 (1983).
24. D. Turyn, R. M. Attar, and J. M. Dellacha, Characteristics of insulin receptors in a clonal line of rat pituitary tumor cells in culture, Acta Phsiol. Pharmacol. Latinoam. 34:199 (1984).
25. J. Havrankova, J. Roth, and M. Brownstein, Insulin receptors are widely distributed in the central nervous system of the rat, Nature 272:827 (1978).
26. V. R. Sara, K. Hall, H. Von Holtz, R. Humbel, B. Sjogren, and L. Wetterberg, Evidence for the presence of specific receptors for insulin-like growth factors 1 (IGF-1) and 2 (IGF-2) and insulin throughout the adult human brain, Neurosci. Lett. 34:39 (1982).
27. N. J. Bohannon, D. P. Figlewicz, E. S. Corp, B. J. Wilcox, D. Porte, Jr., and D. C. Baskin, Identification of binding sites for an insulin-like growth factor (IGF-I) in the median eminence of the rat brain by quantitative autoradiography, Endocrinology 119:943 (1986).
28. L. S. Phillips, R. Vassilopoulou-Sellin. Somatomedins. N. Eng. J. Med. 302:371;438 (1980).
29. A. J. D'Ercole, G. T. Applewhite and L. E. Underwood, Evidence that somatomedin is synthesized by multiple tissues in the fetus, Devlop. Biol., 75:315 (1980).
30. M. Binoux, P. Hossenlopp, C. Lassare and N. Hardouin, Production of insulin-like growth factors and their carrier by rat pituitary gland and brain explants in cultue, FEBS Lett., 124:178 (1981).
31. A. J. D'Ercole, A. D. Stiles, and L. E. Underwood, Tissue concentrations of somatomedin-C: Further evidence for multiple sites of synthesis and paracrine or autocrine mechanisms of action, Proc. Natl. Acad. Sci. USA, 81:935 (1984).
32. M. Binoux, A. Faivre-Bauman, C. Lassarre, A. Barret and A. Tixier-Viddal, Triiodothyronine stimulates the production of insulin-like growth factor (IGF) by fetal hypothalamus cells cultured in serum-free medium, Dev. Brain Res., 21:319 (1985).

33. G. Haselbacher and R. Humbel, Evidence for two species of insulin-like growth factor II (IGF-II and "big" IGF-II) in human spinal fluid. Endcorinology 110:1822, (1982).
34. M. Backstrom, K. Hall, and V. Sara, Somatomedin levels in cerebrospinal fluid from adults with pituitary disorders. Acta Endocrinol (Kbh) 107:171 (1984)
35. P. P. Zumstein, C. Luthi, and R. E. Humbel, Amino acid sequence of a variant pro-form of insulin-like growth factor II, Proc. Natl. Acad. Sci. USA 82:3169 (1985).
36. G. K. Haselbacher, M. E. Schwab, O. Pasi, and R. E. Humbel, Insulin-like growth factor II (IGF-II) in human brain: regional distribution of IGF II of higher molecular mass forms. Proc. Natl. Acad. Sci. USA 82:2153 (1985).
37. V. R. Sara, C. Carlsson-Skwirut, C. Andersson, E. Hall, B. Sjogren, and A. Holmgren, and H. Jornvall, Characterization of somatomedins from human fetal brain: Identification of a variant form of insulin-like growth factor I. Proc. Natl. Acad. Sci. USA 83:4904 (1986).
38. M. B. Soares, D. N. Ishii and A. Efstratiadis, Developmental and tissue-specific expression of a family of transcripts related to rat insulin-like growth factor II mRNA, Nuc. Acids. Res., 13:1119 (1985).
39. A. L. Brown, D. E. Graham, S. P. Nissley, D. J. Hill, A. J. Strain, and M. M. Rechler, Developmental regulation of insulin-like grwoth factor II mRNA in different rat tissues. J. Biol. Chem. 261:13144 (1986).
40. P. K. Lund, B. M. Moats-Staats, M. A. Hynes, J. G. Simmons, M. Jansen, A. J. D'Ercole, and J.J. Van Wyk, Somatomedin-C/insulin-like growth factor-I and insulin-like growth factor-II mRNAs in rat fetal and adult tissues. J. Biol. Chem. 261:14539 (1986).
41. D. C. Baskin, S. C. Woods, D. B. West, M. Van Houten, B. I. Posner, D. M. Dorsa, and D. Porte, Jr., Immunocytochemical detection of insulin in rat hypothalamus and its possible uptake from cerebrospinal fluid. Endocrinology 113:1818 (1983).
42. W. S. Young III, Periventricular hypothalamic cells in the rat brain contain insulin mRNA, Neuropeptides 8:93 (1986).
43. M. Berelowitz, M. Szabo, L. A. Frohman, S. Firestone, L. Chu, and R. L. Hintz, Somatomedin-C mediates growth hormone negative feedback by effects on both the hypothalamus and the pituitary. Science 212:1279 (1981).
44. T. Shibasaki, N. Yamauchi, M. Hotta, A. Masuda, T. Imaki, H. Demura, N. Ling and K. Shizume, In vitro release of growth hormone-releasing factor from rat hypothalamus: Effect of insulin-like growth factor-I, Regulatory Peptides, 15:47 (1986).
45. G. S. Tannenbaum, H. J. Guyda, and B. I. Posner, Insulin-like growth factors: A role in growth hormone negative feedback and body weight regulation via brain. Science 220:77 (1983).
46. H. Abe, M. E. Molitch, J. J. Van Wyk, and L. E. Underwood, Human growth hormone and somatomedin C suppress the spontaneous release of growth hormone in unanesthetized rats. Endocrinology 113:1319 (1983).

47. P. Brazeau, R. Guillemin, N. Ling, J. Van Wyk, and R. Humbel, Inhibition par le somatomedines de la secretion de l'hormone de croissance stimuleepar le facteur hypothalamique somatocrinine (GRF) ou le peptide de synthese hpGRF. C.R. Acad. Sci. [D] (Paris) T295:651 (1982).
48. C. G. Goodyer, L. DeStephano, H. J. Guyda, and B. I. Posner, Effects of insulin-like growth factors on adult male rat pituitary function in tissue culture. Endocrinology 115:1568 (1984).
49. M. S. Sheppard, and R. M. Bala, Insulin-like growth factor inhibition of growth hormone secretion. Can. J. Physiol. Pharmacol. 64:525 (1986).
50. S. Melmed, Insulin suppresses growth hormone secretion by rat pituitary cells. J. Clin. Invest. 73:1425 (1984).
51. S. Melmed, and S. M. Slanina, Insulin suppresses triiodothyronine-induced growth hormone secretion by GH_3 rat pituitary cells, Endocrinology 117:532 (1985).
52. S. Melmed, L. Nielson, and S. Slanina, Insulin suppresses rat growth hormone messenger ribonucleic acid levels in rat pituitary tumor cells, Diabetes 34:409 (1985).
53. S. Yamashita, and S. Melmed, Insulin regulation of rat growth hormone gene transcription, J. Clin. Invest. 78:1008 (1986).
54. S. Yamashita and S. Melmed, Insulin-like growth factor I action on rat anterior pituitary cells: Suppression of growth hormone secretion and messenger ribonucleic acid levels, Endocrinology 118:176 (1986).
55. S. Yamashita and S. Melmed, Effects of insulin on rat anterior pituitary cells. Inhibition of growth hormone secretion and mRNA levels, Diabetes 35:440 (1986).
56. S. Melmed and S. Yamashita, Insulin-like growth factor-I action on hypothyroid rat pituitary cells: Suppression of triiodothyrionine-induced growth hormone secretion and messenger ribonucleic acid levels, Endocrinology 118:1483 (1986).
57. G. P. Ceda, R. G. Davis, R. G. Rosenfeld, and A. R. Hoffman, The growth hormone (GH) releasing hormone (GHRH)-GH-Somatomedin axis: Evidence for rapid inhibition of GHRH-elicited GH release by insulin-like growth factors I and II. Endocrinology (in press).
58. G. P. Ceda, B. Narog, R. G. Rosenfeld, and A. R. Hoffman, The role of insulin-like growth factors and insulin in the regulation of growth hormone secretion, in "Endocrinology '85", G. M. Molinatti and L. Martini, eds., Elsevier Science Publishers, Amsterdam (1986).
59. C. G. Goodyer, S. Marcovitz, J. Hardy, Y. Lefebre, H. Guyda, and B. I. Posner, Effect of insulin-like growth factors on human fetal, adult normal and tumor pituitary function in tissue culture. Acta Endocrinol. (Kbh) 112:49 (1986).
60. S. Yamashita, M. Weiss, and S. Melmed, Insulin-like growth factor I regulates growth hormone secretion and messenger ribonucleic acid levels in human pituitary tumor cells, J. Clin. Endocrinol. Metab. 63:730 (1986).
61. D. M. Wilson, J. A. Thomas, T. E. Hamm, Jr., J. Wyche, R. L. Hintz, and R. G. Rosenfeld, Transplantation of insulin-like growth factor-II secreting tumors into nude rodents. Endocrinology (in press).

TWO TYPES OF RECEPTOR FOR INSULIN-LIKE GROWTH FACTORS ARE EXPRESSED ON NORMAL AND MALIGNANT CELLS FROM MAMMALIAN BRAIN

Steen Gammeltoft[1], Robert Ballotti[2], Finn Cilius Nielsen[1], Aline Kowalski[2], and Emmanuel Van Obberghen[2]

[1]Department of Clinical Chemistry, Bispebjerg Hospital
DK 2400 Copenhagen, Denmark
[2]INSERM U 145, Faculté de Médicine, Université de Nice
F 06034 Nice, France

SUMMARY

Insulin-like growth factors (IGFs) I and II stimulate cell growth in several mammalian tissues. The cellular actions are mediated by interactions with two types of IGF receptor, which have been characterized by their protein structure, binding specificity, and intrinsic tyrosine kinase activity. Recently, expression of IGF I and IGF II genes and production of IGFs have been demonstrated in mammalian brain. In search for the function of IGF I and IGF II in the central nervous system, we have looked for the presence of IGF receptors on normal and malignant cells from fetal and adult mammalian brain and the growth-promoting effects of IGFs on primary cultures of fetal rat astrocytes.

We have shown that two types of IGF receptor are present on plasma membranes from adult rat brain, on fetal rat astrocytes and on human glioma cells. Type I IGF receptor is composed of 2 types of subunits: α-subunits which binds IGF I and IGF II with high affinity and insulin weakly, and β-subunits which show tyrosine kinase activity and autophosphorylation stimulated by IGF I and IGF II with almost similar potency. The molecular size of the type I IGF receptor α-subunit is larger in cultured fetal rat astrocytes and human glioma cells than in normal adult brain (Mr ∿ 130 000 *versus* 115 000), whereas the β-subunit has the same electrophoretic mobility (Mr ∿ 94 000). The type II IGF receptor is a monomeric protein (Mr ∿ 250 000), which binds IGF II 5 times better than IGF I, and does not recognize insulin. The amounts of type II IGF rceptor are significantly higher in fetal and malignant cells than in adult brain. Based on these findings we suggest that IGF receptors in brain undergo developmental changes, which may have functional implications.

The presence of two types of IGF receptor on brain cells strongly suggests regulatory functions of IGFs in mammalian brain. Results in different laboratories including our own have shown that IGFs stimulate growth of cultured fetal rat astrocytes indicating a role of IGF I and IGF II as growth promotors in the central nervous system. It seems possible that the growth effect is mediated by activation of the type I IGF receptor tyrosine kinase.

INTRODUCTION

Insulin-like growth factors (IGFs) I and II belong to the insulin family of peptides and act as growth promotors on several mammalian cells (Humbel, 1984; Froesch et al., 1985). IGF I induces skeletal growth under the control of growth hormone and is identical with somatomedin C (Van Wyk, 1984). In contrast, the physiological role of IGF II is less clear. Immunoreactive IGF II have been discovered in the cerebrospinal fluid and brain of man, whereas no significant amounts of IGF I-like immunoreactivity could be found (Haselbacher and Humbel, 1982; Haselbacher et al., 1985). Binoux et al. (1981) have reported production of IGFs by rat brain explants in culture. The sequencing of cDNA's encoding IGF I and IGF II precursors (Jansen et al., 1983; Bell et al., 1984; Jansen et al., 1986) has been followed by the demonstration of IGF I and IGF II mRNAs in fetal and adult rat brain using rat and human hybridization probes (Scott et al., 1985; Brown et al., 1986; Lund et al., 1986; Hynes et al., 1987). These observations suggest that gene expression and production of IGFs occur in mammalian brain which raises questions about the functions of IGFs in the central nervous system.

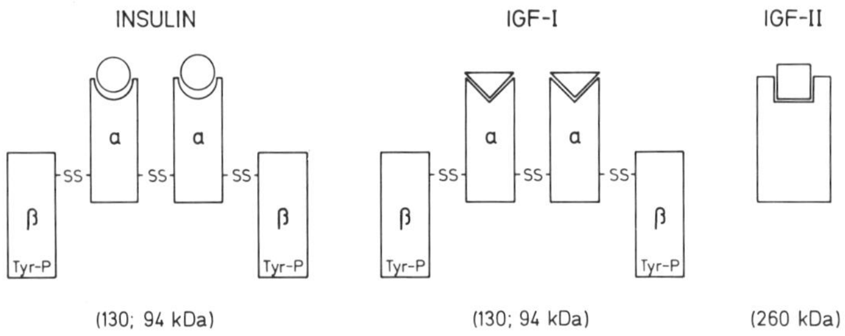

Fig. 1 Subunit structures of receptors for insulin, IGF I and IGF II in mammalian cells. Insulin and IGF I receptors are composed of α-subunits (Mr 130 000), which bind their respective ligands and β-subunits (Mr 94 000) which are autophosphorylated on tyrosine residues. IGF II receptors are monomeric proteins (Mr 260 000) which bind IGF II with high affinity.

In many cells two types of IGF receptor have been identified by their subunit structure, peptide specificity pattern and protein kinase activity (Czech, 1985; Rechler and Nissley, 1985). The type I IGF receptor is an oligomeric glycoprotein composed of two types of subunits (*Fig. 1*). The α-subunits (Mr ∿ 130 000) bind preferentially IGF I, but also IGF II, and insulin weakly. The β-subunits (Mr ∿ 94 000) have intrinsic tyrosine kinase activity, and show IGF-sensitive autophosphorylation (Jacobs et al., 1983; Rubin et al., 1984; Sasaki et al., 1985). Thus, type I IGF receptors are structurally homologous with insulin receptors (Czech, 1985). The homology between insulin and IGF I receptors has recently been documented by the determination of the complete amino acid sequences of the human receptor precursors deduced from cloned cDNA (Ullrich et al., 1985; Ebina et al., 1985; Ullrich et al., 1986).

The type II IGF rceptor is a monomer (Mr ∿ 260 000), which binds IGF II with higher affinity than IGF I and does not recognize insulin. Although the type II receptor is phosphorylated *in vivo* in cultured cells (Haskell et al., 1985a), it seems devoid of intrinsic kinase activity (Corvera et al., 1986). The cellular role of two types of IGF receptor is not clear although it seems possible that type I IGF receptor tyrosine protein kinase mediates the growth actions of IGFs in analogy with the tyrosine protein kinases of other growth factor receptors and retroviral oncogene proteins (Hunter and Cooper, 1985).

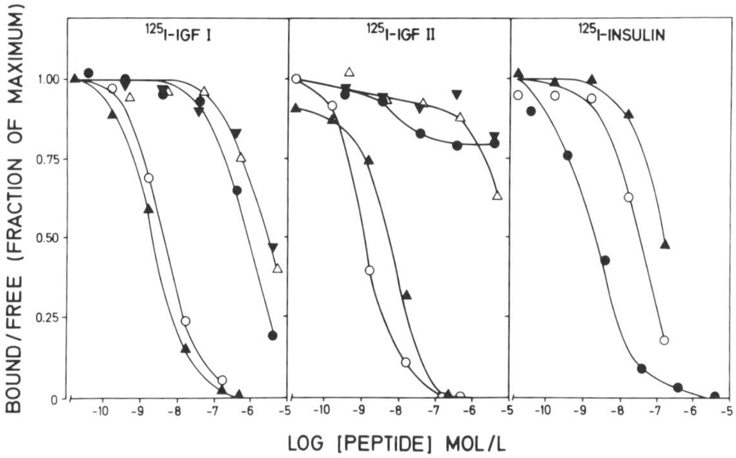

Fig. 2 Competitive binding assay of receptors on adult rat brain cortical plasma membranes. Binding of ^{125}I-labelled IGF I, IGF II or insulin was measured after addition of unlabelled peptides: IGF I (Δ), IGF II (O), porcine insulin (O), coypu insulin (∇) or porcine proinsulin (Δ). Data from Gammeltoft et al. (1985a).

In human and rat brain, receptor binding of ^{125}I-labelled IGF I and IGF II has been observed by several authors (Sara et al., 1982; 1983; Goodyer et al., 1984), but the molecular nature of brain IGF receptors remained unsolved. Our work reviewed here was initiated to describe the structural and functional properties of IGF receptors in different subcellular and cellular preparations of human and rat brain (Gammeltoft et al., 1985a; 1987; Ballotti et al., 1987). The ultimate goal of our studies is to elucidate the possible roles of IGFs in the regulation of normal and malignant cell growth and metabolism as well as neurotransmission in mammalian brain. Recent studies in several laboratories present evidence that IGFs act as growth promotors on astrocytes and oligodendrocytes (Lenoir and Honegger, 1983; McMorris et al., 1986; Schoenee et al., 1986; Ballotti et al., 1987; Han et al., 1987), and as neurotrophic factors on neurons (Burgess et al., 1987).

TWO TYPES OF IGF RECEPTOR ARE PRESENT IN MAMMALIAN BRAIN

The identification of IGF and insulin receptors in rat and human brain is based on competitive receptor binding assay and receptor labelling technique using chemical cross linking of ^{125}I-labelled IGFs or insulin (for experimental details see Gammeltoft et al. 1984a; 1984b; 1985a). Competitive binding assays using purified brain cortical plasma membranes and ^{125}I-labelled IGF I, IGF II or insulin showed distinct receptors for IGF I, IGF II and insulin (*Fig. 2*). Type I IGF receptors recognize IGF I and IGF II with almost similar affinity whereas different insulin analogs are bound with a binding affinity of approximately 1% of that of IGF I. Type II IGF receptors bind IGF II with 5 x higher affinity than IGF I, and do not interact with various insulins. Insulin receptors recognize insulin with 10-100 x higher affinity than IGF II and IGF I, respectively (Gammeltoft et al., 1985a). These patterns are similar to IGF and insulin receptors described in several other tissues (Czech, 1985; Rechler and Nissley, 1985).

Molecular identification of IGF receptors in brain was achieved by the affinity labelling technique. Cross-linking of ^{125}I-IGF I to receptors on adult rat brain cortical membranes, followed by solubilization in SDS and polyacrylamide gel electrophoresis under reducing conditions showed a type I IGF receptor α-subunit with a molecular size of Mr ∿ 115 000, whereas cross-linking of ^{125}I-IGF II preferentially labelled a type II IGF receptor with Mr ∿ 250 000 (Gammeltoft et al., 1985a). The α-subunit of the type I IGF receptor in brain has the same electrophoretic mobility as that of the insulin receptor α-subunit (*Fig. 3*), but the two receptors are clearly distinguished by the specificity towards their respective ligands as well as interaction with specific antibodies to IGF I and insulin receptors (Gammeltoft et al., 1985a). In conclusion, two types of IGF receptors have been identified in adult rat brain by their binding specifity and subunit structure. The IGF receptors are clearly distinguished from insulin receptors in brain.

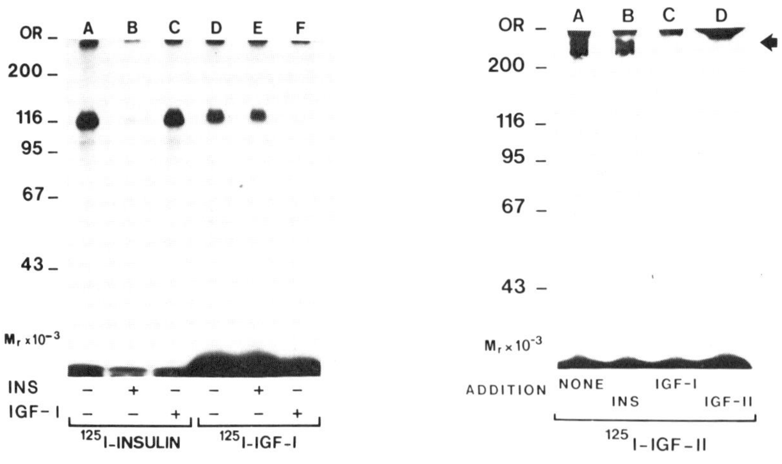

Fig. 3 Affinity labelling of receptors on adult rat brain cortical plasma membranes. Bound ^{125}I-labelled insulin, IGF I or IGF II in the absence or presence of 10^{-6} mol/l of unlabelled insulin, IGF I or IGF II was cross-linked by addition of 10^{-4} mol/l disuccinimidyl suberate. ^{125}I-labelled proteins were analyzed by SDS-polyacrylamide gel electrophoresis under reducing conditions followed by autoradiography. Data from Gammeltoft et al. (1985a).

Table I. Distribution of immunoreactive IGF II and receptor-bound IGF I and IGF II in various regions of adult human and rat brain. Data from Haselbacher et al.(1985) and Gammeltoft et al. (1985a).

Brain region	Immunoreactive IGF II (ng/g wet weight) in human brain	Receptor-bound IGF I and IGF II (pmol/g membrane protein) in rat brain	
Cerebral cortex	1-13	3.2	2.9
Hippocampus	11	3.8	2.6
Forebrain nuclei	4-7	2.7/3.1	1.9/4.1
Thalamus	6	2.3	1.0
Hypothalamus	<1	1.6	1.4
Cerebellum	3/4	4.2	2.6
Pons	2	0.8	1.4

CELLULAR LOCALIZATION OF IGF RECEPTORS AND INSULIN RECEPTORS IN BRAIN

In rat brain, receptors for IGFs and for insulin are present in all the regions investigated including cerebral cortex, olfactory bulb and tubercle, hippocampus, amygdala, corpus striatum, thalamus, hypothalamus, cerebellum and pons (Havrankova et al., 1981; Gammeltoft et al., 1984a; 1985a). The pattern of distribution of receptors in rat brain in membrane binding studies is strikingly similar to that determined recently in quantitative autoradiographic studies of insulin receptors (Hill et al., 1986; Werther et al., 1987) and of IGF I receptors (G.A. Werther, personal communication).

The distribution of immunoreactive IGF II has previously been determined in human brain although the cellular site of synthesis is not clear (Haselbacher et al., 1985). *Table I* shows the regional distribution of IGF II immunoreactivity in human brain and of IGF I and IGF II receptor binding in rat brain. A comparison between these two sets of data obtained in two different mammalian species (Haselbacher et al., 1985; Gammeltoft et al., 1985a) reveals that the relative distribution of IGF II peptide in human brain is in good agreement with the relative distribution of the two types of IGF receptors in rat brain. This may suggest that IGF II acts as an intrinsic paracrine growth factor in different mammalian brain regions, and is not transported by the circulation, cerebrospinal fluid or long-distance neurons in order to exert its actions.

The cellular location of IGF receptors and insulin receptors in the central nervous system cannot be resolved from membrane binding or autoradiographic studies, but in recent studies by ourselves and others, the receptors have been located on cultured brain cells. IGF receptors are expressed on primary cultures of fetal rat astrocytes (Ballotti et al., 1987; Han et al., 1987), human glioma cell lines (Gammeltoft et al., 1987), primary neuronal cultures of rat brain (Burgess et al., 1987), and cultured bovine retinal capillary endothelial cells (King et al., 1985) suggesting that the receptors are ubiquitous in the central nervous system. The same is true for insulin receptors, which have been identified on fetal rat astrocytes and neurons (Lowe et al., 1986), retinal capillary endothelial cells (King et al., 1985) and human cerebral gliomas (Grunberger et al.,

1986; Gammeltoft et al., 1987). These results show that IGF receptors and insulin receptors are widely distributed in mammalian brain on different cellular components: neuronal, glial and vascular cells suggesting that the peptides play a fundamental role in regulation of brain functions.

HETEROGENEITY OF IGF RECEPTORS AND INSULIN RECEPTORS IN MAMMALIAN TISSUES

In adult brain the molecular size of α-subunits of type I IGF receptors is significantly smaller than the value described in several other tissues (Mr 115 000 *versus* 130 000) (Gammeltoft et al., 1985a; Heidenreich et al., 1986). This represents an example of the heterogenity among IGF receptors in different tissues (Nissley and Rechler, 1984). In contrast, the size of the type II IGF receptor in brain is similar to that in other cells (Nissley and Rechler, 1984). Several authors have previously demonstrated that insulin receptors in brain represent a structural subtype regarding the smaller size of their α-subunits in comparison with other tissues (Yip et al., 1980; Heidenreich et al. 1983; Gammeltoft et al., 1984b; Rees-Jones et al., 1984; Cieraldi et al., 1985; Haskell et al., 1985). It has been proposed that the structural heterogeneity of the IGF receptors and insulin receptors may result from differences in N-linked glycosylation (Heidenreich et al., 1983; 1986). It is also possible that the size variations may arise from alternative splicing of the proreceptor mRNA in brain compared with other tissues. Thus, in human placenta two insulin proreceptor mRNAs, which differ in length by 36 nucleotides, have been identified from the cDNA sequences (Ebina et al., 1985; Ullrich et al., 1985).

In a recent study, however, Roth et al. (1986) were unable to confirm the observation by other authors, that insulin receptors in brain are different from those in other tissues regarding their molecular size. Insulin receptors were purified to homogeneity from postmortem human brain cortex by immunoaffinity chromatography, and on SDS-polyacrylamide gel electrophoresis the α-subunit showed a molecular mass of 130 000 similar to that in other tissues (Roth et al., 1986). Apart from differences in methodology, the reason for this discrepancy is not understood. Roth et al. (1986) purified insulin receptors using a monoclonal antibody raised against human placental receptors, whereas other authors analyzed brain insulin receptors by the affinity labelling technique (Yip et al., 1980; Heidenreich et al., 1983; Gammeltoft et al., 1984b). One possible explanation is that the electrophoretic mobility of α-subunits of purified receptors is slower than that of affinity labelled receptors. Alternatively, it may be argued that different insulin receptor populations in brain are analyzed by the two methods. Thus, insulin receptor α-subunits on cerebral microvessels are significantly larger than those on brain cortical membranes (Mr 130 000 *versus* 115 000) (Haskell et al., 1985b). Furthermore, α-subunits of insulin receptors on cultured rat astrocytes show a molecular size of Mr 130 000 (Lowe et al., 1986), whereas those on postmitotic neuronal cultures from rat brain have a Mr value of 115 000 (Burgess et al., 1987).

The structural variation displayed by rat brain insulin receptors compared with other tissues is accompanied by functional changes. These include the absence of negatively co-operative interactions between binding sites (Gammeltoft et al., 1984a; Van Schravendijk et al., 1984), and a different insulin specificity (Gammeltoft et al., 1984a; Hendricks et al., 1984). In rat brain, IGF I, IGF II and insulin from a histricomorph rodent, the coypu, are bound with higher affinity to the insulin receptor than in liver and fat cells (Gammeltoft et al., 1984a). Based on the peptide specificity it

Table II. Concentrations of type I and type II IGF receptors and insulin receptors in adult and fetal brain. Data from Gammeltoft et al. (1985a; 1987) and Ballotti et al. (1987).

	Receptor concentration (pmol/g membrane or cell protein) estimated by Scatchard analysis.		
	Type I IGF	Type II IGF	Insulin
Adult rat brain cortex membranes	120	40	100
Adult human glioma cells	120	250	30
Fetal rat glial cells	100	500	<10

has been suggested that the insulin receptor variant in brain mediate growth activity of insulin rather than metabolic activity (Gammeltoft et al., 1984a; 1985b). Other studies have suggested that atypical insulin receptors with high affinity for IGFs are also present in human placenta and the human IM-9 lymphoid cell line (Hintz et al., 1984; Jonas et al., 1986). In brain placenta and lymphoid cells it may be speculated that insulin exerts growth and metabolic effects via two different subtypes of receptors.

Recent studies by Casella et al. (1986) suggest that two different forms of the type I IGF receptor, designated type IA and IB, are present in human placenta. Type IA binds IGF I with highest affinity and is blocked by antibody to IGF I receptor, αIR-3, whereas type IB binds IGF II with higher affinity than IGF I and is not blocked by αIR-3. It has been speculated that the two different forms of type I IGF receptor are linked to different effects like growth activation and stimulation of amino acid transport, respectively (Casella et al., 1986). In rat soleus muscle IGFs stimulate uptake of xylose and aminoisobutyric acid by interaction with the type I IGF receptor (Yu and Czech, 1984), and in L6 myoblasts the pleiotypic actions of IGFs are mediated by the type I receptor (Ewton et al., 1987). In conclusion, accumulating evidence points to a significant heterogeneity among receptors for insulin and IGFs in mammalian tissues, and that different receptor subtypes may be linked to different cellular responses to insulin and IGFs (Gammeltoft et al. 1984a; Nissley and Rechler, 1984; Gammeltoft and Van Obberghen, 1986).

DEVELOPMENTAL CHANGES OF IGF RECEPTORS AND INSULIN RECEPTORS IN BRAIN

In fetal and adult rat brain the two types of IGF receptor have similar binding characteristics (*c.f. Fig. 2)*, whereas their concentrations show marked variations (*Table II*). In fetal astrocytes the cellular amount of type II IGF receptors is about twice that of type I IGF receptors (Ballotti et al., 1987). On adult rat brain cortical membranes the concentration of type I IGF receptors is significantly higher than that of type II receptors

(Gammeltoft et al., 1985a). Human glioma cells show higher amounts of type II than type I IGF receptor (Gammeltoft et al., 1987). Furthermore, the amounts of insulin receptors are significantly higher in normal adult brain than on fetal and malignant brain cells. These observations suggest that the expression of IGF and insulin receptors undergo significant changes during fetal development and malignant transformation of cells in mammalian brain. Similar changes have been reported for IGF receptors and insulin receptors during development of the central nervous system of the human fetus (Sara et al., 1983) and of the chick embryo (Bassas et al., 1985) as well as during differentiation of cultured myoblasts into myotubes (Beguinot et al., 1985).

Table III. Molecular masses of IGF receptors and insulin receptors in mammalian brain. Data from Gammeltoft et al. (1984b; 1985a; 1987) and Ballotti et al. (1987).

	Molecular weights (10^3 daltons) estimated on SDS-polyacrylamide gel electrophoresis under reducing conditions		
	Type I IGF	Type II IGF	Insulin
Adult rat brain cortex membranes	115,94	250	115,94
Adult human glioma cells	130,98	250	130,98
Fetal rat glial cells	130,94	250	130,94

Analysis of receptor structure revealed significant changes between fetal and adult brain concerning the molecular size of the type I IGF receptor (*Table III*). In primary cultures of undifferentiated fetal rat astrocytes the Mr value of the α-subunit of the IGF I receptor is 130 000 (Ballotti et al., 1987; Han et al., 1987) compared with a value of 115 000 obtained in whole adult brain (Gammeltoft et al., 1985a; Heidenreich et al., 1986). In primary cultures of postmitotic neurons from rat brain cortex the type I IGF receptor α-subunit show a Mr value of 115 000 (Burgess et al., 1987).

A decrease in the molecular size of the brain insulin receptor during development of the fetal and postnatal rat brain has also been demonstrated (Grizzard et al., 1984; Brennan et al., 1986; Lowe et al., 1986). As mentioned above human glioma cells express IGF I receptors and insulin receptors, the molecular size of which is similar to that observed in fetal brain (Grunberger et al., 1986; Gammeltoft et al., 1987). Thus, the structure and cellular concentrations of IGF and insulin receptors show marked changes during fetal development as well as malignant transformation of cells in rat and human brain. The cellular mechanism of these developmental changes and their functional significances are not yet known.

TYPE I IGF RECEPTOR IN BRAIN IS A TYROSINE KINASE

IGF I receptors in human placenta and IM-9 lymphoid cells show intrinsic tyrosine kinase activity, and IGF I-sensitive autophosphorylation of its β-subunit (Jacobs et al., 1983; Rubin et al., 1983; Sasaki et al., 1985; Yu et al., 1986). The elucidation of the IGF I receptor primary structure showed, that its β-subunit portion contains a 257-residue region with tyrosine kinase features which are homologous with the members of the *src* family of tyrosine kinase oncogene proteins, as well as the hormone receptors of this family (Ullrich et al., 1986). The highest degree of sequence homology is found with the insulin receptor tyrosine kinase ($\sim$ 84%) (Ullrich et al., 1985). The structural homology is reflected by the observation that the biochemical characteristics of the IGF I receptor-associated kinase (Sasaki et al., 1985; Yu et al., 1986) are closely similar to those of the insulin receptor kinase (Gammeltoft and Van Obberghen, 1986).

Phosphorylation of the type I IGF receptor β-subunit in human brain has been demonstrated by incubation of solubilized, lectin-purified receptors with (γ-^{32}P) ATP followed by immunoprecipitation with a specific monoclonal antibody to IGF I receptor (αIR-3), and SDS-polyacrylamide gel electrophoresis under reducing conditions (*Fig. 4*). This protocol revealed a protein (M_r $\sim$ 94,000), the phosphorylation of which is stimulated twice by IGF I (10^{-7} mol/l) (Gammeltoft et al., 1985a). Its electrophoretic mobility is similar to that observed in other tissues suggesting that the β-subunit of the IGF I receptor is more conserved than its α-subunit. It has previously been shown that the β-subunit of the insulin receptor in brain is highly conserved in contrast to the α-subunit (Gammeltoft et al., 1984b; Rees-Jones et al., 1984).

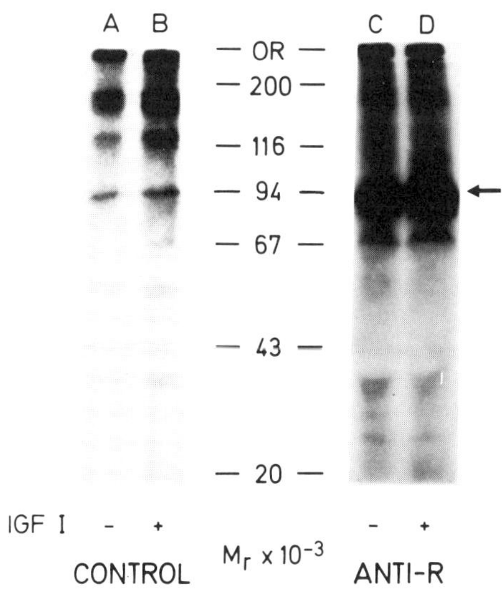

Fig. 4 Phosphorylation of type I IGF receptors on adult and human brain cortical plasma membranes. Partially purified receptors were incubated in the absence or presence of 10^{-7} mol/l of IGF I and phosphorylated with (γ-^{32}P) ATP. Phosphoproteins were immunoprecipitated with antibody αIR-3 to IGF I receptors (anti-R) or mouse IgG (control), and analysed by SDS-polyacrylamide gel electrophoresis under reducing conditions followed by autoradiography. Data from Gammeltoft et al. (1985a).

The high degree of conservation of insulin and IGF I receptor β-subunits suggests that the associated kinase activity may play a fundamental role in the cellular mechanism of action of insulin and IGFs. Apart from ligand binding and kinase activation, the signal transmission is poorly comprehended. Two questions are particular intriguing: the mechanism of receptor transmembrane signalling, and the nature of cellular substrates for the receptor tyrosine kinases. For the dimeric insulin receptor as well as the monomeric receptor for epidermal growth factor it has been suggested that receptor aggregation plays an important role in signal transfer across the plasma membrane (Kahn et al., 1977; Heffetz and Zick, 1986; Schlessinger, 1987). In different cell types insulin-sensitive phosphorylation of membrane and cytosolic proteins has been demonstrated, and it has been suggested that they may play a role in insulin action (Gammeltoft and Van Obberghen, 1986). One of these phosphoproteins (Mr ∿ 120 000) has also been found in brain although its functional role remains to be established (Shemer et al., 1986). So far, endogenous protein substrates for the IGF receptor kinase have not been demonstrated in brain or other tissues.

Recent studies in our laboratory have demonstrated that the type I IGF receptor tyrosine kinase is expressed on glioma cell lines originating from primary human brain tumors, suggesting a role of IGF-stimulated tyrosine protein phosphorylations in brain tumor promotion (Gammeltoft et al., 1987). Furthermore, primary cultures of fetal rat brain cortical glial cells show IGF-sensitive autophosphorylation of tyrosine residues on type I IGF receptor β-subunits. The specificity and dose-response of this effect is similar to that of IGF stimulated thymidine incorporation in cultured astrocytes suggesting a possible role of type I IGF receptor kinase activation in IGF-stimulated glial cell growth (Ballotti et al., 1987). It should be added that in fetal glial cells, the molecular size of the IGF receptor β-subunit is identical to that observed in adult brain (Mr ∿ 94 000), whereas in malignant glioma the size seems to be slightly larger (Mr ∿ 98 000), presumably due to increased degree of glycosylation (*c.f. Table III*).

In conclusion, the type I IGF receptor in brain is a tyrosine kinase, which show IGF-sensitive autophosphorylation of its β-subunit and phosphorylation of exogenous substrates like histones and synthetic peptides. Studies in fetal glial cells suggest that activation of the receptor kinase may possibly play a role in IGF-stimulated cell growth.

IGFs STIMULATE CELL GROWTH IN MAMMALIAN BRAIN

The expression of IGF I and IGF II genes and production of IGF-like immunoreactivity in mammalian brain suggest that IGFs are synthesized in the central nervous system. At present the physiological role of brain IGFs is not clear, but the presence of two types of IGF receptor on neuronal and glial cells suggests that IGFs exert their action within the brain.

Several observations suggest that IGFs exert trophic effects on cells in the central nervous system. IGF I and IGF II increase DNA synthesis in primary glial cell cultures of fetal rat brain (Lenoir and Honegger, 1983; McMorris et al., 1986; Ballotti et al., 1987, Han et al., 1987). In addition, IGF II levels in the frontal cortex of a 3-month old infant with megaencephaly were about ten times higher than in a normal control whereas the amounts of IGF receptors were unchanged. The increase in brain size was mainly due to hypertrophy of cortical glial cells (Schoenle et al., 1986).

Thus, IGFs seem to be active in stimulating glial cell division in developping and postnatal brain. It may be speculated that IGF I and IGF II act as glial promoting factors in adult brain.

IGFs increase RNA synthesis in primary cultures of postmitotic neurons from rat brain (Burgess et al., 1987). This is the first observation that IGF I and IGF II may act as neurotrophic factors in mammalian brain. Furthermore, IGFs may exert regulatory actions on microvascular endothelial cells in the central nervous system. Primary cultures of retinal vascular endothelial cells express two types of IGF receptor as well as insulin receptors, which may be involved in transendothelial transport of their peptide ligands across the blood-brain barrier (King et al., 1985; Haskell et al., 1985b; Frank et al., 1986). It is possible that IGFs are identical with yet unidentified factors which induce formation of intercellular tight junctions during development of the blood-brain barrier in vertebrates (Janzer and Raff, 1987; Abott, 1987).

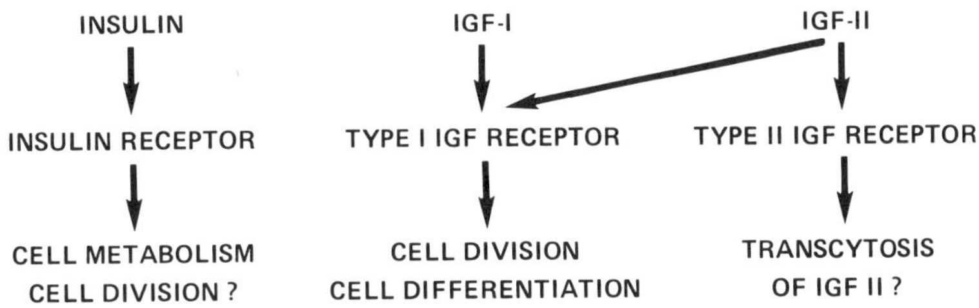

Fig. 5 Model of the cellular mechanism of action of IGF I, IGF II and insulin in mammalian brain. Three types of receptors for insulin, and IGFs are present on neuronal, glial and endothelial cells. Insulin interacts with its own receptor shich stimulates cell metabolism and/or cell division. IGF I or IGF II bind to type I IGF receptor which induces cell division and differentiation. The type II IGF receptor may be involved in transcytosis of IGF II.

The cellular mechanism of IGF effects on glial, neurons and endothelia in mammalian brain is not clear (*Fig. 5*). It is tempting to speculate that the type I IGF receptor with its intrinsic tyrrosine kinase activity mediates IGF effects on cell division, in analogy with the tyrosine kinases of receptors for other growth factors like epidermal growth factor, platelet-derived growth factor and colony-stimulating factor and of several cellular and retroviral oncogene proteins (Heldin and Westermark, 1984). Recently, it has been demonstrated that IGF I induces expression of c-fos in L6 rat skeletal muscle cells, suggesting that IGF I action at least in part may be mediated by c-fos, a cellular oncogene thought to play a role in cell proliferation (Stumpo and Blachshear, 1986; Ong et al., 1987).

In contrast the function of type II IGF receptor seems less clear, but it has been speculated that the type II receptor may have a role in cellular uptake of IGFs (Czech, 1985). This model is based on the observation that insulin increases the apparent affinity of the IGF II receptor (King et al., 1982), and causes a redistribution of the receptor between plasma membranes and low density microsomes in rat adipocytes (Oppenheimer et al., 1983; Wardzala et al., 1984). The effect is similar to the insulin-induced translocation of glucose transporters from an intracellular compartment to the cell surface in fat cells (Cushman and Wardsala, 1980), and the insulin-stimulated redistribution of transferrin receptors in fat cells (Davis et al., 1986). Based on these analogies it may be speculated that IGF II receptors on glial cells and microvascular endothelial cells in brain are involved in cellular uptake and transcytosis of IGFs. A role of this process in intracerebral transport of peptides is possible.

CONCLUSIONS AND PERSPECTIVES

In the present review we have discussed the physiological role and cellular mechanism of action of IGFs in the central nervous system. The concept that IGF I and IGF II may act as growth factors in mammalian brain is based on four kinds of experimental evidence, which has been obtained reecently in different laboratories. (a) Brains of fetal and adult rat contain multiple IGF I and IGF II mRNAs when analyzed by Northern blot hydridizations of poly(A^+) mRNAs. (b) Immunoreactive IGF II and its putative precursors are present in acidic extracts of adult human brain, and IGFs are produced by rat brain explants in culture. (c) Two types of IGF receptor have been identified on membranes and cells from fetal and adult brain. (d) IGF I and IGF II stimulate cell division of rat astrocytes in primary culture, and IGF I induce RNA synthesis of postmitotic neuronal cultures.

The cellular sites of synthesis of IGF I and IGF II in brain are not clear, but it seems possible that both neurons and astrocytes produce IGFs. In addition, IGF I and IGF II in the circulation may be accumulated in the brain by transport across the blood-brain-barrier. IGF II is significantly more abundant in brain than IGF I as judged from concentrations of mRNAs and immunoreactive peptides. It is generally believed that IGF II is a fetal growth-promoting factor based on the higher amounts of IGF II mRNAs in fetal tissues compared with adult tissues of the rat and the higher circulating levels of IGF II in the fetal rat. In rat tissues the expression of the IGF II gene vanishes postnatally with the exception of the central nervous system suggesting a role for IGF II in the adult brain.

In addition to IGF I and IGF II, a number of polypeptide growth factors have been identified in the central nervous system. These include platelet-derived growth factor, nerve growth factor, fibroblast growth factor, and interleukins. This novel observation points to an important role of growth factors in regulation of cell replication and differentiation during development and regeneration of the central nervous system. It may be speculated that the different cellular components of the brain: neurons, astrocytes and endothelial cells communicate in a complex manner through growth factor production, receptor expression and induction of cell division and differention in analogy with the cells of the immune system. Furthermore, growth factors may be associated with the formation of malignant brain tumors. Future research should be directed to define the cellular origins and targets of the polypeptide growth factors to understand their role in the central nervous system.

ACKNOWLEDGEMENTS

Institut National de la Santé et de la Récherche, Paris, France, and European Molecular Biology Organization, Heidelberg, West-Germany are thanked for supporting Steen Gammeltoft during short-term fellowships in INSERM U 145, Nice, France 1984-86. The studies were supported by grants from the Danish Medical Research Council, INSERM, France, NOVO Foundation, Denmark, and the National Cancer Societies of Denmark, Switzerland and Sweden.

REFERENCES

Abbott, N.J., 1987, Glia and the blood-brain barrier. Nature, 325:195.

Ballotti, R., Nielsen, F.C., Kowalski, A., Heldin, C.-H., Van Obberghen, E., and Gammeltoft, S., 1987, Insulin-like growth factors stimulate growth of cultured fetal rat glial cells: possible role of type I receptor tyrosine kinase activation. EMBO J., in press.

Bassas L., Pablo, F. de, Lesniak, M.A., and Roth, J., 1985, Ontogeny of receptors for insulin-like peptides in chick embryo tissues: Early dominance of insulin-like growth factor over insulin receptors in brain. Endocrinology, 117:2321.

Beguinot, F., Kahn, C.R., Moses, A.C., and Smith R.J., 1985, Distinct biologically active receptors for insulin, insulin-like growth factor I, and insulin-like growth factor II in cultured skeletal muscle cells. J. Biol. Chem., 260:15892.

Bell, G.I., Merryweather, J.P., Sanchez-Pescador, R., Stempien, M.M., Priestly, L, Scott, J., and Rall, L.B., 1984, Sequence of a cDNA clone encoding human preproinsulin-like growth factor II. Nature, 310:775.

Binoux, M., Hossenlopp, P., Lasarre, C., and Hardouin, N., 1981, Production of insulin-like growth factors and their carrier by rat pituitary gland and brain explants in culture. FEBS Lett., 124:178.

Brennan, W.A., 1986, Developmental aspects of the rat brain insulin receptor, in: III International Symposium on Insulin Receptors and Insulin Action - Molecular and Clinical Aspects, Madrid. p. 69.

Brown, A.L., Graham, D.E., Nissley S.P., Hill, D.J., Strain, A.J., and Rechler M.M., 1986, Developmental regulation of insulin-like growth factor II mRNA in different rat tissues. J. Biol. Chem., 261:13144.

Burgess, S.K., Jacobs, S., Cuatrecasas, P., and Sahyoun, N., 1987, Characterization of a neuronal subtype of insulin-like growth factor I receptor. J. Biol. Chem., in press.

Casella, S.J., Han, V.K., D'Ercole, J., Svoboda, M.E., and Van Wyk, J., 1986, Insulin-like growth factor II binding to the type I somatomedin receptor. J. Biol. Chem., 261:9268.

Ciaraldi, T., Robbins, R., Leidy, J.W., Thamm, P., and Bernhanu, P., 1985, Insulin receptors on cultured hypothalamic cells: Functional and structural differences from receptors on peripheral target cells. Endocrinology, 116:2179.

Corvera, S., Whitehead, R.E., Mottola, C., and Czech, M.P., 1986, The insulin-like growth factor II receptor is phosphorylated by a tyrosine kinase in adipocyte plasma membranes. J. Biol. Chem., 261:7675.

Cushman, S.W., and Wardzala, L.J., 1980, Potential mechanism of insulin action on glucose transport in the isolated rat adipose cell. J. Biol. Chem., 255:4758.

Czech, M.P., 1985, The nature and regulation of the insulin receptor: Structure and function. Ann. Rev. Physiol., 47:357.

Davis, R.J., Corvera, S., and Czech, M.P., 1986, Insulin stimulates cellular iron uptake and causes the redistribution of intracellular transferrin receptors to the plasma membrane. J. Biol. Chem., 261:8708.

Ebina, Y., Ellis, L., Jarnagin, K., Edery, M., Graf, L., Clauser, E., Ou, J.-h., Masiarz, F., Kan, Y.W., Goldfine, I.D., Roth, R.A., and Rutter, W.J., 1985, The human insulin receptor cDNA: The structural basis for hormone-activated transmembrane signalling. Cell, 40:747.

Ewton, D.Z., Falen, S.L., and Florini, J.R., 1987, The type II insulin-like growth factor (IGF) receptor has low affinity for IGF-I analogs: Pleiotypic actions of IGFs on myoblasts are apparently mediated by the type I receptor. Endocrinology, 120:115.

Frank, H.J.L., Pardridge, W.M., Morris, W.L., Rosenfeld, R.G., and Choi, T.B., 1986, Binding and internalization of insulin and insulin-like growth factors by isolated brain microvessels. Diabetes, 35:654.

Froesch, E.R., Schmid, Chr., Schwander, J., and Zapf, J., 1985, Actions of insulin-like growth factors. Ann. Rev. Physiol., 47:443.

Gammeltoft, S., Staun-Olsen, P., Ottesen, B., and Fahrenkrug, J., 1984a, Insulin receptors in rat brain cortex. Kinetic evidence for a receptor subtype in the central nervous system. Peptides, 5:937.

Gammeltoft, S., Kowalski, A., Fehlmann, M., and Van Obberghen, E., 1984b, Insulin receptors in rat brain: insulin stimulates phosphorylation of its receptor β-subunit. FEBS Lett., 172:87.

Gammeltoft, S., Haselbacher, G.K., Humbel, R.E., Fehlmann, M., and Van Obberghen, E., 1985a, Two types of receptor for insulin-like growth factors in mammalian brain. EMBO J., 4:3407.

Gammeltoft, S., Fehlmann, M., and Van Obberghen, E., 1985b, Insulin receptors in the mammalian central nervous system: binding characteristics and subunit structure. Biochimie, 67:1147.

Gammeltoft, S., and Van Obberghen, E., 1986, Protein kinase activity of the insulin receptor. Biochem. J., 235:1.

Gammeltoft, S., Ballotti, R., Kowalski, A., Westermark, B., and Obberghen, E. van, 1987, Expression of two types of receptor for insulin-like growth factors in human malignant glioma. Cancer Res., in press.

Goodyer, C.G., Stéphano, L. de, Lai, W.H., Guyda, H.J., and Posner, B.I., 1984, Characterization of insulin-like growth factor receptors in rat anterior pituitary, hypothalamus, and brain. Endocrinology, 114:1187.

Grizzard, J.D., D'Ercole, A.J., Wilkins, J.R., Moats-Staats, B.M., and Williams, R.W., 1984, Affinity-labeled somatomedin-c receptors and binding proteins from the human fetus. J. Clin. Endocrinol. Metab., 58:535.

Grunberger, G., Lowe, W.L. Jr., McElduff, A., and Glick, R.P., 1986, Insulin receptor of human cerebral gliomas. Structure and function. J. Clin. Invest., 77:997.

Han, V.K.M., Lauder, J.M., and D'Ercole, J., 1987, Characterization of somatomedin/insulin-like growth factor receptors and correlation with biologic action in cultured neonatal rat astroglial cells. J. Neurosci., in press.

Haselbacher, G., and Humbel, R., 1982, Evidence for two species of insulin-like growth factor II (IGF II and "big" IGF II) in human spinal fluid. Endocrinology, 110:1822.

Haselbacher, G.K., Schwab, M.E., Pasi, A., and Humbel, R.E., Insulin-like growth factor II (IGF II) in human brain: Regional distribution of IGF II and of higher molecular mass forms. Proc. Natl. Acad. Sci. (USA), 82:2153.

Haskell, J.F., Nissley, S.P., Rechler, M.M., Sasaki, N., Greenstein, L., and Lee, L., 1985a, Evidence for the phosphorylation of the type II insulin-like growth factor receptor in cultured cells. Biochem. Biophys. Res. Comm., 130:793.

Haskell, J.F., Meezan, E., and Pillion, D.J., 1985b, Identification of the insulin receptor of cerebral microvessels. Am. J. Physiol., 248:E115.

Havrankova, J., Brownstein, M., and Roth, J., 1981, Insulin and insulin receptors in rodent brain. Diabetologia, 20:268.

Heffetz, D., and Zick, Y., 1986, Receptor aggregation is necessary for activation of the soluble insulin receptor kinase. J. Biol. Chem., 261:889.

Heidenreich, K.A., Zahniser, N.R., Berhanu, P., Brandenburg, D., and Olefsky, J.M., 1983, Structural differences between insulin receptors in the brain and peripheral target tissues. J. Biol. Chem., 258:8527.

Heidenreich, K.A., Freidenberg, G.R., Figlewicz, D.P., and Gilmore, P.R., 1986, Evidence for a subtype of insulin-like growth factor I receptor in brain. Regul. Peptides, 15:301.

Heldin, C.-H., and Westermark, B., 1984, Growth factors: Mechanism of action and relation to oncógenes. Cell, 37:9.

Hendricks, S.A., Roth, J., Rishi, S., and Becker, K.L., 1983, Insulin in the nervous system, in: "Brain Peptides", D. Krieger, M. Brownstein, and J.B. Martin, eds. John Wiley & Sons, New York. p. 903.

Hill, J.M., Lesniak, M.A., Pert, C.B., and Roth, J., Autoradiographic localization of insulin receptors in rat brain: Prominence in olfactory and limbic areas. Neurosci., 17:1127.

Hintz, R.L., Thorsson, A.V., Enberg, G., and Hall, K., 1984, IGF-II binding on human lymphoid cells: Demonstration of a common high affinity receptor for insulin like peptides. Biochem. Biophys. Res. Comm., 118:774.

Humbel, R.E., 1984, Insulin-like growth factors, somatomedins, and multiplication stimulating activity: Chemistry, in: "Hormonal proteins and peptides", vol. XII, C.H. Li, ed. Academic Press, New York. p. 57

Hunter, T., and Cooper, J.A., 1985, Protein-tyrosine kinases. Ann. Rev. Biochem., 54:897.

Hynes, M.A., Van Wyk, J.J., Brooks, P.J., d'Ercole, A.J., Jansen, M., and Lund, P.K., 1987, Growth hormone dependence of somatomedin-C/insulin-like growth factor-I and insulin-like growth factor-II mRNAs. Molec. Endocrinol., in press.

Jacobs, S., Kull, F.C., Earps, H.S., Svoboda, M.E., Van Wyk, J.J., and Cuatrecasas, P., 1983, Somatomedin-C stimulates the phosphorylation of the β-subunit of its own receptor. J. Biol. Chem., 258:9581.

Jansen, M., Van Schaik, F.M.A., Ricker, A.T., Bullock, B., Woods, D.E., Gabbay, K.H., Nussbaum, A.L., Sussenbach, J.S., and Van den Brande J.L., 1983, Sequence of cDNA encoding human insulin-like growth factor I precursor. Nature, 306:609.

Jansen, M., Van Schaik, F.M.A., Van Tol, H., Van den Brande, J.L., and Sussenbach, J.S., 1985, Nucleotide sequences of cDNAs encoding precursors of human insulin-like growth factor II (IGF-II) and an IGF-II variant. FEBS Lett., 179:243.

Janzer, R.C., and Raff, M.C., 1987, Astrocytes induce blood-brain barrier properties in endothelial cells. Nature, 325:253.

Jonas, H.A., Newman, J.D., and Harrison, L.C., An atypical insulin receptor with high affinity for insulin-like growth factors copurified with placental insulin receptors. Proc. Natl. Acad. Sci. (USA), 83:4124.

Kahn, C.R., Baird, K.L., Jarrett, D.B., and Flier, J.S., 1978, Direct demonstration that receptor crosslinking or aggregation is important in insulin action. Proc. Natl. Acad. Sci. (USA), 75:4209.

King, G.L., Rechler, M.M., and Kahn, C.R., 1982, Interactions between the receptors for insulin and the insulin-like growth factors on adipocytes. J. Biol. Chem., 258:10001.

King, G.L., Goodman, A.D., Buzney, S., Moses, A., and Kahn, C.R., 1985, Receptors and growth-promoting effects of insulin and insulinlike growth factors on cells from bovine retinal capillaries and aorta. J. Clin. Invest., 75:1028.

Lenoir, D., and Honegger, P., 1983, Insulin-like growth factor I (IGF I) stimulates DNA synthesis in fetal rat brain cell cultures. Devel. Brain Res. 7:205.

Lowe, W.L., Boyd, F.T., Clarke, D.W., Raizada, M.K., Hart, C., and LeRoith, D., 1986, Development of brain insulin receptors: Structural and functional studies of insulin receptors from whole brain and primary cell cultures. Endocrinology, 119:25.

Lund, P.K., Moats-Staats, B.M., Hynes, M.A., Simmons, J.G., Jansen, M., D'Ercole, A.J., and Van Wyk, J.J., 1986, Somatomedin-C/insulin-like growth factor-I and insulin-like growth factor-II mRNAs in rat fetal and adult tissues. J. Biol. Chem., 261:14539.

McMorris, F.A., Smith, T.M., DeSalvo, S., and Furlanetto, R.W., 1986, Insulin-like growth factorI/ somatomedin C: A potent inducer of oligodendrocyte development. Proc. Natl. Acad. Sci. (USA), 83:822.

Nissley, S.P., and Rechler, M.M., 1984, Insulin-like growth factors: Biosynthesis, receptors, and carrier proteins, in: "Hormonal proteins and peptides", vol. XII, C.H. Li, Academic Press, New York. p. 127.

Ong, J., Yamashita, S., and Melmed, S., 1987, Insulin-like growth factor I induces c-fos messenger ribonucleic acid in L6 rat skeletal muscle cells. Endocrinology, 120:353.

Oppenheimer, C.L., Pessin, J.E., Massague, J., Gitomer, W., and Czech, M.P., 1983, Insulin action rapidly modulates the apparent affinity of the insulin-like growth factor II receptor. J. Biol. Chem., 258:4824.

Rechler, M.M., and Nissley, S.P., 1985, The nature and regulation of the receptors for insulin-like growth factors. Ann. Rev. Physiol., 47:425.

Rees-Jones, R.W., Hendricks, S.A., Quarum, M., and Roth, J., 1984, The insulin receptor of rat brain is coupled to tyrosine kinase activity. J. Biol. Chem., 259:3470.

Roth, R.A., Morgan, D.O., Beaudoin, J., and Sara, V., 1986, Purification and characterization of the human brain insulin receptor. J. Biol. Chem., 261, 3753.

Rubin, J.B., Shia, M.A., and Pilch, P.F., 1983, Stimulation of tyrosine-specific phosphorylation in vitro by insulin-like growth factor I. Nature, 305:438.

Sara, V.R., Hall, K, Holtz, H. von, Humbel, R., Sjögren, B., and Wetterberg, L., 1982, Evidence for the presence of specific receptors for insulin-like growth factors 1 (IGF-1) and 2 (IGF-2) and insulin throughout the adult human brain. Neurosci. Lett., 34:39.

Sara, V.R., Hall, K., Misaki, M., Fryklund, L., Christensen, N., and Wetterberg, L., 1983, Ontogenesis of somatomedin and insulin receptors in the human fetus. J. Clin. Invest., 71:1084.

Sasaki, N., Rees-Jones, R.W., Zick, Y., Nissley, S.P., and Rechler, M.M., 1985, Characterization of insulin-like growth factor I-stimulated tyrosine kinase activity associated with the β-subunit of type I insulin-like growth factor receptors of rat liver cells. J. Biol. Chem., 260:9793.

Schlessinger, J., 1986, Allosteric regulation of the epidermal growth factor receptor kinase. J. Cell Biol., 103:2067.

Schoenle, E.J., Haselbacher, G.K., Briner, J., Janzer, R.C., Gammeltoft, S., Humbel, R.E., and Prader, A., 1986, Elevated concentration of IGF II in brain tissue from an infant with macrencephaly. J. Pediat., 108:737.

Scott, J., Cowell, J., Robertson, M.E., Priestley, L.M., Wadey, R., Hopkins, B., Pritchard, J., Bell, G.I., Rall, L.B., Graham, C.F., and Knott, T.J., 1985, Insulin-like growth factor-II gene expression in Wilms' tumour and embryonic tissues. Nature, 317:260.

Shemer, J., Penhos, J.C., and LeRoith, D., 1986, Insulin receptors in lizard brain and liver: structural and functional studies of and subunits demonstrate evolutionary conservation. Diabetologia, 29:321.

Stumpo, D.J., and Blackshear, P.J., 1986, Insulin and growth factor effects on c-fos expression in normal and protein kinase C-deficient 3T3-L1 fibroblasts and adipocytes. Proc. Natl. Acad. Sci. (USA), 83:9453.

Ullrich, A., Bell, J.R., Chen, E.Y., Herrera, R., Petruzzelli, L.M., Dull, T.J., Gray, A., Coussens, L., Liao, Y.-C., Tsubokawa, M., Mason, A., Seeburg, P.H., Grunfeld, C., Rosen, O.M. & Ramachandran, J., 1985, Human insulin receptor and its relationship to the tyrosine kinase family of oncogenes. Nature, 313:756.

Ullrich, A., Gray, A., Tam, A.W., Yang-Feng, T., Tsubokawa, M., Collins, C., Henzel, W., Le Bon, T., Kathuria, S., Chen, E., Jacobs, S., Francke, U., Ramachandran, J., and Fujita-Yamaguchi, Y., 1986, Insulin-like growth factor I receptor primary structure: comparison with insulin receptor suggests structural determinants that define functional specificity. EMBO J., 5:2503.

Van Schravendijk, C.F.H., Hooghe-Peters, E.L., De Meyts, P., and Pipeleers, D.G., 1984, Identification and characterization of insulin receptors on foetal-mouse brain-cortical cells. Biochem. J., 220:165.

Van Wyk, J.J., 1984, The somatomedins: Biological actions and physiologic control mechanisms, in: "Hormonal proteins and peptides", vol. XII, C.H. Li, ed., Academic Press, New York. p. 81

Wardzala, L.J., Simpson, I.A., Rechler, M.M., and Cushman, S.W., 1984, Potential mechanism of the stimulatory action of insulin on insulin-like growth factor II binding to the isolated rat adipose cell. Apparent redistribution of receptors cycling between a large intracellular pool and the plasma membrane. J. Biol. Chem., 259:8378.

Werther, G.A. Hogg, A., Oldfield, B.J., McKinley, M.J., Figdor, R., Allen, A.M., and Mendelsohn F.A.O., 1987, Localisation and characterisation of insulin receptors in rat brain and pituitary gland using in vitro autoradiography and computerised densitometry. Endocrinology, in press.

Yip, C.C., Moule, M.L., and Yeung, C.W.T., 1980, Characterization of insulin receptor subunits in brain and other tissues by photoaffinity labeling. Biochem. Biophys. Res. Comm., 96:1671.

Yu, K.-T., and Czech, M.P., 1984, The type I insulin-like growth factor receptor mediates the rapid effects of multiplication-stimulating activity on membrane transport systems in rat soleus muscle. J. Biol. Chem., 259:3090.

Yu, K.-T., Peters, M.A., and Czech, M.P., 1986, Similar control mechanisms regulate the insulin and type I insulin-like growth factor receptor kinases. J. Biol. Chem., 261:11341.

ROLE OF INSULIN, INSULINLIKE GROWTH FACTORS, AND NERVE GROWTH FACTOR IN NEURITE FORMATION

Douglas N. Ishii[*] and Esperanza Recio-Pinto[**]

[*]Departments of Physiology and Biochemistry, Colorado State University, Fort Collins, Colorado 80523

[**]Department of Physiology and Anesthesiology, Cornell University Medical Center, 1300 York Ave. New York, NY 10021

INTRODUCTION

The formation of proper connections between nerve cells and their targets is an important determinant of the behavioral repertoire of higher animals. Old connections may be broken and new ones established, adding to plasticity for response to a changing environment. Among the many and complex variables contributing to the structure of the neural network are the neurotrophic polypeptides. For decades nerve growth factor (NGF) stood alone as the only identified representative of this class. More recently, evidence has begun to emerge supporting the hypothesis (Recio-Pinto and Ishii, 1984; Ishii et al., 1985) that insulin and the insulinlike growth factors (IGFs) are members of a broad family of structurally related neuritogenic polypeptides. Here we review and extend the experimental observations supporting this hypothesis.

INSULIN AND IGFs ARE MEMBERS OF A SUPERGENE FAMILY

Amino acid sequence data show homologies between insulin (Sanger et al., 1955), IGF-I (Rinderknecht and Humbel, 1978a), IGF-II (Rinderknecht and Humbel, 1978b), mouse NGF (Frazier et al., 1972), human relaxin (Schwabe et al., 1977; James et al., 1977), and insect prothoracicotropic hormone (Nagasawa et al., 1986). Somatomedin A (Engberg et al., 1984) and somatomedin C (Klapper et al., 1983) are the same as IGF-I. Rat IGF-I has been partially sequenced (Rubin et al., 1982). Multiplication stimulating activity (Marquardt et al., 1981) is most likely rat IGF-II.

Nucleotide sequence data further support the concept that these proteins are encoded by an extended gene family. cDNA clones encoding rat (Ullrich et al., 1977; Villa-Komaroff et al., 1978) and other vertebrate preproinsulins have been isolated and sequenced. In other vertebrates only a single gene is observed, but the rat and mouse express two functional, nonallelic genes. Gene I appears to have arisen as a retroposon in the rat (Soares et al., 1986).

Human (Dull et al., 1984; Bell et al., 1984; Bell et al., 1985) and rat (Dull et al., 1984; Whitfield et al., 1984; Soares et al., 1985) pre-pro-IGF-II nucleotide sequences have been determined from cDNA and genomic DNA clones, and share the same size and domain structure: signal peptide/B chain/C chain/A chain/D chain/trailer polypeptide. Domains B and C have been re-defined (Soares et al., 1986). Only a single IGF-II gene is detected in human (Dull et al., 1984) and rat (Soares et al., 1986) DNA. It is located downstream from the human insulin (Bell et al., 1985) and the rat insulin-II (Soares et al., 1986) genes. These data support the suggestion for gene duplication followed by a divergent, rather than convergent, mode of evolution (Blundell and Humbel, 1980).

A similar organizational structure is observed for the human IGF-I nucleotide sequences (Jansen et al., 1983; Bell et al., 1985; de Pagter-Holthuizen et al., 1986). There is but a single human IGF-I gene (Bell et al., 1985). The A and B domains of IGFs are homologous to those of proinsulin, but there is no D domain in proinsulin. The C domain of the IGFs is not cleaved out as occurs in the processing of insulin.

It is, therefore, not surprising that insulin and IGFs have overlapping biological activities and can cross-occupy one another's receptors at high concentrations (Zapf et al., 1978; Rechler et al., 1980). A review is available comparing the actions of insulin and IGFs in peripheral tissues (Froesch and Zapf, 1985).

cDNA clones encoding rat, pig, and human relaxin have been sequenced (Hudson et al., 1983). The relaxin gene codes a single polypeptide (signal peptide/B chain/C peptide/A chain) which ultimately is processed to the biologically active form containing the A and B chains linked by disulfide bonds (James et al., 1977). The sequence homology in the A and B chains is somewhat limited between the human relaxin and insulin (Bell et al., 1980) genes. However, introns are located at similar positions in the C peptide. Overall, the suggestion of evolutionary divergence is tentatively supported. A more detailed discussion of the gene structure of the insulin/IGF/relaxin family may be found in Soares et al. (1986).

Considerable amino acid sequence homology is found between the A and B chains of the insect prothoracicotropic hormone (Nagasawa et al., 1986), human insulin, and porcine relaxin. The melanization and reddish coloration hormone (MRCH) is found in the brain and ganglia of armyworms in which pigmentation is regulated by population density (Iwao, 1968; Ogura, 1975). The N-terminal amino acid sequence of MRCH has homology with the C-terminal sequence of IGF-II (Matsumoto et al., 1985). The common ancestral gene must have existed long ago to account for the common sequences observed between insects and mammals. Of course, a comparison of the nucleotide sequences is necessary to establish the nature of these relationships.

There is a suggestion that NGF may more distantly belong to the insulin/IGF/relaxin grouping because the mouse NGF amino acid sequence is about 25% homologous to proinsulin's sequence (Frazier et al., 1972; Bradshaw, 1978). The nucleotide sequences of mouse (Scott et al., 1983) and human (Ullrich et al., 1983) pre-pro-NGF show an even greater degree of homology to that of proinsulin. Nevertheless, it is not yet possible to decide whether convergent or divergent evolution is involved, due to marked differences in the overall organization of their nucleotide sequences. The 3-dimensional structures of NGF and insulin are very different.

RELATIONSHIP BETWEEN GENE EXPRESSION AND REGULATION OF THE NERVOUS SYSTEM

The expression of NGF and IGF-II genes in effector organs is consistent with the expected distribution for neurotrophic factors. However, their distributions are not the same. For example, in adult heart NGF mRNA levels are high (Shelton and Reichardt, 1984) but IGF-II mRNA levels are low (Soares et al., 1987). A large body of evidence supports the current view that NGF is produced in sensory and sympathetic nerve target tissues and attracts the advancing growth cone up a concentration gradient during development. Once synapse formation has occured, the high concentrations of NGF may no longer be required. Smaller amounts of NGF released from tissues are internalized at the nerve terminals and are transported in a retrograde fashion back to the nerve cell body, there to exert its effects. A number of informative reviews are available (Mobley et al., 1977; Bradshaw, 1978; Vinores and Guroff, 1980; Harper and Thoenen, 1980; Shooter et al., 1981).

NGF Gene Expression

An extensive survey reveals that only a single band of 1.3 kb is expressed in various tissues (Shelton and Reichardt, 1984). Adult tissues with extensive sympathetic innervation, such as heart, are found to have higher levels of NGF mRNA than tissues with little innervation, such as skeletal muscle. There is a positive correlation between transcript and catecholamine levels in tissues. The correlation is not exact because brain is found to have high transcript levels, but little sympathetic innervation.

Explanted irides show an increase in NGF mRNA content (Shelton and Reichardt, 1984; Heumann and Thoenen, 1986). However, this phenomenon does not appear to be related to denervation *per se*, because mRNA levels are not elevated in irides denervated *in vivo* (Shelton and Reichardt, 1986).

IGF-II Gene Expression

The unique rat IGF-II gene gives rise to a multitranscript family whose members are distributed with different ratios in different tissues (Soares et al., 1985). The transcripts differ in the presence of alternate 5' noncoding exons, and also in the length of the fourth exon due either to differential splicing or differential polyadenylation. Two promoters have been found, both of which appear to be active. Gene expression is tissue-specific and developmentally regulated. High levels of transcripts are observed in a number of fetal tissues, but only brain and spinal cord are found to have demonstrable levels in the adult (Soares et al., 1987). This is in agreement with a preliminary report that cerebrospinal fluid contains much higher levels of IGF-II activity than serum (Widmer et al., 1985). These data support the hypothesis that IGF-II has an important function in nervous tissue.

The high level of IGF-II gene expression in developing tissues may reflect a state receptive to innervation. The developmental down-regulation of IGF-II transcript levels in rat skeletal muscle (Soares et al., 1985) suggests that gene expression might be regulated by maturation events following synaptogenesis. To test this possibility, the sciatic nerve on the left side was transected in young rats (Fig. 1). The level of IGF-II transcripts in denervated muscle was high, in contrast to that in intact muscle from the contralateral side. Only the 3.4 kb transcript is evident here, but with longer exposure of the autoradiogram the 1.1 kb and other transcripts are revealed. The results show that innervation regulates IGF-II gene expression. These interesting findings will be presented in greater detail elsewhere (D.N. Ishii, M.B. Soares, and A. Efstratiadis, submitted).

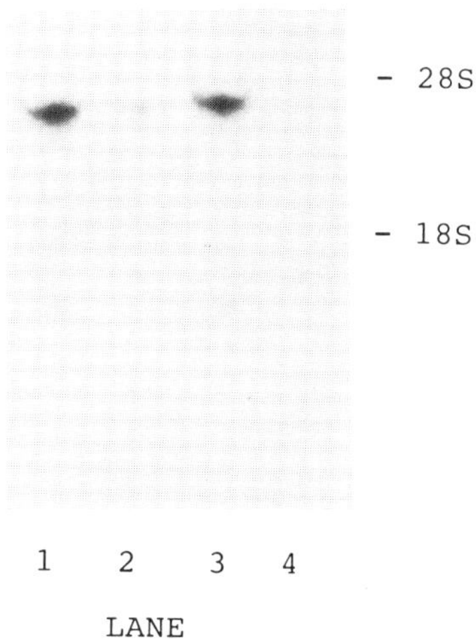

Fig. 1. Denervation causes up regulation of the IGF-II gene in rat muscle. Two littermate rats (11-day-old) were anesthesized with ketamine and phenobarbital, and the sciatic nerve was transected high up in the left hind legs. The right hind legs were unoperated. Muscle RNA samples from the hind right and left legs (gastrocnemius, anterial tibial, peroneus longus, peroneus brevus, and extensor digitorum longus) were isolated from 19-day-old (8 days postoperative) and 24-day-old (13 days postoperative) rats. Equivalent amounts of RNA (40 µg) were electrophoresed in agarose gels containing formaldehyde then transferred to nitrocellulose as described (Soares et al., 1985). The nitrocellulose blots were hybridized to nick translated rat IGF-II cDNA clone 27. Lane 1, operated left hind leg of 19 day-old rat; lane 2, unoperated right hind leg of the same rat; lane 3, operated left leg of 24 day-old rat; lane 4, unoperated right leg. The coding region probe detects a major band in the region of 3.5 kb. For a more complete discussion of the IGF-II multitranscript family consult Soares et al. (1987).

Intact adult muscle will not accept additional innervation. However, denervated muscle returns to a state resembling that of developing muscle and regains the capacity to accept innervation. The level of expression of the IGF-II gene correlates positively with the state receptive to innervation. The expression of the IGF-I gene following denervation has not yet been studied, but IGF-I activity is increased in regenerating sciatic nerves (Hansson et al., 1986). Gene up-regulation following injury to peripheral nerves may be an important event stimulating regeneration.

These results suggest the roles of NGF and IGF-II may be somewhat different during peripheral nerve regeneration. Other data to be presented below support the overview that NGF and insulin/IGFs have complementary and overlapping neurophysiologic actions.

NEURITE GROWTH AND SURVIVAL OF NEURONS

Effects of NGF

The administration of NGF to young vertebrates can cause extensive overgrowth (Levi-Montalcini and Angeletti, 1968), whereas the specific antiserum can lead to destruction of the sensory (Johnson et al., 1980) and sympathetic (Cohen, 1960) nervous system. Neurites can be induced in cultured ganglia (Levi-Montalcini et al., 1954). The capacity of NGF to chemotactically attract growing neurites can be shown *in vitro* (Campenot, 1977; Gunderson and Barrett, 1980) and *in vivo* (Menesini-Chen et al., 1978). The retrograde axonal transport of NGF (Hendry et al., 1974) is believed to be of physiological significance partly because the interruption of transport by axotomy can lead to neuron death, which is preventable by the simultaneous administration of NGF (Hendry and Campbell, 1976).

The overgrowth of the peripheral nervous system produced by administration of excess NGF is not the result of increased neuroblast proliferation. Rather, NGF supports the survival of young neurons during a critical period in development (Charlwood et al., 1974). Neuroblasts are overproduced, probably to ensure all target tissues become innervated, and surplus neurons are destined to die. It is believed that neurons successful in forming synapses may secure a source of the essential NGF through retrograde axonal transport, and unsuccessful neurons are pruned (Hamburger and Oppenheim, 1982).

Insulin and IGFs Stimulate Neurite Formation

The half-maximally (ED50) effective IGF-II concentration is approximately 0.1-0.4 nM for the induction of neurite growth in cultured sensory and sympathetic neurons (Recio-Pinto et al., 1986). Supraphysiological insulin concentrations were earlier reported to induce neurites in cultured dorsal root ganglia cultures (Snyder and Kim, 1980). Under improved culture conditions, physiological concentrations of insulin are now found to be active (Recio-Pinto et al., 1986). Insulin has roughly the same ED50 as IGF-II in sympathetic cultures, but is 300 times lower in potency in sensory cells. It is possible that the low potency of insulin in sensory, parasympathetic (Collins and Dawson, 1983), and brain (Bhat, 1983; Aizenman et al., 1986) neurons is due to cross-occupancy of IGF receptors. Neither the presence of other serum factors, nor of non-neuronal cells, is required for the neurite response (Recio-Pinto et al., 1986). The response to insulin is inhibited by anti-insulin antiserum, but not by anti-NGF antiserum. High concentrations of insulin and IGF-II do not displace NGF from its high affinity receptor, and recombinant insulin is as potent as preparations from tissue sources. The potential that insulin/IGFs may act on brain neurons is of considerable interest, because NGF does not appear to regulate neurite growth within the CNS.

Certain human neuroblastoma cell lines have properties attractive for the study of the effects of neuritogenic factors (for review see Ishii et al., 1985). SH-SY5Y is a cloned cell line in which both the average neurite length and proportion of neurite-bearing cells are increased by insulin and IGF-II (Recio-Pinto and Ishii, 1984). IGF-I also induced neurites at physiological concentrations, and had an ED50 of about 0.5 nM (Fig. 2). For purposes of comparison the dose response to insulin was studied. Insulin's ED50 of about 5 nM compares favorably with the 4 nM previously reported (Recio-Pinto and Ishii, 1984). It is worth noting that this ED50 is reduced to 0.5 nM when bacitracin, an inhibitor of insulin degradation, is added to cultures. Cycloheximide, an inhibitor of protein synthesis, is found to reversibly inhibit insulin-dependent neurite growth and leucine incorporation. Several inhibitors of RNA synthesis, such as actinomycin D, can antagonize the response to insulin. It appears both transcription and translation are important for the insulin effect.

An important aspect of neurite development is the maturation of synapses. Functional synapses can form between cultured retinal ganglion cells and muscle cells (Puro et al., 1982). There is a precocious induction of evocable synaptic transmission in the presence of low concentrations of insulin (Puro and Agardh, 1984).

The incidence of electrotonic coupling between pairs of cultured sympathetic neurons is increased by insulin (Kessler et al., 1984; Wolinsky et al., 1985). Although electrotonic synapses are not known to occur in sympathetic ganglia, it is possible that plasticity may be involved.

Insulin and IGFs Support Neuron Survival

Like NGF, insulin and IGF-II can support the survival of sensory and sympathetic neurons (Recio-Pinto et al., 1986). Their effect on survival is direct on neurons, and not mediated through effects on non-neurons. These factors are not as efficacious as NGF in capacity to support survival. The effect of neurotrophic factors on survival is independent of the effect on neurite formation (Campenot, 1977).

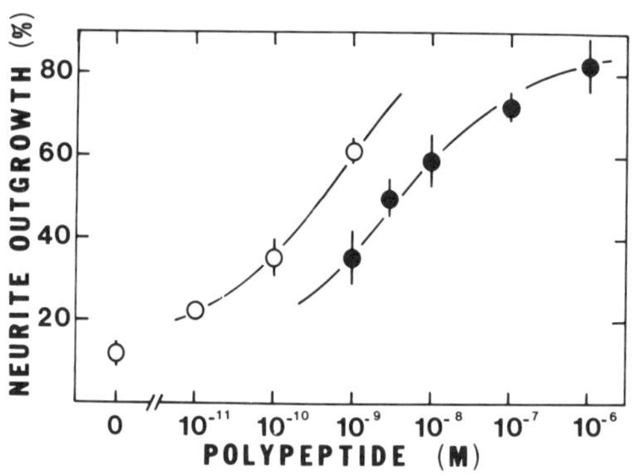

Fig. 2. Effect of various concentrations of IGF-I and insulin on neurite outgrowth in SH-SY5Y cells. Cells were cultured for 3 days in serum-free RPMI 1640 medium containing the indicated concentrations of ligand. (○), IGF-I; (●), insulin. Values are means ± S.D. (N = 3 cultures; 95-180 cells scored per culture). For additional details on methods consult Recio-Pinto and Ishii, (1984).

STIMULATION OF CELL GROWTH AND PROLIFERATION

Insulin can increase thymidine incorporation in human neuroblastoma cells (Recio-Pinto and Ishii, 1984). It appears to do so in certain human neuroblastoma cell lines such as SH-SY5Y, LA-N-5, CHP-100, and CHP-270, but not in IMR-32, MC-IXC, and SH-EP1 cells (Table 1). There appears to be a rough correlation with the capacity for responsiveness with respect to neurite outgrowth (Recio-Pinto and Ishii, 1984). IMR-32 can respond by neurite outgrowth to NGF, but is resistant (Sonnenfeld and Ishii, 1982). Its neurite response to insulin has not been tested. The reason for the

Table 1. Effect of Insulin on ^{3}H-Thymidine Incorporation in Various Human Neuroblastoma Cell Lines

Cell Line	Serum (%)	^{3}H-Thymidine Incorporation[a] (cpm/flask x 10^{-3})	
		Control	Insulin
SH-SY5Y	10	114.4 ± 3.7	146.2 ± 5.4[b]
LA-N-5	1	7.9 ± 0.3	20.5 ± 0.6[b]
CHP-100	1	66.1 ± 10.4	99.6 ± 7.7[c]
LA-N-1	1	18.5 ± 0.7	18.2 ± 0.9
	10	7.7 ± 0.2	8.4 ± 0.2[c]
CHP-270	1	13.1 ± 0.1	17.7 ± 1.5[c]
IMR-32	1	54.5 ± 5.2	55.3 ± 7.8
	10	25.4 ± 1.8	28.1 ± 1.7
MC-IXC	1	82.0 ± 12.6	96.3 ± 11.6
	15	8.9 ± 0.7	9.4 ± 0.4
SH-EP1	1	12.1 ± 1.1	12.4 ± 0.7

[a] Cells were cultured for 1 day in RPMI 1640 medium with the indicated concentration of serum. The incorporation of 3H-thymidine into the trichloroacetic acid insoluble fraction was determined after a 2 hour pulse (Recio-Pinto and Ishii, 1984). The values are means ± S.E.M. (N = 4 cultures). The data are from several experiments.

[b] $P < 0.01$ between treated and untreated cultures.

[c] $P < 0.05$ between treated and untreated cultures.

heterogeneity in response to neuritogenic polypeptides is not understood. Sonnenfeld and Ishii (1982) and Recio-Pinto and Ishii (1984) may be consulted for references to the various cell lines.

The ED50 for the insulin concentration-dependent increase in SH-SY5Y cell population density was about 0.6 nM (Fig. 3). This potency indicates that insulin is acting through its own receptors, rather than through IGF sites in SH-SY5Y cells. Insulin by itself was unable to sustain the population growth rate under serum-free conditions.

IGF-II increased the protein content per cell and the population density (Table 2). The ED50 of about 3 nM indicates that the IGF receptors mediate these effects. These results agree with those of Mattsson et al. (1986) who report that low concentrations of IGF-I and IGF-II can stimulate thymidine incorporation and proliferation of SH-SY5Y cells.

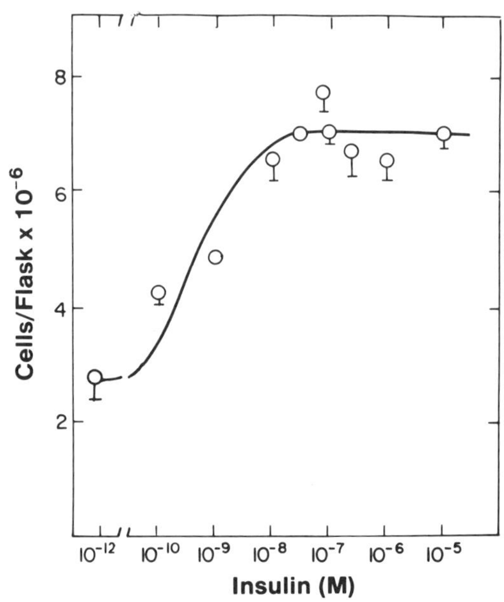

Fig. 3. Effect of various concentrations of insulin on SH-SY5Y cell population density. Cells were incubated for 4 days in RPMI 1640 medium containing 1% serum and the indicated concentrations of insulin. The lowest concentration corresponds to that endogenous to the serum. The number of cells in each culture was determined. Values are means ± S.E.M. (N = 3 cultures). For additional details on methods consult Sonnenfeld and Ishii (1982).

Table 2. Effect of IGF-II on SH-SY5Y Cell Proliferation and Protein Content.

Treatment	Cell Density[a] (cells/flask x 10^{-6})	Protein Content (μg per 10^6 cells)
None	3.64 $\pm$ 0.12	123 $\pm$ 4
IGF-II, 3 nM	6.23 $\pm$ 0.21[b]	152 $\pm$ 6[b]

[a]Cells were cultured for 4 days in serum-free RPMI 1640 medium with and without IGF-II. The cell density and protein content were measured as described by Sonnenfeld and Ishii (1982). The values are means $\pm$ S.E.M. (N = 5 cultures).

[b]$P < 0.01$ between treated and untreated cultures.

One interpretation of these results is that human neuroblastoma cells are arrested in, or have reverted to, an early developmental stage in which the proliferative response to insulin/IGFs is retained.

The studies in neuroblastoma cells support the possibility that insulin/IGFs may regulate survival and/or proliferation of young neurons. For example, insulin can increase ornithine decarboxylase activity (Roger and Fellows, 1980), and uridine and thymidine uptake (Raizada et al., 1980; Yang and Fellows, 1980) in preparations of rat brain. Cerebellar cell survival is supported by insulin (Huck, 1982). IGF-I is more potent than insulin in stimulating thymidine incorporation in rat telencephalon cultures (Lenoir and Honegger, 1983). Unqualified support for the hypothesis is, however, not yet possible, because these studies with brain cells did not distinguish between effects on neurons and glia. This caveat is real because insulin can stimulate protein, RNA, and DNA synthesis in brain glial cultures (Clarke et al., 1985).

Insulin's effects on neurite growth are independent of its effects on cell proliferation (Recio-Pinto and Ishii, 1984; Recio-Pinto et al., 1986). For example, insulin can stimulate neurite outgrowth in SH-SY5Y cells whether during exponential growth in medium with serum, or quiescent in serum-free medium. Moreover, sensory and sympathetic neurons in the postmitotic stage of development are able to respond with neurites.

In contrast, NGF is not a mitogen (reviewed in Mobley et al., 1977). Neither thymidine uptake nor the population growth rate is enhanced in various human neuroblastoma cell lines (Sonnenfeld and Ishii, 1982). NGF does, however, stimulate protein and RNA synthesis, and precocious maturation of neuroblasts.

COOPERATIVE INTERACTIONS BETWEEN INSULIN, IGFs, AND NGF

Insulin, IGFs, and NGF can promote neurite growth in the same SH-SY5Y cell (Recio-Pinto and Ishii, 1984) and overlapping populations of sensory and sympathetic neurons (Recio-Pinto et al., 1986). This suggests the possibility for cooperative interactions in the regulation of neurite formation.

Insulin and IGFs can Modulate NGF Binding and Response

SH-SY5Y cells can survive for at least a week in serum-free medium without a decrease in the population density (Sonnenfeld and Ishii, 1982). Growth resumes upon reintroduction of serum.

NGF's capacity to induce neurites is lost in serum-free SH-SY5Y cell cultures (Recio-Pinto et al., 1984). There is no generalized loss in capacity of cells to extend neurites under serum-free conditions, because the cells retain responsiveness to insulin, IGF-II, and tumor promoters (Spinelli and Ishii, 1983). The combination of insulin or IGF-II together with NGF causes a synergistic potentiation of neurite formation. Because 1 nM insulin, and 0.1 nM IGF-II, are active, evidently each ligand causes potentiation through its own receptor. Synergistic potentiation is also observed in PC12 cells (Recio-Pinto et al., 1984).

Synergistic potentiation in SH-SY5Y cells is due, in part, to the capacity of insulin and IGF-II to modulate NGF binding. The properties of the high affinity (Slow) and low affinity (Fast) NGF sites are described in the following section. Under serum-free culture, the capacity of SH-SY5Y cells to bind NGF to high affinity receptors and respond with neurites are concurrently lost (Recio-Pinto et al., 1984). Both functions can be regained by adding serum, insulin, or IGF-II to cultures. Insulin can increase the number but not affinity of Slow NGF receptors.

The effect of insulin on the acute time-course of ^{125}I-NGF binding is shown in Fig. 4. Cells were harvested, then ^{125}I-NGF binding was studied in incubations with or without insulin supplementation. The left panel shows the time course of binding immediately following cell harvest. Down modulation of ^{125}I-NGF binding to Slow receptors was seen, as previously reported (Sonnenfeld and Ishii, 1985). Binding in the presence of insulin was slightly greater.

When cells were preincubated for 6.5 hours prior to assay of NGF binding, there was a substantial decay in binding capacity, which was prevented by insulin (right panel). Insulin maintained the NGF receptor binding capacity (left panel) at the same level as that immediately following the acute down regulation (right panel).

Curiously, preincubation eliminated down modulation of NGF binding (compare left and right panels, Fig. 4). We can think of two explanations. Down modulation may represent decay of NGF activity due to

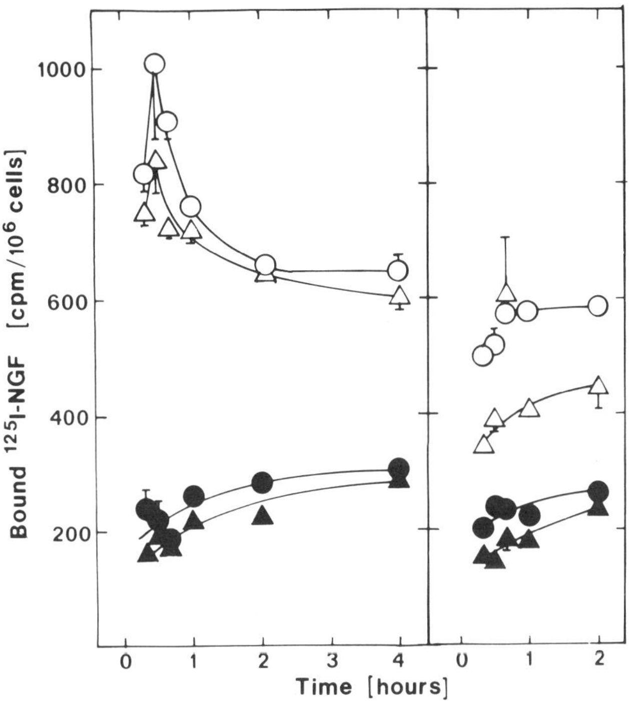

Fig. 4. Effect of preincubation and insulin on the time course of ^{125}I-NGF binding in SH-SY5Y cells. Cells were harvested and incubated at 37°C without or with 0.1 µM insulin in serum-free RPMI 1640. Left Panel: Immediate addition of 0.1 nM ^{125}I-NGF without or with 10 nM NGF. Right panel: Preincubation for 6.5 hours prior to addition of ^{125}I-NGF. (△), no addition; (○), plus insulin; (corresponding solid symbols), nonspecific binding found with 10 nM NGF. Binding was assayed as described (Sonnenfeld and Ishii, 1985). Values are means ± S.E.M. (N = 3).

release from various hormonal influences endogenous to serum. Alternatively, down modulation may represent a redistribution of NGF receptors perturbed during cell harvest. Other receptors are internalized and cycle even in the absence of ligand (Anderson et al., 1982; Oka and Czech, 1986). Whatever the cause, down modulation does not appear to be initiated solely as a result of occupancy of NGF receptors. The widespread interpretation that down regulation is the result of internalization triggered primarily by formation of NGF-receptor complexes may profit from re-examination.

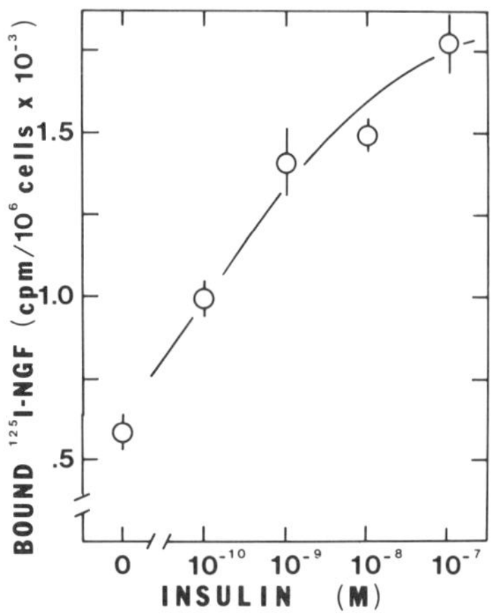

Fig. 5. Effect of various concentrations of insulin on binding capacity of Slow NGF receptors in SH-SY5Y cells. Cells were cultured for two days in RPMI 1640 medium containing 12% serum and the indicated concentrations of insulin. Following harvest, cells were incubated for 3 hours with the same concentrations of insulin, 0.1 nM ^{125}I-NGF, and without or with 10 nM NGF. Binding was assayed as described (Sonnenfeld and Ishii, 1985). Only specific binding to the high affinity Slow NGF receptor is shown. Values are percentages of untreated cultures and are means $\pm$ S.E.M. (N = 3 replicate determinations).

The relationship between insulin concentration and capacity to bind ^{125}I-NGF to Slow receptors is shown in Fig. 5. The cells were cultured for 2 days with various concentrations of insulin, then ^{125}I-NGF binding was studied. The dose-response relationship was broad and had the same shape as the curve for insulin-dependent neurite growth (Recio-Pinto and Ishii, 1984). It is likely that NGF binding and response is modulated through the insulin receptors at physiological concentrations, because insulin was active at 1 nM. NGF receptor binding capacity may be further activated through cross-occupancy of IGF receptors at high insulin concentrations.

Table 3. Effect of Cell Density, Serum, and Insulin on ^{125}I-NGF Binding in LA-N-1 Cells

Treatment	Specifically Bound ^{125}I-NGF (cpm/10^6 cells) Fast	Slow
A.		
Confluent	1424 ± 195	979 ± 191
Non-confluent	0 ± 0	1452 ± 183
B.		
Serum	836 ± 107	1811 ± 93
Serum plus insulin	2153 ± 130	2103 ± 174
Serum-free	0 ± 0	1472 ± 732
Serum-free plus insulin	791 ± 166	4110 ± 136

Part A: Nonconfluent or confluent cultures were grown in RPMI 1640 medium with 12% serum. Cells were harvested and incubated for 1 hour at 37C with 0.1 nM radioactive NGF (177 cpm/pg) alone and with 0.1 μM NGF. Fast and Slow NGF binding was measured (Sonnenfeld and Ishii, 1985).

Part B: Confluent cultures were grown for 3 days in RPMI 1640 medium in some cases supplemented with 12% serum, 0.1 μM insulin, or both, as indicated. Cells were assayed for Fast and Slow NGF sites as above (radioactive NGF, 59 cpm/pg).

Only specific binding is shown. Values are means ± S.E.M. (N = 3).

Some human neuroblastoma cells have both Fast and Slow NGF sites (Sonnenfeld and Ishii, 1982; 1985). ^{125}I-NGF binding to the Fast NGF sites in LA-N-1 cells was also increased by insulin or serum (Table 3).

Fast and Slow sites appear to be independently regulated: (a) Fast but not Slow sites were lost in non-confluent cell cultures (Table 3, Part A). Potential contributory influences may include cell-cell contact or release of a diffusible substance. The greater activity of Slow NGF receptors in non-confluent cultures is probably due to reduced degradation of insulin and IGFs. (b) Under serum-free conditions, Fast sites were completely lost but there was little change in the Slow sites (Table 3, Part B). These results show that Fast and Slow NGF sites may both be modulated by insulin, but have distinct responses to signals such as cell density and serum-free environment. For a discussion of other differences between Fast and Slow sites, see Sonnenfeld and Ishii (1985).

Insulin increases Slow NGF receptor binding in LA-N-1 cells grown in the presence or absence of serum, as it does in SH-SY5Y cells (Table 4, Part B). Under serum-free conditions the loss of Slow NGF receptor binding capacity was incomplete compared to the more complete loss observed in SH-SY5Y cells (Recio-Pinto et al., 1984). In the latter cell line, binding was always studied under conditions in which the cell density was much sparcer (Recio-Pinto et al., 1984). Hence, whether the quantitative difference in response is due to density, or other causes such as heterogeneity between cell lines, is not known.

A MODEL FOR NEURITE FORMATION REGULATED BY INSULIN, IGFs AND NGF

The model for neurite formation under multiple regulatory control in SH-SY5Y cells (Ishii et al., 1985) may be extended as shown in Fig. 6. This model is concerned with long-term events such as those involved in development or regeneration.

Receptors for Neuritogenic Polypeptides

Two types of NGF binding sites have been detected (Sutter et al., 1979). High affinity (also referred to as Type I, or Slow) NGF sites have a K_d value of about 1-3 x 10^{-11} M in sensory (Sutter et al., 1979), sympathetic (Olender and Stach, 1980), human neuroblastoma (Sonnenfeld and Ishii, 1982; 1985), and PC12 (Ishii and Mill, 1987) cells. The K_d of the low affinity (Type II, or Fast) NGF sites is about 0.5-2 x 10^{-9} M. The association rate constants for Fast and Slow NGF sites are indistinguishable (Sutter et al., 1979; Sonnenfeld and Ishii, 1985), and differences in affinities are due largely to separate dissociation rate constants. Curvilinear Scatchard plots are best explained by two types of sites, and there is no evidence for negative cooperative interactions (Sutter et al., 1979; Sonnenfeld and Ishii, 1985; Ishii and Mill, 1987). It does not appear that NGF mediates the conversion of low affinity to high affinity NGF sites (Sonnenfeld and Ishii, 1985), but other relationships have not been convincingly ruled out. Fast sites, unlike Slow sites, may be found on non-neurons as well as neurons (Zimmermann and Sutter, 1983).

The K_d value of the high affinity sites correlates with neurite outgrowth within the limited context of simple occupancy theory, but a role for the low affinity sites is not ruled out when modern "spare receptor" theory (Stephenson, 1956) is considered (Ishii and Mill, 1987). High affinity, saturable, and "specific" binding may be found even on non-receptor materials (Cuatrecasas and Hollenberg, 1975; Goldstein et al., 1971). This is particularly a problem with a highly charged molecule like NGF which readily adsorbs to a variety of surfaces. Therefore, it is important to obtain additional evidence that the sites are receptors. It is comforting that antagonists can reversibly inhibit both NGF binding to these sites and neurite outgrowth (Ishii, 1982), indicating that at least

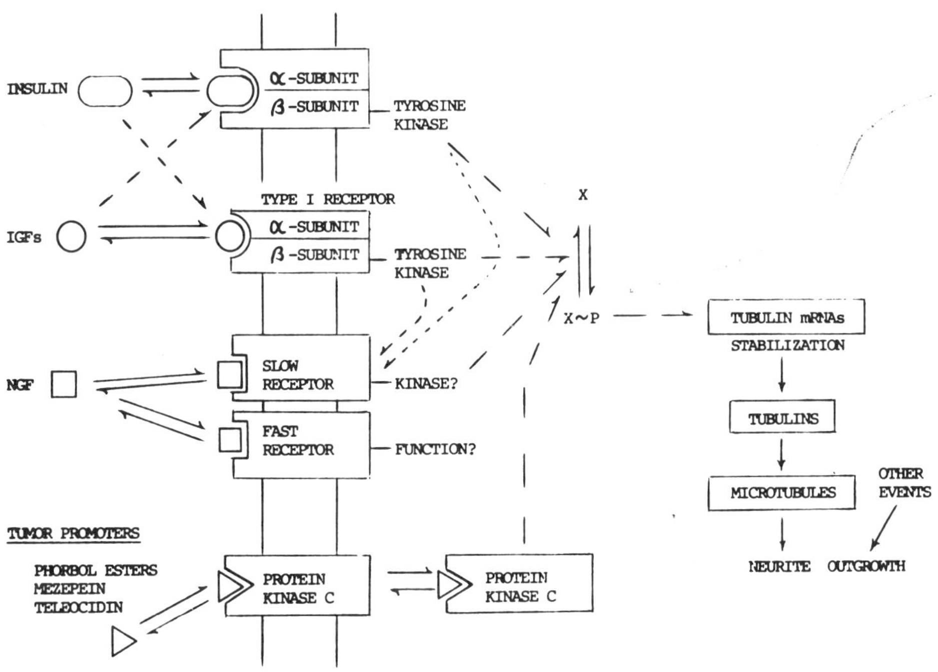

Fig. 6. A model of neurite outgrowth under regulation by multiple neuritogenic factors in SH-SY5Y cells. See text for details.

one of the sites is the receptor. Certain human neuroblastoma cell lines, such as SH-SY5Y, have only the high affinity NGF sites, but, nevertheless, retain the capacity for neurite formation (Sonnenfeld and Ishii, 1982; Sonnenfeld and Ishii, 1985). Moreover, binding to high affinity sites and neurite outgrowth can be concommitantly inactivated and reactivated in SH-SY5Y cells (Recio-Pinto et al., 1984), providing the most convincing evidence supporting the initial speculation by Sutter et al. (1979) that the high affinity NGF sites are the receptors mediating neurite formation. Ishii and Mill (1987) may be consulted for a more complete discussion of NGF binding sites.

Insulin (Posner et al., 1974; Havrankova et al., 1978; Pacold and Blackard, 1979) and IGF (Sara et al., 1981; Goodyer et al., 1984; Rosenfeld et al., 1984) binding sites are present in crude homogenates and particulate preparations derived from brain. Sites are also present on microvessels (van Houten and Posner, 1979) and glia (Clarke et al., 1984). It is difficult to make correlations between average binding parameters in a complex tissue with specific neuronal functions.

The cloned SH-SY5Y cell provides an unusual opportunity to study the relationship between binding of insulin and its homologs and a function of understood neuronal importance, namely neurite formation (Recio-Pinto et al., 1987). Equilibrium and kinetic data indicate there are two types of insulin sites. Neither negative cooperativity nor cross-occupancy of IGF sites can account for the observed heterogeneity in insulin binding. Insulin and IGF-II do not compete for binding to NGF receptors on SH-SY5Y cells (Recio-Pinto and Ishii, 1984). The high affinity insulin site has a K_d of 3 nM, which fits closely the ED50 of 4 nM for neurite outgrowth (in the absence of bacitracin).

The brain insulin receptors are smaller than receptors in peripheral tissues (Yip et al., 1980), due to decreased glycosylation (Heidenreich and Brandenburg, 1986). Furthermore, negative cooperativity is not observed (Van Schravendijk et al., 1984; Gammeltoft et al., 1984). Preliminary reports indicate that the insulin receptors on human neuroblastoma cells are of the brain type (Ota et al., 1986). These observations additionally support the hypothesis that insulin may play a special role in the nervous system.

Type I IGF receptors (Kasuga et al., 1981; Rechler et al., 1983) are additionally present on SH-SY5Y cells (Recio-Pinto et al., 1987). At physiologic concentrations it is evident that insulin and IGFs are acting through their own receptors to induce neurites. At supraphysiological concentrations, cross occupancy may explain insulin's broad dose response curves for increased neurite growth (Recio-Pinto and Ishii, 1984) and tubulin mRNA levels (Mill et al., 1985).

Kinase Activity Associated with Receptors

The phosphorylation of key cellular constituents is a potential common event in the initiation of neurite formation mediated by NGF, insulin, IGFs, and tumor promoters (Ishii et al., 1985; Ishii and Mill, 1987).

NGF can promote phosphorylation of substrates in superior cervical ganglion (Yu et al., 1980) and PC12 (Halegoua and Patrick, 1980) cells. Various NGF sensitive kinases and their substrates have been described (End et al., 1983; Nakanishi and Guroff, 1985; Hama and Guroff, 1985). It is not yet clear whether the high affinity NGF receptor is itself a kinase.

The insulin receptor is comprised of alpha and beta-subunits (Jacobs et al., 1979). An examination of the nucleotide domains of the cDNA encoding the insulin receptor (Ebina et al., 1985) revealed its intrinsic kinase activity on the beta subunit. Insulin can cause phosphorylation of a number of substrates (Cohen, 1982; Burns et al., 1984; Kadowaki et al., 1985), and autophosphorylation of its own receptor (Kasuga et al., 1982). The IGF type I receptor is structurally quite similar to the insulin receptor (Massague and Czech, 1982), and contains kinase activity (Jacobs et al., 1983; Sasaki et al., 1985). Insulin-mediated phosphorylation of a 34 kD protein in SH-SY5Y cells is reversible and correlates with neurite outgrowth (Ishii and Mill, 1987).

The ability of tumor promoters to modulate any neuronal function was first demonstrated in cultured sensory ganglia (Ishii, 1978). Brain has the highest concentration of tumor promoter receptors of any tissue (Blumberg et al., 1981). The tumor promoting phorbol esters, mezerein, and teleocidin can specifically and reversibly induce neurites in SH-SY5Y cells (Spinelli et al., 1982; Spinelli and Ishii, 1983; Ishii et al., 1985). Neither insulin nor NGF can compete for binding to these sites. The tumor promoter receptor is most likely protein kinase C (Castagna et al., 1982; Niedel et al., 1983), and cycles between the plasma membrane and the cell interior.

The direct or indirect phosphorylation of a common intermediate, X~P, may be the transmembrane event shared by the neuritogenic polypeptides and tumor promoting phorbol esters in SH-SY5Y cells. These ligands can cause a similar but not identical pattern of phosphorylation (Halegoua and Patrick, 1980; Hama et al., 1986). We speculate that the various actions of the neuritogenic polypeptides may be mediated through phosphorylation of more than one "second messenger". The commonly phosphorylated intermediate involved in the neurite growth pathway remains to be identified. Biochemical events such as phosphorylation may drive the rapid morphological changes observed in the growth cone and cell surface in response to NGF (Seeley and Greene, 1983; Connolly et al., 1984).

Regulation of Tubulin mRNA Levels

The incorporation of structural proteins into the cytoskeleton of axons and dendrites is a fundamental process in the construction of neurites. Microtubules are important fibrillar elements formed by the polymerization of alpha- and beta-tubulin protein subunits. Excess microtubule production is observed in NGF-induced neurites (Levi-Montalcini, 1966), and neurites disassemble in the presence of drugs that depolymerize microtubules (Yamada et al., 1971).

The capacity of insulin to enhance neurite outgrowth correlates closely with its ability to enhance tubulin mRNA levels in SH-SY5Y cells (Mill et al., 1985). Physiological concentrations of IGF-II are also active. NGF can elevate tubulin mRNA levels in cultured sensory neurons (Ishii and Mill, 1987). It increases tubulin mRNA (Fernyhough and Ishii, 1987), tubulin (Drubin et al., 1985), and microtubule (Luckenbille-Edds et al., 1979) levels in PC12 cells. Interestingly, insulin by itself can neither induce neurites nor increase tubulin mRNA levels in PC12 cells. However, both responses are potentiated when cells are treated with the combination of insulin and NGF, providing another biochemical basis for cooperative interactions (Fernyhough and Ishii, 1987). These results support the important generalization that tubulin transcript levels are specifically elevated whenever neurite elongation is initiated by polypeptide neuritogenic factors (Fernyhough and Ishii, 1987).

The mechanism for elevation appears to involve the stabilization of tubulin transcripts by NGF (Fernyhough and Ishii, 1987) and insulin (J.F. Mill, J.L. Roberts, and D.N. Ishii, in preparation). This suggests that the stabilization of transcripts may be important for maintenance of neurites. This possibility was tested as shown in Fig. 7. When translation was inhibited by cycloheximide in insulin-treated SH-SY5Y cells, neurites were lost with a half-life of less than 5 hours. When transcription was inhibited with actinomycin D, the neurites had a half-

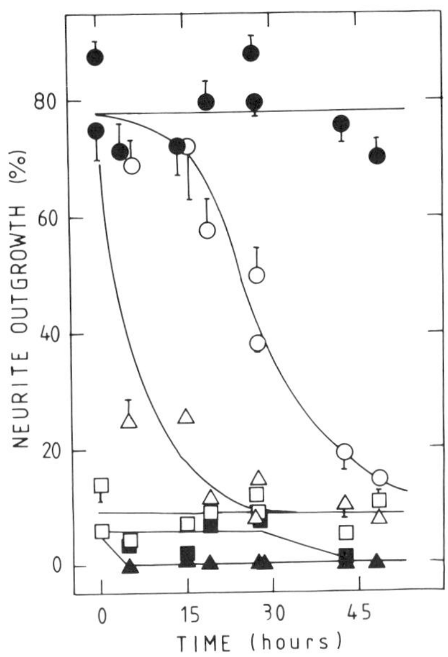

Fig. 7. Effect of cycloheximide and actinomycin D on rate of destabilization of insulin-dependent neurites in SH-SY5Y cells. Cells were cultured for 3 days in RPMI 1640 medium with 1 µM insulin. The cultures subsequently were untreated or treated with 2 µg/ml cycloheximide or actinomycin D as follows: (●), insulin; (△), insulin plus cycloheximide; (○), insulin plus actinomycin D. Cells cultured for 3 days without insulin were subsequently treated as follows: (□), untreated; (▲), cycloheximide; (■), actinomycin D. Neurite outgrowth was scored as described (Recio-Pinto and Ishii, 1984). Two separate experiments are indicated by the direction of the error bars. Values are means ± S.E.M. (N = 4 replicate cultures, 100 cells scored per culture).

life of about 30 hours, suggesting that mRNA loss is rate-limiting for destabilization of neurites. Ongoing translation from pre-existing transcripts continue to support neurites. On the other hand, when insulin was simply washed out effectively reducing putative transcript stabilization, neurites had a shorter half-life of less than 12 hours (Fig. 8). Together, the results are consistent with insulin-mediated stabilization of transcripts as having a functionally important role in the maintenance of neurites.

The data supports the hypothesis that insulin and IGFs are members of an extended family of neuritogenic polypeptides (Recio-Pinto and Ishii, 1984; Ishii et al., 1985). The high levels of IGF gene expression and NGF activity, found during development or following nerve injury, may

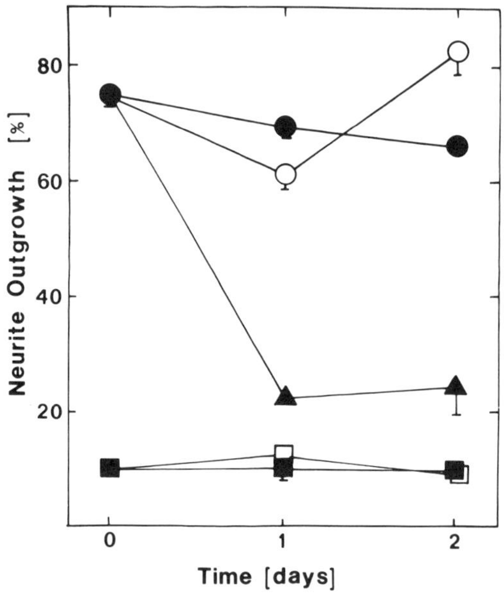

Fig. 8. Reversibility of neurite outgrowth following washout of insulin in SH-SY5Y cells. Cells were cultured for 3 days in RPMI 1640 medium with 0.1 μM insulin, then treated as follows: (●), no treatment; (▲), washed 3 times; (○), washed 3 times and insulin added back. Other cells were cultured for 3 days in RPMI 1640 only, then treated as follows: (■), no treatment; (□), washed 3 times. Neurite outgrowth was scored (Recio-Pinto and Ishii, 1984). Values are means ± range (N = 2).

stimulate the accumulation of tubulin mRNAs in neurons essential for production of additional microtubules for neurite elongation. The neuritogenic polypeptides may cooperate in neurite formation in certain cells, but differences in distribution and actions suggest distinct roles in different populations of neurons.

ACKNOWLEDGEMENTS

This work was supported in part by an award from the Diabetes Research and Education Foundation and grant R01 NS 24787 from the National Institute of Neurological and Communicative Disorders and Stroke to DNI. E. R-P is a postdoctoral fellow supported by NIH grant 2T32 DK07152.

REFERENCES

Aizenman, Y., Weichsel, M.E. Jr., and de Vellis, J., 1986, Changes in insulin and transferrin requirements of pure brain neuronal cultures during embryonic development. Proc. Natl. Acad. Sci. USA, 83: 2263.

Anderson, R.G.W., Brown, M.S., Beisiegel, U., and Goldstein, J.L., 1982, Surface distribution and recycling of the low density lipoprotein receptor as visualized with antirecepter antibodies. J. Cell Biol., 93: 523.

Bell, G.I., Merryweather, J.P., Sanchez-Pescador, R., Stempien, M.M., Priestley, L., Scott, J. and Rall, L.B., 1984, Sequence of a cDNA clone encoding human preproinsulin-like growth factor II. Nature, 310: 775.

Bell, G.I., Gerhard, D.S., Fong, N.M., Sanchez-Pescador, R. and Rall, L.B., 1985, Isolation of the human insulin-like growth factor genes: Insulin-like growth factor II and insulin genes are contiguous. Proc. Natl. Acad. Sci. USA, 82: 6450.

Bhat, N.R., 1983, Insulin dependent neurite outgrowth in cultured embryonic mouse brain cells. Dev. Brain Res., 11: 315.

Blumberg, P. M., Declos, K. B., and Jaken, S., 1981, Tissue and species specificity for phorbol ester receptors. In: "Organ and species specificity in chemical carcino-genesis", R. Langenbach, S. Nesnow, and J.M. Rice, eds., pp. 201-227, Plenum Publishing Corp., New York, New York.

Blundell, T. L., and Humbel, R. E., 1980, Hormone families: pancreatic hormones and homologous growth factors. Nature, 287: 781.

Bradshaw, R. A., 1978, Nerve growth factor. Ann. Rev. Biochem., 47: 191.

Burns, R. G., Islam, K., and Chapman, R., 1984, The multiple phosphorylation of the microtubule-associated protein MAP2 controls the MAP2:tubulin interaction. Eur. J. Biochem., 141: 609.

Campenot, R. B., 1977, Local control of neurite development by nerve growth factor. Proc. Natl. Acad. Sci. USA, 74: 4516.

Castagna, M., Takai, Y., Kaibuchi, K., Sano, K., Kikkawa, U., and Nishizuka, Y., 1982, Direct activation of calcium-activated, phospholipid-dependent protein kinase by tumor-promoting phorbol esters. J. Biol. Chem., 257: 7847.

Charlwood, K. A., Griffith, M. J., Lamont, M. D., Vernon, C. A.,and Wilcock, J. C., 1974, Effects of nerve growth factor from the venom of Vipera russelli on sensory and sympathetic ganglia from the embryonic chick in culture. J. Embryol. Exp. Morphol., 32: 239.

Clarke, D.W., Boyd, F.T. Jr., Kappy, M.S. and Raizada, M.K., 1984, Insulin binds to specific receptors and stimulates 2-deoxy-D-glucose uptake in cultured glial cells from rat brain. J. Biol. Chem., 259: 11672.

Clarke, D.W., Boyd, F.T. Jr., Kappy, M.S. and Raizada, M.K., 1985, Insulin stimulates macromolecular synthesis in cultured glial cells from rat brain. Am. J. Physiol., 249: 484.

Cohen, P., 1982, The role of protein phosphorylation in neural and hormonal control of cellular activity. Nature, 296: 613.

Cohen, S., 1960, Purification of a nerve-growth promoting protein from the mouse salivary gland and its neuro-cytotoxic antiserum. Proc. Natl. Acad. Sci. USA, 46: 302.

Collins, F. and Dawson, A., 1983, An effect of nerve growth factor on parasympathetic neurite outgrowth. Proc. Natl. Acad. Sci. USA, 80: 2091.

Connolly, J.L., Green, S.A. and Greene, L.A., 1984, Pit formation and rapid changes in surface morphology of sympathetic neurons in response to nerve growth actor. J. Cell Biol., 90: 176.

Cuatrecasas, P., and Hollenberg, M. D., 1975, Binding of insulin and other hormones to non-receptor materials: saturability, specificity and apparent "negative cooperativity". Biochem. Biophys. Res. Commun., 62: 31.

De Pagter-Holthuizen, P., van Schaik, F.M.A., Verduijn, G.M., van Ommen, G.J.B., Bouma, B.N., Jansen, M. and Sussenbach, J.S., 1986,

Organization of the human genes for insulin-like growth factors I and II. FEBS Lett., 195: 179.

Drubin, D.G., Feinstein, S.C., Shooter, E.M. and Kirschner, M.W., 1985, Nerve growth factor-induced neurite outgrowth in PC12 cells involves the coordinate induction of microtubule assembly and assembly-promoting factors. J. Cell Biol., 101: 1799.

Dull, T. J., Gray, A., Hayflick, F. S., and Ullrich, A., 1984, Insulin-like growth factor II precursor gene organization in relation to the insulin gene family. Nature, 310: 777.

Ebina, Y., Ellis, L., Jarnagin, K., Edery, M., Graf, L., Clauser, E., Ou, J., Masiarz, F., Kan, Y. W., Goldfine, I. D., Roth, R. A., and Rutter, W. J., 1985, The human insulin receptor cDNA: the structural basis for hormone-activated transmembrane signalling. Cell, 40: 747.

End, D., Tolson, N., Hashimoto, S., and Guroff, G., 1983, Nerve growth factor-induced decrease in the cell-free phosphorylation of a soluble protein in PC12 cells. J. Biol. Chem., 258: 6549.

Engberg, G., Carlquist, M., Jornball, H., Hall, K., 1984, The characterization of somatomedia A, isolated by microcomputer-controlled chromatography, reveals an apparent identity to insulin-like growth factor I. Europ. J. Biochem., 143: 117.

Fernyhough, P. and Ishii, D.N., 1987, Nerve growth factor modulates tubulin transcript levels in pheochromocytoma PC12 cells. Neurochem. Res., In press.

Frazier, W.A., Angeletti, R.H. and Bradshaw, R.A., 1972, Nerve growth factor and insulin: Structural similarities indicate an evolutionary relationship reflected by physiological action. Science, 176: 482.

Froesch, E.R. and Zapf, J., 1985, Insulin-like growth factors and insulin: comparative aspects. Diabetologia, 28: 485.

Gammeltoft, S., Stâun-Olsen, P., Ottensen, B. and Fahrenkrug, J., 1984, Insulin receptors in rat brain cortex. Kinetic evidence for a receptor subtype in the central nervous system. Peptides, 5: 937.

Goldstein, A., Lowney, L. I., and Pal, B. K., 1971, Stereospecific and non-specific interactions of the morphine congener levorphanol in subcellular fractions of mouse brain. Proc. Natl. Acad. Sci. USA, 69: 1742.

Goodyer, C.G., De Stephano, L., Lai, W.H., Guyda, H.J., and Posner, B. I., 1984, Characterization of insulin-like growth factor receptors in rat anterior pituitary, hypothalamus, and brain. Endocrinology, 114: 1187.

Gundersen, R. W., and Barrett, J. N., 1980, Characterization of the turning response of dorsal root neurites toward nerve growth factor. J. Cell Biol., 87: 546.

Halegoua, S., and Patrick, J., 1980, Nerve growth factor mediates phosphorylation of specific proteins. Cell, 22: 571.

Hama, T. and Guroff, G., 1985, Distribution of Nsp100 and Nsp100 kinase, a nerve growth factor-sensitive phosphorylation system, in rat tissues. J. Neurochem., 45: 1279.

Hama, T., Huang, K.-P., and Guroff, G., 1986, Protein kinase C as a component of a nerve growth factor-sensitive phosphorylation system in PC12 cells. Proc. Natl. Acad. Sci. USA, in press.

Hamburger, V., and Oppenheim, R. W., 1982, Naturally occurring neuronal death in vertebrates. Neurosci. Commentaries, 1: 39.

Hansson, H.A., Dahlin, L.B., Danielsen, N., Fryklund, L., Nachemson, A.K., Polleryd, P., Rozell, B., Skottner, A., Stemme, S. and Lundborg, G., 1986, Evidence indicating trophic importance of IGF-I in regenerating peripheral nerves. Acta Physiol. Scand., 126: 609.

Harper, G. P., and Thoenen, H., 1980, Nerve growth factor: biological significance, measurement, and distribution. J. Neurochem., 34: 5.

Havrankova, J., Roth, J., and Brownstein, M., 1978a, Insulin receptors are widely distributed in the central nervous system of the rat. Nature, 272: 827.

Heidenreich, K.A. and Brandenberg, D., 1986, Oligosaccharide heterogeneity of insulin receptors. Comparison of N-linked glycosylation of insulin receptors in adipocytes and brain. Endocrinology, 118: 1835.

Hendry, I.A. and Campbell, J., 1976, Morphometric analysis of rat superior cervical ganglion after axotomy and nerve growth factor treatment. J. Neurocytol., 5: 351.

Hendry, I. A., Stockel, K., Thoenen, H., and Iversen, L. L., 1974, The retrograde axonal transport of nerve growth factor. Brain Res., 68: 103.

Heumann, R. and Thoenen, H., 1986, Comparison between the time course of changes in nerve growth factor protein levels and those of its messenger RNA in the cultured rat iris. J. Biol. Chem., 261: 9246.

Huck, S., 1982, Serum-free medium for cultures of the postnatal mouse cerebellum: Only insulin is essential. Brain Res. Bulletin, 10: 667.

Hudson, P., Haley, J., John, M., Cronk, M., Crawford, R., Haralambidis, J., Tregear, G., Shine, J. and Niall, H., 1983, Structure of a genomic clone encoding biologically active human relaxin. Nature, 301: 628.

Ishii, D. N., 1978, Effect of tumor promoters on the response of cultured embryonic chick ganglia to nerve growth factor. Cancer Res., 38: 3886.

Ishii, D. N., 1982, Inhibition of iodinated nerve growth factor binding by the suspected tumor promoters saccharin and cyclamate. J. Natl. Cancer Inst., 68: 299.

Ishii, D. N., Recio-Pinto, E., Spinelli, W., Mill, J. F., and Sonnenfeld, K.H., 1985, Neurite formation modulated by nerve growth factor, insulin, and tumor promoter receptors. Internat. J. Neurosci., 26: 109.

Ishii, D.N. and Mill, J.F., 1987, Molecular mechanisms of neurite formation stimulated by insulinlike factors and nerve growth factor. Curr. Topics Membrane Res., In press.

Iwao, S., 1968, Some effect of grouping in lepidopterous insects. Colloques. int. Cent. natn. Rech. scient., 173: 185.

Jacobs, S., Hazum, E., Schechter, Y., and Cuatrecasas, P., 1979, Insulin receptor: covalent labeling and identification of subunits. Proc. Natl. Acad. Sci. USA, 76: 4918.

Jacobs, S., Kull, F. C., Earp, H. S., Svoboda, M. E., van Wyk, J. J., and Cuatrecasas, P., 1983, Somatomedin-C stimulates the phosphorylation of the beta subunit of its own receptor. J. Biol. Chem., 258: 9581.

James, R., Niall, H., Kwok, S. and Bryant-Greenwood, G., 1977, Primary structure of porcine relaxin: homology with insulin and related growth factors. Nature, 267: 544.

Jansen, M., van Schaik, F.M., Ricker, A.T., Bullock, B., Woods, D.E., Gabbay, K.H., Nussbaum, A.L., Sussenbach, J.S., and Van den Brande, J.L., 1983, Sequence of cDNA encoding human insulin-like growth factor I precursor. Nature, 306: 609.

Johnson, E. M., Gorin, P. D., Brandeis, L. D., and Pearson, J., 1980, Dorsal root ganglion neurons are destroyed by exposure in utero to maternal antibody to nerve growth factor. Science, 210: 916.

Kadowaki, T., Fujita-Yamaguchi, Y., Nishida, E., Takaku, F., Akiyama, T., Kathuria, S., Akanuma, Y., and Kasuga, M., 1985, Phosphorylation of tubulin and microtubule-associated proteins by the purified insulin receptor kinase. J. Biol. Chem., 260: 4016.

Kasuga, M., Van Obberghens, E., Nissley, S. P., and Rechler, M. M., 1981, Demonstration of two subtypes of insulin-like growth factor receptors by affinity cross-linking. J. Biol. Chem., 256: 5305.

Kasuga, M., Karlsson, F. A., and Kahn, C. R., 1982, Insulin stimulates phosphorylation of the 95,000-dalton subunit of its own receptor. Science, 215: 185.

Kessler, J.A., Spray, D.C., Saez, J.C. and Bennett, M.V.L., 1984, Determination of synaptic phenotype: Insulin and cAMP independently initiate development of electrotonic coupling between cultured sympathetic neurons. Proc. Natl. Acad. Sci. USA, 81: 6235.

Klapper, D.G., Svoboda, M.E., van Wyk, J.J., 1983, Sequence analysis of somatomedin C: Confirmation of identity with insulin-like growth factor I. Endocrinology, 112: 2215.

Lenoir, D. and Honegger, P., 1983, Insulin-like growth factor I (IGF I) stimulates DNA synthesis in fetal rat brain cell cultures. Dev. Brain Res., 7: 205.

Levi-Montalcini, R., 1966, The nerve growth factor: Its mode of action on sensory and sympathetic nerve cells. Harvey Lect., 60: 217.

Levi-Montalcini, R. and Angeletti, P. U., 1968, Nerve growth Factor. Physiol. Rev., 48: 534.

Levi-Montalcini, R., Meyer, H., and Hamburger, V., 1954, In vitro experiments on the effects of mouse sarcomas 180 and 37 on the spinal and sympathetic ganglia of the chick embryo. Cancer Res., 14: 49.

Luckenbille-Edds, L., Van Horn, C., and Greene, L.A., 1979, Fine structure of initial outgrowth processes induced in a pheochromocytoma cell line (PC12) by nerve growth factor. J. Neurocytol. 8: 493.

Marquardt, H., Todaro, G. J., Henderson, L. E., and Oroszlan, S., 1981, Purification and primary structure of a polypeptide with multiplication stimulating activity from rat liver cell cultures. J. Biol. Chem., 256: 6859.

Massague, J., and Czech, M. P., 1982, The subunit structures of two distinct receptors for insulin-like growth factors I and II and their relationship to the insulin receptor. J. Biol. Chem., 257: 5038.

Matsumoto, S., Isogai, A. and Suzuki, A., 1985, N-terminal amino acid sequence of an insect neurohormone, melanization and reddish coloration hormone (MRCH): heterogeneity and sequence homology with human insulin-like growth factor II. FEBS Lett., 189: 115.

Mattsson, M.E.K., Enberg, G., Ruusala, A-I., Hall, K. and Pahlman, S., 1986, Mitogenic response of human SH-SY5Y neuroblastoma cells to insulin-like growth factor I and II is dependent on the stage of differentiation. J. Cell Biol., 102: 1949.

Menesini-Chen, M.G.M., Chen, J.S., and Levi-Montalcini, R., 1978, Sympathetic nerve fibers ingrowth in the central nervous system of neonatal rodent upon intracerebral NGF injections. Arch. Ital. Biol., 116: 53.

Mill, J. F., Chao, M. V., and Ishii, D. N., 1985, Insulin, insulin-like growth factor II, and nerve growth factor effects on tubulin mRNA levels and neurite formation. Proc. Natl. Acad. Sci. USA, 82: 7126.

Mobley, W. C., Server, A. C., Ishii, D. N., Riopelle, R. J., and Shooter, E. M., 1977, Nerve growth factor. New Eng. J. Med., 297: 1096 (Part I), 1149 (Part II), and 1211 (Part III).

Nagasawa, H., Kataoka, H., Isogai, A., Tamura, S., Suzuki, A., Mizoguchi, A., Fukiwara, Y., Suzuki, A., Takahashi, S.Y., and Ishizaki, H., 1986, Amino acid sequence of a prothoracicotropic hormone of the silkworm Bombyx mori. Proc. Natl. Acad. Sci. USA, 83: 5840.

Nakanishi, N., and Guroff, G., 1985, Nerve growth factor-induced increase in the cell-free phosphorylation of a nuclear protein in PC12 cells. J. Biol. Chem., 260: 7791.

Niedel, J. E., Kuhn, L. J., and Vanderbark, G. R., 1983, Phorbol diester receptor copurifies with protein kinase C. Proc. Natl. Acad. Sci. USA, 80: 36.

Ogura, N., 1975, Hormonal control of larval coloration in the armyworm, Leucania separata. J. Insect Physiol., 21: 559.

Oka, Y. and Czech, M.P., 1986, The type II insulin-like growth factor receptor is internalized and recycles in the absence of ligand. J. Biol. Chem. 261: 9090.

Olender, E. J., and Stach, R. W., 1980, Sequestration of ^{125}I-labeled nerve growth factor by sympathetic neurons. J. Biol. Chem., 255: 9338.

Ota, A., Pruss, B.M., Shemer, J., Lowe, W.L., Shepard, A. and LeRoith, D., 1986, Characterization of the insulin receptors in neuroblastoma cell lines. Soc. Neurosci. Abs., 12(Part 1): 371.

Pacold, S. T., and Blackard, W. G., 1979, Central nervous system insulin receptors in normal and diabetic rats. Endocrinology, 105: 1452.

Pilch, P.F., Rubin, J.B. and Shia, M.A., 1983, Insulin-like growth factor dependent protein kinase activity. Fed. Proc., 42: 2252a.

Posner, B. I., Kelly, P. A., Shiu, R. P. C., and Friesen, H. G., 1974, Studies of insulin, growth hormone and prolactin binding: tissue distribution, species variation and characterization. Endocrinology, 95: 521.

Puro, D. G., and Agardh, E., 1984, Insulin-mediated regulation of neuronal maturation. Science, 225: 1170.

Puro, D. G., Battelle, B. -A., and Hansmann, K. E., 1982, Development of cholinergic neurons of the rat retina. Dev. Biol., 91: 138.

Raizada, M.K., Yang, F.W. and Fellows, R.E., 1980, Binding of ^{125}I-insulin to specific receptors and stimulation of nucleotide incorporation in cells cultured from rat brain. Brain Res., 200: 389.

Raizada, M. K., Stamler, J. F., Quinlan, J. T., Landas, S., and Phillips, M. I., 1982, Identification of insulin receptor-containing cells in primary cultures of rat brain. Cell. Molec. Neurobio., 2: 47.

Rechler, M.M., Zapf, J., Nissley, S.P., Froesch, E.R., Moses A.C., Podskalny, J.M., Schilling, E.E., and Humbel, R.E., 1980, Interactions of insulin-like growth factors I and II and multiplication-stimulating activity with receptors and serum carrier proteins. Endocrinology, 107: 1451.

Rechler, M. M., Kasuga, M., Sasaki, N., de Vroede, M. A., Romanus, J. A. and Nissley, S. P., 1983, Properties of insulin-like growth factor receptor subtypes. In: "Insulin-like growth factors/Somatomedins: Basic chemistry, biology, and clinical importance", E.M. Spencer, ed., pp. 459-490. W. de Gruyter, New York, NY.

Recio-Pinto, E., and Ishii, D. N., 1984, Effects of insulin, insulinlike growth factor-II, and nerve growth factor on neurite outgrowth in cultured human neuroblastoma cells. Brain Res., 302: 323.

Recio-Pinto, E., Lang, F. F., and Ishii, D. N., 1984, Insulin and insulin-like growth factor II permit nerve growth factor binding and the neurite formation response in cultured human neuroblastoma cells. Proc. Natl. Acad. Sci. USA, 81: 2562.

Recio-Pinto, E., Rechler, M. M. and Ishii, D. N., 1986, Effects of Insulin, Insulinlike Growth Factor-II, and Nerve Growth Factor on Neurite Formation and Survival in Cultured Sympathetic and Sensory Neurons. J. Neurosci., 6: 1211.

Recio-Pinto, E., Ishii, D.N. and Rechler, M.M., 1987, Insulin and insulinlike growth factor receptors regulating neurite formation in cultured human neuroblastoma cells. J. Neurosci. Res., Submitted.

Rinderknecht, E., and Humbel, R. E., 1978a, Primary structure of human insulin-like growth factor-II. Fed. Eur. Biochem. Soc. Lett., 89: 283.

Rinderknecht, E., and Humbel, R. E., 1978b, The amino acid sequence of human IGF-I and its structural homology with proinsulin. J. Biol. Chem., 253: 2769.

Roger, L.J. and Fellows, R.E., 1980, Stimulation of ornithine decarboxylase activity by insulin in developing rat brain. Endocrinology, 106: 619.

Rosenfeld, R. G., Ceda, G., Wilson, D. M., Dollar, L. A., and Hoffman, A. R., 1984, Characterization of high affinity receptors for insulin-like growth factors I and II in rat anterior pituitary cells. Endocrinology, 114: 1571.

Rubin, J.S., Mariz, I., Jacobs, J.W., Daughaday, W.H. and Bradshaw, R.A., 1982, Isolation and partial sequence analysis of rat basic somatomedin. Endocrinol., 110: 734.

Sanger, F., Thompson, E.O.P., and Kital, R., 1955, The amide groups of insulin. Biochem. J., 59: 509.

Sara, V.R., Hall, K., Misaki, M., Fryklund, L., Christensen, N. and Wetterberg, L., 1983, Ontogenesis of somatomedin and insulin receptors in the human fetus. J. Clin. Invest., 71: 1084.

Sasaki, N., Rees-Jones, R.W., Zick, Y., Nissley, S.P. and Rechler, M.M., 1985, Characterization of insulin-like growth factor I-stimulated tyrosine kinase activity associated with the beta-subunit of type I insulin-like growth factor receptor of rat liver cells. J. Biol. Chem., 260: 9793.

Schwabe, C., and McDonald, J.K., 1977, Primary structure of the B-chain of porcine relaxin. Biochem. biophys. Res. commun., 75: 503.

Scott, J., Selby, M., Urdea, M., Quiroga, M., Bell, G.I., and Rutter, W.J., 1983, Isolation and nucleotide sequence of a cDNA encoding the precursor of mouse nerve growth factor. Nature, 302: 538.

Seeley, P.J. and Greene, L.A., 1983, Short-latency local actions of nerve growth factor at the growth cone. Proc. Natl. Acad. Sci. USA, 80: 2789.

Shelton, D. L. and Reichardt, L. F., 1984, Expression of the beta-nerve growth factor gene correlates with the density of sympathetic innervation in effector organs. Proc. Natl. Acad. Sci. USA, 81: 7951.

Shelton, D.L. and Reichardt, L.F., 1986, Studies on the regulation of beta-nerve growth factor gene expression in the rat iris: The level of mRNA-encoding nerve growth factor is increased in irises placed in explant cultures in vitro, but not in irises deprived of sensory or sympathetic innervation in vivo. J. Cell Biol., 102: 1940.

Shooter, E. M., Yanker, B. A., Landreth, G. E., and Sutter, A., 1981, Biosynthesis and mechanism of action of nerve growth factor. Recent Prog. Horm. Res., 37: 417.

Snyder, E.Y. and Kim, S.U., 1980, Insulin: Is it a nerve survival factor? Brain Res., 196: 565.

Soares, M. B., Ishii, D. N., and Efstratiadis, A., 1985, Developmental and tissue specific expression of a family of transcripts related to rat insulin-like growth factor II mRNA. Nuc. Acids Res., 13: 1119.

Soares, M.B., Schon, E., Henderson, A., Karathansis, S.K., Cate, R., Zeitlin, S., Chirgwin, J. and Efstratiadis, A., 1986, RNA-mediated gene duplication: The rat preproinsulin 1 gene is a functional retroposon. Mol. Cell. Biol., 5: 2090.

Soares, M.B, Turken, A., Ishii, D.N., Mills, L., Episkopou, V., Cotter, S., Zeitlin, S. and Efstratiadis, A., 1987, The rat insulin-like growth factor II gene: A single gene with two promoters expressing a multitranscript family. In press.

Sonnenfeld, K. H., and Ishii, D. N., 1982, Nerve growth factor effects and receptors in cultured human neuroblastoma cell lines. J. Neurosci. Res., 8: 375.

Sonnenfeld, K. H., and Ishii, D. N., 1985, Fast and slow nerve growth factor binding sites in human neuroblastoma and rat pheochromocytoma cell lines: Relationship of sites to each other and to neurite formation. J. Neurosci., 5: 1717.

Spinelli, W., and Ishii, D. N., 1983, Tumor promoter receptors regulating neurite formation in cultured human neuroblastoma cells. Cancer Res., 43: 4119.

Spinelli, W., Sonnenfeld, K. H., and Ishii, D. N., 1982, Paradoxical effect of phorbol ester tumor promoters on neurite outgrowth in cultured human neuroblastoma cells. Cancer Res., 42: 5067.

Stephenson, R. P., 1956, A modification of receptor theory. Brit. J. Pharmacol. Chemother., 11: 379.

Sutter, A., Riopelle, R. J., Harris-Warrick, R. M., and Shooter, E. M., 1979, Nerve growth factor receptors: Characterization of two distinct classes of binding sites on chick embryo sensory ganglia cells. J. Biol. Chem., 254: 4972.

Ullrich, A., Shine, J., Chirgwin, J., Pictet, R., Tischer, E., Rutter,

W.J. and Goodman, H.M., 1977, Rat insulin genes: Construction of plasmids containing the coding sequences. Science, 196: 1313.

Ullrich, A., Gray, A., Berman, C. and Dull, T. J., 1983, Human beta-nerve growth factor gene sequence highly homologous to that of mouse. Nature, 303: 821.

Van Houten, M. and Posner, B.I., 1979, Insulin binds to brain blood vessels in vivo. Nature, 282: 623.

Van Schravendijk, C.F.H., Hooghe-Peters, E.L., DeMeyts, P. and Pipeleers, D.G., 1984, Identification and characterization of insulin receptors on foetal-mouse brain cortical cells. Biochem. J., 220: 165.

Villa-Komaroff, L., Efstratiadis, A., Broome, S., Lomedico, P., Tizard, R., Naber, S.P., Chick, W.L. and Gilbert, W., 1978, A bacterial clone synthesizing proinsulin. Proc. Natl. Acad. Sci. USA, 75: 3727.

Vinores, S. and Guroff, G., 1980, Nerve growth factor: mechanism of action. Ann. Rev. Biophys. Bioeng., 9: 223.

Whitfield, H. J., Bruni, C. B., Frunzio, R., Terrell, J. E., Nissley, S. P., and Rechler, M. M., 1984, Isolation of a cDNA clone encoding rat insulin-like growth factor-II precursor. Nature, 312: 277.

Widmer, U., Zapf, J. and Froesch, E.R., 1984, Insulin-like growth factors and their carrier protein in cerebrospinal fluid of normals and acromegalics. In: "Seventh International Congress of Endocrinology", p1413, Quebec, Canada.

Wolinsky, E.J., Patterson, P.H. and Willard, A.L., 1985, Insulin promotes electrical coupling between cultured sympathetic neurons. J. Neurosci., 5: 1675.

Yamada, K. M., Spooner, B. S., and Wessells, N. K., 1971, Ultrastructure and function of growth cones and axons of cultured nerve cells. J. Cell Biol., 49: 614.

Yang, J.W. and Fellows, R.E., 1980, Characterization of insulin stimulation of the incorporation of radioactive precursors into macromolecules in cultured rat brain cells. Endocrinology, 107: 1717.

Yip, C.C., Moule, M.L. and Yeung, C.W.T., 1980, Characterization of insulin receptor subunits in brain and other tissues by photoaffinity labeling. Biochem. Biophys. Res. Commun., 96: 71.

Yu, M. W., Tolson, N. W., and Guroff, G., 1980, Increased phosphorylation of specific nuclear proteins in superior cervical ganglia and PC12 cells in response to nerve growth factor. J. Biol. Chem., 255: 10481.

Zapf, J., Schoenle, E. and Froesch, E.R., 1978, Insulin-like growth factors I and II. Some biological actions and receptor binding characteristics of two purified constituents of nonsuppressible insulin-like activity of human serum. Europ. J. Biochem., 87: 285.

Zimmermann, A. and Sutter, A., 1983, Beta-nerve growth factor (β-NGF) receptors on glial cells. Cell-cell interaction between neurons and Schwann cells in cultures of chick sensory ganglia. EMBO J., 2: 879.

CONTRIBUTORS

ROBERT BALLOTTI
INSERM V145
Faculte de Medicine
Universite de Nice
F06034 Nice, France

DENIS G. BASKIN
Department of Biological Structure
University of Washington
Seattle, Washington 98195

JOHN J.M. BERGERON
Department of Anatomy
McGill University
Montreal, Canada H3A 1A1

MICHEL BERNIER
Department of Biological Chemistry
Johns Hopkins University
School of Medicine
Baltimore, Maryland 21205

NANCY J. BOHANNON
Department of Biological Structure
University of Washington
Seattle, Washington 98195

DONALD P. BOTTARO
Joslin Diabetes Center
One Joslin Place
Boston, Massachusetts 02215

FREDERICK T. BOYD
Department of Biochemistry
University of Massachusetts Medical School
55 Lake Avenue North
Worcester, Massachusetts 06510

WILLIAM A. BRENNAN, JR.
Department of Biochemistry and Molecular Biology
Harvard University
Cambridge, Massachusetts

G. COLIN BUDD
Departments of Physiology and Anatomy
Medical College of Ohio
Toledo, Ohio 43699

C.P. CHAN
Howard Hughes Medical Institute
University of Washington
Mail Stop SL-15
Seattle, Washington 98195

DERREL W. CLARKE
Department of Pediatrics
University of Florida
College of Medicine
Gainesville, Florida 32610

DAVID L. COOPER
Department of Pathology
University of Florida
College of Medicine
Gainesville, Florida 32610

DENISE R. COOPER
University of South Florida
College of Medicine
J.A. Haley Veterans Hospital
Tampa, Florida

SHERIN DEVASKAR
Department of Pediatrics
St. Louis University
St. Louis, Missouri

DANIEL M. DORSA
Department of Pharmacology
University of Washington
Seattle, Washington 98195

ROBERT V. FARESE
University of South Florida
College of Medicine
J.A. Haley Veterans Hospital
Tampa, Florida

LAURA M. MUDD
Department of Physiology
University of Florida
College of Medicine
Gainesville, Florida 32610

FINN CILIUS NIELSEN
Department of Clinical Chemistry
Bispebjerg Hospital
DK-2400 Copenhagen, Denmark

YUTAKA OOMURA
Department of Physiology
Faculty of Medicine
Kyushu University 60
Fukuoka 812, Japan

BEN PANSKY
Departments of Physiology
and Anatomy
Medical College of Ohio
Toledo, Ohio 43699

S.L. PELECH
Howard Hughes Medical Institute
University of Washington
Mail Stop SL-15
Seattle, Washington 98195

C.B. PERT
Clinical Neuroscience Branch
NIMH, NIH
Bethesda, Maryland 20892

M. IAN PHILLIPS
Department of Physiology
University of Florida
College of Medicine
Gainesville, Florida 32610

CARLOS R. PLATA-SALAMAN
Department of Physiology
Faculty of Medicine
Kyushu University 60
Fukuoka 812, Japan

DANIEL PORTE, JR.
Department of Medicine
University of Washington
and
Division of Metabolism
and Endocrinology
VA Medical Center
1660 South Columbian Way
Seattle, Washington 98108

BARRY I. POSNER
Department of Medicine
McGill University
Montreal, Canada H3A 1A1

JENNIFER J. POULAKOS
Department of Pediatrics
University of Florida
College of Medicine
Gainesville, Florida 32610

MOHAN K. RAIZADA
Department of Physiology
University of Florida
College of Medicine
Gainesville, Florida 32610

ESPERANZA RECIO-PINTO
Department of Physiology
and Anesthesiology
Cornell University Medical Center
1300 York Avenue
New York, New York 10021

ELAINE M. RICHARDS
Department of Physiology
University of Florida
College of Medicine
Gainesville, Florida 32610

CHARLES T. ROBERTS, JR.
Section of Molecular and Cellular
Physiology
Diabetes Branch, NIDDK, NIH
Bethesda, Maryland 20892

M. ROJESKI
Diabetes Branch, NIDDK, NIH
Bethesda, Maryland 20892

RON G. ROSENFELD
Department of Pediatrics
Stanford University
Medical Center
Stanford, California

J. ROTH
Diabetes Branch, NIDDK, NIH
Bethesda, Maryland 20892

RUBEN SCHECHTER
Department of Pediatrics
St. Louis University
St. Louis, Missouri

KATHLEEN SHIVERICK
Department of Pharmacology and
Experimental Therapeutics
University of Florida
College of Medicine
Gainesville, Florida 32610

DIANNE P. FIGLEWICZ
Department of Psychology
University of Washington
Seattle, Washington 98195

SUSAN C. FROST
Department of Biochemistry
University of Florida
College of Medicine
Gainesville, Florida 32610

STEEN GAMMELTOFT
Department of Clinical Chemistry
Bispebjerg Hospital
DK-2400 Copenhagen, Denmark

W. TIMOTHY GARVEY
Department of Medicine
University of California, S.D.
La Jolla, California 92093

KIM A. HEIDENREICH
Department of Medicine, M023E
University of California, S.D.
La Jolla, California 92093

J.M. HILL
Clinical Neuroscience Branch
NIH, NIMH
Bethesda, Maryland 20892

ANDREW R. HOFFMAN
Department of Medicine
Stanford University
Medical Center
Stanford, California

DOUGLAS N. ISHII
Departments of Physiology
and Biochemistry
Colorado State University
Ft. Collins, Colorado 80523

ARNOLD KAHN
Department of Pediatrics
St. Louis University
St. Louis, Missouri

EDDY KARNIELI
Faculty of Medicine
Technion and Rambam
Medical Center
Haifa, Israel

MASOOD N. KHAN
Department of Medicine
McGill University
Montreal, Canada H3A 1A1

GEORGE L. KING
Joslin Diabetes Center
One Joslin Place
Boston, Massachusetts 02215

RONALD A. KOHANSKI
Department of Biological
Chemistry
Johns Hopkins University
School of Medicine
Baltimore, Maryland 21205

ALINE KOWALSKI
INSERM V145
Faculte de Medicine
Universite de Nice
F06034 Nice, France

E.G. KREBS
Howard Hughes Medical Institute
University of Washington
Mail Stop SL-15
Seattle, Washington 98195

DON M. LAIRD
Department of Biological
Chemistry
Johns Hopkins University
School of Medicine
Baltimore, Maryland 21205

M. DANIEL LANE
Department of Biological
Chemistry
Johns Hopkins University
School of Medicine
Baltimore, Maryland 21205

DEREK LE ROITH
Section of Molecular and
Cellular Physiology
Diabetes Branch, NIDDK, NIH
Bethesda, Maryland 20892

M.A. LESNIAK
Diabetes Branch, NIDDK, NIH
Bethesda, Maryland 20892

WILLIAM L. LOWE, JR.
Section of Molecular and Cellular
Physiology
Diabetes Branch, NIDDK, NIH
Bethesda, Maryland 20892

LAURANE G. MENDELSOHN
Central Nervous System Research
Lilly Research Laboratories
Indianapolis, Indiana 46285

LESLIE J. STEIN
Department of Psychology
University of Washington
Seattle, Washington 98195

COLIN SUMNERS
Department of Physiology
University of Florida
College of Medicine
Gainesville, Florida 32610

D.A. TINKER
Howard Hughes Medical Institute
University of Washington
Mail Stop SL-15
Seattle, Washington 98195

EMMANUEL VAN OBBERGHEN
INSERM V145
Faculte de Medicine
University de Nice
F06034 Nice, France

SHOOU-LIH WANG
Department of Pharmacology and Experimental Therapeutics
University of Florida
College of Medicine
Gainesville, Florida 32610

BARBARA J. WILCOX
Division of Metabolism and Endocrinology
Va Medical Center
1660 South Columbian Way
Seattle, Washington 98108

STEPHEN C. WOODS
Departments of Psychology and Medicine
University of Washington
Seattle, Washington 98195

AUTHOR INDEX

SUBJECT INDEX